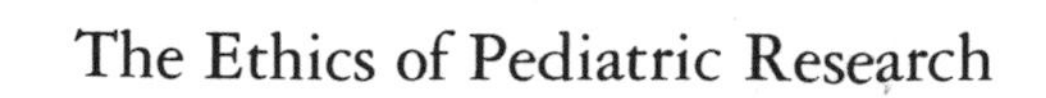

The Ethics of Pediatric Research

DAVID S. WENDLER

The Ethics of Pediatric Research

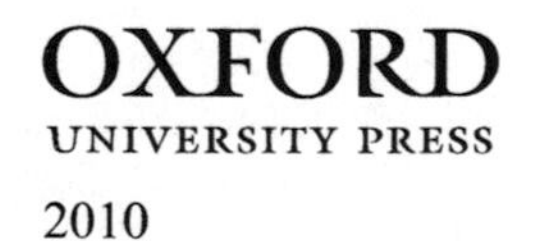

2010

OXFORD
UNIVERSITY PRESS

Oxford University Press, Inc., publishes works that further
Oxford University's objective of excellence
in research, scholarship, and education.

Oxford New York
Auckland Cape Town Dar es Salaam Hong Kong Karachi
Kuala Lumpur Madrid Melbourne Mexico City Nairobi
New Delhi Shanghai Taipei Toronto

With offices in
Argentina Austria Brazil Chile Czech Republic France Greece
Guatemala Hungary Italy Japan Poland Portugal Singapore
South Korea Switzerland Thailand Turkey Ukraine Vietnam

Published by Oxford University Press, Inc.
198 Madison Avenue, New York, New York 10016

www.oup.com

Library of Congress Cataloging-in-Publication Data

Wendler, David.
The ethics of pediatric research / David S. Wendler.
p. ; cm.
Includes bibliographical references.
ISBN 978-0-19-973008-7
1. Pediatrics—Research—Moral and ethical aspects. I. Title.
[DNLM: 1. Pediatrics—ethics. 2. Ethics, Medical. 3. Ethics, Research. WS 21 W471e 2010]
RJ85.W46 2010
618.9200072—dc22
2009024070

9 8 7 6 5 4 3 2 1

Printed in the United States of America
on acid-free paper

ACKNOWLEDGMENTS

The bulk of the present manuscript was written while I was a faculty fellow in ethics at the Safra Center for Ethics, Harvard University. Thanks to the Center's then-director, Dennis Thompson, for being such an astute and accommodating host, and to Dr. John Gallin and Dr. Ezekiel Emanuel for allowing me the time necessary to pursue the fellowship.

My thinking on the ethics of pediatric research has benefited greatly from the writings of others in the field and the discussions I have had with countless individuals over the course of the past 5 years, especially my wonderful colleagues in the Department of Bioethics at the National Institutes of Health (NIH).

Special thanks to Alan Wertheimer, Paul Litton, and Franklin Miller who read earlier versions of the manuscript and provided incisive comments. Also thanks for challenging and beneficial comments and criticism along the way from Nir Eyal, Connie Rosati, Leonard Glantz, and two anonymous reviewers for Oxford University Press. Parts of the present work were presented to the 2006–2007 Harvard faculty fellows in ethics, the Harvard Program in Ethics and Health, and the NIH Department of Bioethics. Thanks to all the participants for their input and advice.

CONTENTS

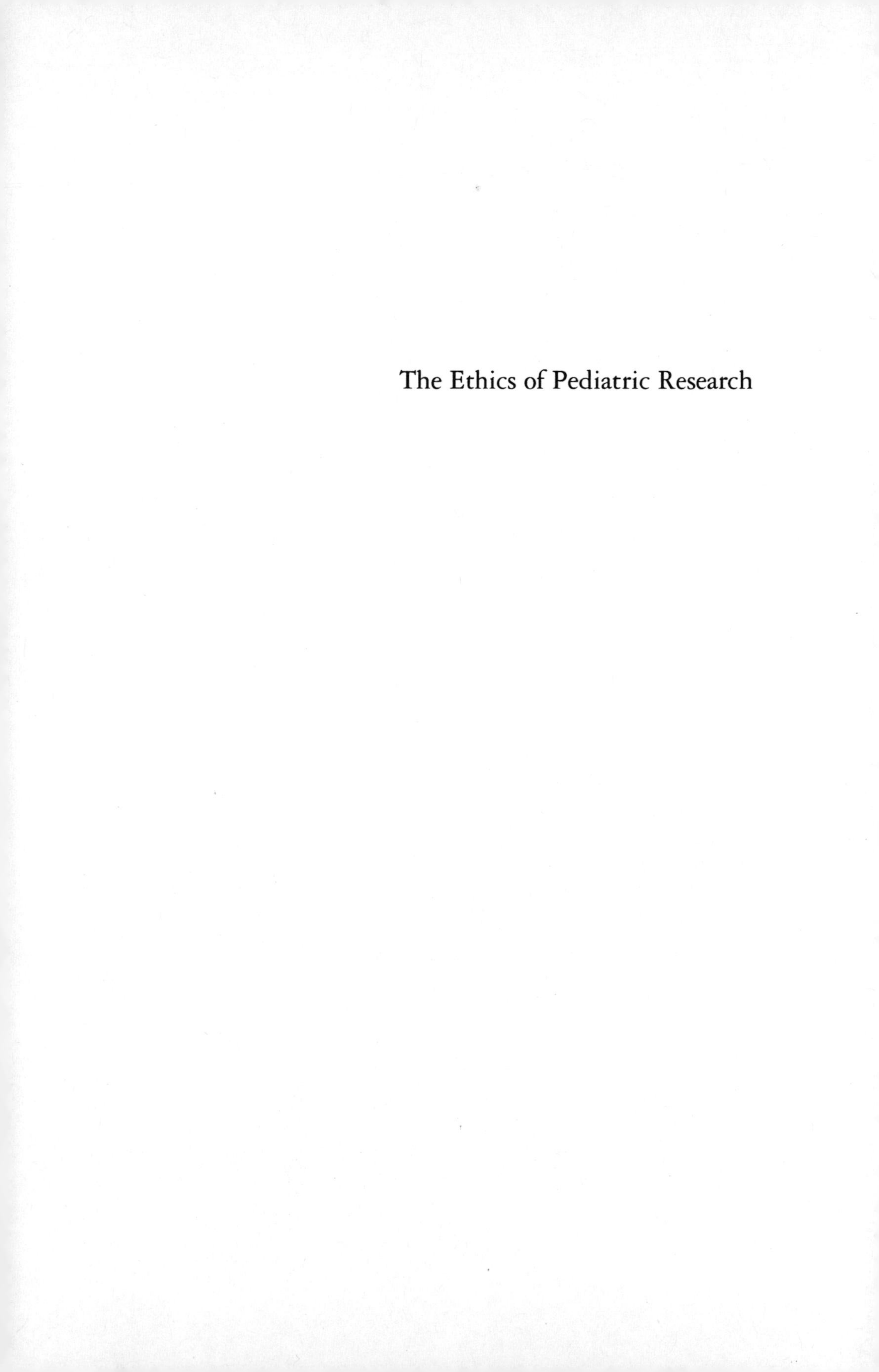

The Ethics of Pediatric Research

ONE | Introduction

A Vaccine for Rotavirus

Rarely has a disease so easily treated killed so many. Rotavirus, a wheel-shaped virus transmitted by ingestion of contaminated food or water and contact with contaminated surfaces, causes inflammation of the stomach and intestines (i.e., gastroenteritis). Affected children experience vomiting and watery diarrhea for 3 to 8 days, accompanied by low-grade fever and abdominal pain.[1] Treatment consists of little more than potable water and, in severe cases, intravenous fluids, with the goal of keeping the child hydrated until the infection runs its course. Rotavirus in higher-income countries results in sick children and cranky parents, along with brief trips to the hospital for some.[2] Rotavirus in countries where children lack access to potable water often leads to severe dehydration and, for over 600,000 children every year, shock and death.[3] Rotavirus kills one in every 200 children in the developing world.

Those diseases that sicken and kill children in lower-income countries—malaria is a good example—tend to be relatively minor problems in higher-income countries. Higher-income countries thus have put relatively little effort into identifying improved methods to prevent, treat, and cure these diseases. Rotavirus turns out to be an important exception because it affects hundreds of thousands of children in higher-income countries every year.[4] Although rotavirus is almost never life-threatening for these children, it does lead to discomfort for the children and unwanted medical bills for their parents. These costs, in markets with the political power to insist on and the resources to pay for new treatments, have led to numerous efforts to find ways to prevent rotavirus infection, including efforts to develop a safe and effective vaccine.

The rotavirus vaccine program produced several vaccines that were abandoned,[5] and then identified what have been described as two of the safest and most effective vaccines ever developed.[6] The rotavirus vaccines, estimated to cost several hundred dollars per child, have the potential, assuming requisite funding is made available, to save the lives of hundreds of thousands of children every year.[7] Development of these vaccines represents an extraordinary accomplishment, possibly one of the most significant developments in medical science over the past several decades. Yet, according to a compelling argument, one that has yet to be fully addressed and will be the focus of the present work, development of the rotavirus vaccines was unethical. It was unethical, it is argued, because the process of developing the vaccines required some children to undergo research procedures that posed risks, but did not offer them any chance for clinical benefit.

The clinical trials that tested the rotavirus vaccines did offer some potential for clinical benefit to the children who received the vaccine. Although unproven at the time, the vaccines offered some chance of protection from rotavirus and posed relatively low risks. Arguably, participation in these studies was in the clinical interests of the children who received the vaccine. However, to determine whether the vaccine produced an immune response in these children, the investigators gave other children placebo injections, and all participating children underwent blood draws purely for research purposes. These blood draws, as well as the placebo vaccine injections, posed some risks without any chance for clinical benefit. As such, these procedures are instances of what I will refer to as "nonbeneficial" research procedures.[8] The focus of the present work is, then, to assess whether it ever can be appropriate to subject children to nonbeneficial research procedures.

A nonbeneficial research procedure is one that poses risks and burdens, but fails to offer a compensating potential for clinical benefit. Although the research blood draws included in the rotavirus vaccine trials posed very low risks, they offered essentially no potential to benefit the children who underwent them. What I am calling nonbeneficial research procedures often are described as procedures that offer no potential for clinical benefit at all. The problem with this characterization is that few, if any, research interventions offer absolutely no chance for clinical benefit. The reasons for this are highlighted by a fascinating study in which radiologists at the U.S. National Institutes of Health (NIH) retrospectively analyzed the records of 1,000 individuals who had undergone research scans of their brains.[9]

All 1,000 individuals had been determined to be healthy and asymptomatic by physician examination and participant history prior to the research scans and, not surprisingly, 82% of the research scan results were normal. More surprising, 18% of the scans identified abnormalities in the brains of these normal volunteers. Of these scans, 15.1% required no referral, 1.8% required a routine referral, and 1.1% necessitated urgent referral. The urgent-referral group included two primary brain tumors, demonstrating a prevalence of at least 0.2% of brain tumors in ostensibly healthy individuals. This frightening possibility is not limited to adults. Analysis of the brain scans of 225 pediatric research participants found 47 abnormalities. Although the vast majority raised little or no concern, one lesion (2%) necessitated urgent referral for medical follow-up.[10]

These findings all arose in the context of clinical research that was not looking for brain tumors and was not designed to benefit participants. The studies were designed to evaluate various aspects of physiology in what were thought to be normal brains. The possibility of what have come to be known as "incidental" findings arises with almost all research interventions. Brains thought to be normal may hide tumors that are uncovered incidentally during research scans. Technicians examining the blood of normal volunteers for purely research purposes may identify possible blood disorders. Simple screening as part of mental health or smoking studies may identify health concerns unrelated to the research.

Fortuitous findings in the research context can lead to treatment that otherwise might have been delayed or denied. Although the chance of such findings tends to be very low, it is not zero, and the potential benefit to individuals of early detection can be dramatic. It is for this reason that limiting our attention to research procedures and studies that offer no potential at all for clinical benefit would yield an analysis of almost no practical import. We will thus expand our coverage to include pediatric research that offers insufficient potential for clinical benefit to compensate for the risks and burdens it poses to the participating children. Put differently, we will focus on pediatric research that poses *net* risks to its participants.

Before leaving the topic of incidental findings, it is important to note that not all incidental findings are beneficial. Typically, the majority of abnormal findings have no known clinical significance. A radiologist who finds that a particular structure in an individual's brain is shaped somewhat differently may have no idea if this difference has, or ever will have any clinical significance, thus leaving her with the dilemma of what, if anything, to tell the individual. Many false-positives also occur. An abnormality on a research scan, initially thought to be a brain tumor, may be found, perhaps only after many months of waiting, worry, and follow-up, to be harmless. The fact that pursuit of incidental findings can yield varying levels of stress, anxiety, costs, and burdens for many, in addition to enormous clinical benefit for a few, has led to an entire literature on how this issue should be addressed in the research context.[11]

The inclusion of nonbeneficial procedures in clinical studies represents the rule, rather than the exception. As we will see in the next section, the process of improving medical treatments for children through pediatric research depends on it.[12–15] This research raises ethical concern because it involves exposing children who cannot consent to some risks for the benefit of others. According to a powerful argument, this practice is unethical, representing a classic instance in which vulnerable individuals are exploited for the benefit of others. This argument has the potential to jeopardize future attempts to improve medical treatments for children and may cast ethical doubt over past attempts, including the rotavirus vaccine trials. This possibility could have enormous social implications. According to the Institute of Medicine, biomedical research "has helped change medical care and public health practices in ways that, each year, save or lengthen the lives of tens of thousands of children around the world, prevent or reduce illness or disability in many more, and improve the quality of life for countless others."[16] These advances offer vital reason to conduct and support nonbeneficial pediatric research. At the same time, we have a strong obligation to protect individual children from abuse and exploitation, even when committed in the service of a valuable cause. This tension underscores the importance of trying to determine under what conditions, if any, it can be appropriate to conduct nonbeneficial pediatric research.

The Prevalence of Nonbeneficial Pediatric Research

To characterize a given disease and identify possible ways to treat it, researchers often need to perform nonbeneficial research procedures—blood draws, biopsies, radiological scans. To determine what, if anything, is abnormal in these results, investigators also may need to conduct the same tests in healthy individuals to establish a baseline set of normal values against which to evaluate findings in patients.[17] Baseline values for height and weight can be obtained from the noninvasive measurements of a range of individuals. Normal values for protein levels in the blood require some healthy children to undergo purely research blood draws, while determining normal functions for aspects of cognitive function might require healthy children to undergo the risks and burdens of radiological scans.

Once the symptoms of a disease have been characterized, and perhaps its cause identified, investigators begin the process of finding a treatment by giving a few individuals single doses of potential therapies. Although these "pharmacokinetic" studies do not offer a compensating potential for clinical benefit, they do provide information regarding which doses children can tolerate—vital information for designing studies of the potential treatment's safety and efficacy. As an example, the combination of lopinavir and ritonavir was found to be effective against HIV infection in adults. At that point, it could simply have been approved for children as well. The problem with this approach is that children differ from adults in medically relevant ways. Children typically weigh less, have different metabolic rates, and different immune systems. These differences highlight the importance of evaluating whether treatments found to be safe and effective in adults also are safe and effective in children.

In the first step of the process of evaluating the use of lopinavir/ritonavir treatment in children, investigators gave a few children single doses to determine how much of the drug combination they could tolerate.[18] These studies, necessary preludes to future efficacy studies, posed some risks to the pediatric participants. Although the risks to the participants from a single dose were very low, the potential for clinical benefit was even less. Once investigators identify an acceptable dose, they conduct trials to assess the toxicity and preliminary efficacy of those doses before initiating treatment trials to evaluate whether the experimental treatment is better than (or, in equivalence trials, at least as good as) existing treatments for the condition in question. These studies, called *phase III studies*, can offer a compensating potential for clinical benefit. They also typically include procedures that do not, such as needle sticks to assess blood levels of a drug, biopsies to determine whether a drug is reaching a tumor, and radiological scans to evaluate a drug's side-effect profile. In this way, 'nonbeneficial' research covers individual studies that do not offer a compensating potential for clinical benefit, as well as the purely research interventions that are included in many clinical trials. Because the question of whether it is acceptable to expose children to research risks for the benefit of others applies equally to nonbeneficial procedures and nonbeneficial studies, this distinction will largely be immaterial to the present discussion. Thus, I often will use the term *nonbeneficial pediatric research* without any further specification.

Absent compelling reason to do otherwise, investigators should conduct nonbeneficial research with adults who can consent, rather than with children who cannot consent (in Chapter 8, we consider what constitutes a compelling reason in this regard). However, for a number of reasons, research intended to improve health care for children often must (eventually) be conducted with children.[19] First, some diseases and conditions affect children only, or affect children in different ways than they do adults (such as certain forms of cancer). Second, children often require forms of medication different from what is used in adults, such as palatable oral medications. Third, the ways in which medicines are absorbed, distributed to organs, and excreted depend on an individual's stage of development.[20] Because absorption depends on development, and because the relative size of children's organs does not match those of adults, calculating pediatric doses by simple extrapolation from adult studies poses risks of both over- and under-dosing. Fourth, some medicines act differently in children, or not at all, because the necessary receptors on which the medicines act are not present in children. Fifth, some adverse effects of medicines are relevant to children only, such as impact on growth.[21] The cumulative effect of these differences on the need for pediatric research is nicely summarized in the CIOMS guidelines:

> The participation of children is indispensable for research into diseases of childhood and conditions to which children are particularly susceptible (cf. vaccine trials), as well as for clinical trials of drugs that are designed for children as well as adults. In the past, many new products were not tested for children though they were directed toward diseases also occurring in childhood; thus children either did not benefit from these new drugs or were exposed to them though little was known about their specific effects or safety in children. Now it is widely agreed that, as a general rule, the sponsor of any new therapeutic, diagnostic, or preventive product that is likely to be indicated for use in children is obliged to evaluate its safety and efficacy for children before it is released for general distribution.[22]

Questioning the Acceptability of Nonbeneficial Pediatric Research

The need for and conduct of pediatric research has focused a good deal of attention on the various ethical issues it raises. These include the extent to which children should have a say in whether they are enrolled in research. Should children be required prospectively to approve their enrollment in research? Should their objections to research participation be respected? And, to what extent do the answers to these questions depend on the age and maturity level of the children, or the possibility that the research will benefit them? Other questions focus on what information should be provided to children and their parents. Should young children be informed that an experimental treatment poses a risk of death, albeit a very low one? Should parents be informed that their daughter was found to be pregnant on a test to determine study eligibility? The present work focuses on the general question, in some sense prior to these, of whether it can be ethically acceptable to expose children to research risks for the benefit of others. This question is more controversial, and more fundamental. If we find that the answer to this question is no, the other questions are rendered largely academic.

The year before he became Chief Justice of the U.S. Supreme Court, Warren E. Berger argued that nonbeneficial pediatric research is indefensible and "no rational social order will or should tolerate it."[23] This view can grant that it is a good thing that the rotavirus vaccines exist, and their existence is even a good thing for the participating children, assuming that those in the placebo group have access to the vaccine. But, on this view, the fact that these children participated in the studies was not, in itself, of value for them. To the contrary, being exposed to nonbeneficial research procedures is against children's interests and involves their being exploited for the benefit of others. For these reasons, it should be prohibited, by rational societies at least. The importance of trying to determine whether nonbeneficial pediatric research can be justified is underscored by the fact that many prominent commentators endorse this view.[24]

Leon Kass, a prominent commentator on issues in bioethics, and one-time chairman of the U.S. President's Council on Bioethics, described nonbeneficial pediatric research in the following terms:

> People who we hope eventually to benefit are for the time being at the very least—and forgive me—to make the point luridly, they are our guinea pigs. It's not a nice way to put it, but they are experimental subjects for the gaining of this knowledge, and we can dress it up any way we like, but that's part of the essence of it, and it's much better if you're going to do it to have that clearly in mind.[25]

The most compelling argument for this view was articulated over 30 years ago by Paul Ramsey, a noted theologian of the time. In a series of articles over the course of a decade, Ramsey argued that individuals may be exposed to the risks of nonbeneficial research only when they consent to it. Since (most) children cannot provide informed consent, Ramsey concluded that nonbeneficial pediatric research is unethical. Over the past several decades, a number of commentators have attempted to rebut Ramsey's arguments and justify at least some nonbeneficial pediatric research.[26,27] Unfortunately, as we shall see in Chapter 4, no one has completely answered Ramsey's challenge.

Tom Murray nicely summarizes this state of the debate, noting that many commentators endorse at least some nonbeneficial pediatric research despite the fact that the arguments offered in its favor have been "notably weaker than the arguments favoring a complete ban on such research."[28] In 2005, Norman Fost, one of the most important commentators on pediatric research ethics, agreed. "In my view," he argued, "the justification for nontherapeutic research on children has never been made. The brilliant work of the National Commission for the Protection of Human Subjects never really, in my view, made the case for allowing nontherapeutic intrusions into children who were incapable of consent."[29] The moral imperative to protect children from unethical treatment provides powerful impetus to consider whether this is still the case, or whether it is possible to justify (some) nonbeneficial pediatric research despite the strong arguments against it.

The commentators and quotations considered thus far reveal that worries regarding the ethical acceptability of nonbeneficial pediatric research often are voiced by ethicists and academics who comment on clinical research from some remove. Skeptics might regard this fact as evidence for the possibility that these concerns are peculiar to those who are not closely involved in and familiar with pediatric research. Thus, one might hope that pediatricians and pediatric researchers have a more congenial and better informed view of the ethics of pediatric research. In fact, many pediatric clinical researchers express precisely the same concerns—and these concerns appear to be shared by many pediatricians. For example, almost half of the respondents to a survey of Canadian and European pediatricians stated that children should not be enrolled in research unless it offers them the potential for clinical benefit.[30]

Method of the Book

The aim of this book is to evaluate under what conditions, if any, it can be ethically acceptable to expose children to research risks for the benefit of others. As such, this book is intended as a work in moral philosophy, applied to the specific question of the normative status of enrolling children in nonbeneficial clinical research. The method used will be to evaluate the ways in which we think about and analyze nonbeneficial pediatric research, as well as the ways in which we think about and analyze related contexts. We will attempt to develop an analysis of the present dilemma that is consistent with the ways we think about and analyze contexts that raise similar questions and issues, with the assumption that, failing compelling reason to do otherwise, we should hold the same view on these issues as they arise in different contexts.

We will consider a range of examples that are related in different ways to the present question. Our views or intuitions regarding what is right and wrong in those cases will be taken as evidence for certain views, and against others. However, our intuitive responses to specific examples, while important, will not provide the only test for a successful view. We also can evaluate the acceptability of the views to which our intuitions lead us by applying a general criterion of plausibility. To what extent does a given view make sense independent of the specific intuitions that led to it? Any view that deserves our consideration should be consistent with (most of) our intuitive judgements in individual cases and make sense once we step back from those intuitions and consider the view in the context of our broader lives and commitments.

A number of authors have preceded us, and we will consider their views here. Because no systematic analysis has been made of previous analyses of nonbeneficial pediatric research, this analysis may be of independent interest. Making clear what considerations and lines of argument have been pursued previously, and why they have not yielded a complete justification for nonbeneficial pediatric research, has its own value. At the same time, we will not attempt to exhaustively catalog all previous efforts on this topic. Instead, we will focus on the most prominent views and supplement them with representatives of any approaches not thereby assayed. While I hope to do justice to each of the views considered here, I will not attempt to provide an exhaustive account of any of them. The goal will be to consider each account in the depth necessary to clarify what works and what does not work with respect to the approach in question; we will be philosophical vultures of a kind, willing to learn from the efforts of others without being able to do full justice to the depth and breadth of those efforts.

We will begin with the writings of Paul Ramsey. Ramsey posed the fundamental ethical challenge for future authors on this topic when he argued that pediatric research can be ethically acceptable only when it is in the interests of the participating children. Ramsey at first assumes that the only type of benefit children might receive in the context of clinical research—the only type of benefit that could compensate for the risks and burdens they face—is medical or clinical benefit. It is the suggestion of a number of authors that children may benefit in other ways that will serve as the foundation on which the present analysis builds.

Other commentators effectively deny Ramsey's claim that pediatric research can be ethically justified only when it is in the interests of participating children. Some argue, for example, that pediatric research can be justified, even when it is not in the children's best interests, by appeal to the choices the children would make if they were competent, or the choices they are likely to make once they become competent. Still others attempt to show that children have an obligation to participate in clinical research, even when it is contrary to their interests.

We will consider these arguments, and others like them, in the coming chapters. I argue that none of them provides a complete justification for nonbeneficial pediatric research. In light of this conclusion, I want to consider the possibility of answering Ramsey's challenge, rather than avoiding it. That is, I want to consider the extent to which we can justify nonbeneficial pediatric research by appeal to the interests of participating children. This approach involves the attempt to continue and extend the work of previous authors who have accepted Ramsey's claim that participation in clinical research is justified only to the extent that it is in the interests of the participating children, but deny his assumption that participation in clinical research can be in children's interests only to the extent that it offers them a compensating potential for clinical benefit. In particular, a number of authors have argued that children might derive educational benefit from their participation in nonbeneficial research.

This line of argument was first articulated, as far as I can tell, by William Bartholome, a pediatrician who participated in the discussions of the U.S. National Commission on pediatric research. Bartholome argued that participation in clinical research can offer at least some children the potential for moral growth.[31] They may learn, in effect, to be better persons, more moral individuals, as the result of participating in nonbeneficial research that is designed to help others. This line of argument has been endorsed and further developed by Terence Ackerman,[32] as well as by Lainie Ross and Robert Nelson.[33] Their arguments provide a way to justify some nonbeneficial pediatric research with older children who have the cognitive abilities necessary to gain such educational benefit. The problem, as the authors themselves recognize, is that this consideration does not apply to very young children, thus providing only a partial justification for nonbeneficial pediatric research. Their work, however, also points to the possibility of considering whether there are other ways in which children might benefit from participation in nonbeneficial research.

The present work will attempt to follow this line of reasoning and thereby extend the work of these authors in a particular way. Because the more obvious and even some less obvious ways in which children might benefit have been evaluated, we will move into less familiar and more contentious terrain. This analysis will require some foundational work in normative ethics and a consideration of approaches that at least initially may seem less than appealing. We will search for a path that leads back from this foundational work to conclusions about the practical questions in pediatric research. This attempt to connect foundational questions in normative ethics with practical concerns in clinical research will necessitate engagement with a number of issues in philosophical ethics. We will need a number of foundation concepts and arguments at our disposal to consider the present issues in the depth they require and deserve. Readers whose main interest lies in bioethics may be less interested in the details of this argument. For them, brief summaries along the way are intended to provide a way to follow the argument without having to explore in depth its every step.

One can analyze the ethical appropriateness of a given action or practice at a number of levels. All are important, but it is a mistake to try to address them all at once. The present work will begin and focus primarily on the level of the ethics of individual behavior and action, in particular, as it occurs in the course of conducting nonbeneficial pediatric research. A second level concerns the institutional policies, and a third the societal regulations, relevant to nonbeneficial pediatric research. The question of what is the right institutional policy or societal regulation is influenced, but not determined solely, by what constititutes appropriate behavior at the individual level. In the present case, developing an account of whether individual instances of nonbeneficial pediatric research can be ethically acceptable does not settle the question of whether institutions should endorse and conduct it, nor whether nonbeneficial pediatric research should be sanctioned by public policy. Although the bulk of the present work focuses on the individual-level question of whether it can be acceptable to expose children to research risks for the benefit of others, I will finish by considering the related policy question of whether society should allow or prohibit nonbeneficial pediatric research in light of the preceding analysis, as well as issues that arise specifically at the policy level.

Lessons Learned

As mentioned, and as we shall consider in greater depth in Chapter 4, many efforts to justify nonbeneficial pediatric research attempt to sidestep Ramsey's challenge by appealing in one way or another to children's potential agency: for example, that the children would consent to it if they could, it is likely that they will retroactively "consent" to it at some point in the future, or that reasonable individuals would give their consent. These approaches often are based on the at least implicit assumption that any justification for nonbeneficial pediatric research must somehow connect up with the participating children's presumed, actual, or future agency. This approach reflects an important strand of philosophical analysis according to which the things we do have implications for us, for our lives, to the extent that they have implications for us as moral agents or persons.

This focus on moral agency is informed by the assumption that, when developing accounts in normative ethics, the subject of the account is the autonomous moral agent and one attempts to determine what counts as acceptable behavior for him, what constitutes a valuable life for him, or what are his rights and obligations. Because one is focused on the autonomous agent, one comes to the view that the goal of moral theory is to develop a set of guidelines or action-guiding principles for how autonomous individuals should act and lead their lives. When thinking of the task in terms of giving instructions of this kind, one inevitably focuses on agency, on giving instructions that people can use to decide how to act and what to do. The paradigm challenge for moral theory is seen as the autonomous moral agent deciding whether to do A or B: eat or not eat, lie or not lie, follow one's heart or one's brain. The solution to be provided by moral theorizing is some account or guidelines that help the agent decide what to do. "Choose the option that maximizes overall pleasure or happiness," some tell him. "Do whatever you want consistent with your obligations and the rights of others," say others.[34]

From this perspective, one might wonder whether there can be any practical implications to moral theorizing that focuses on individuals who lack moral agency. It would be as if someone developed an account of the ways in which the hair color with which we are born is of vital significance to our lives. Unless and until we can do something about it, by genetic engineering say, such advice does nothing and moves no one. This approach to analyzing moral concerns misses a number of important issues, not least of which is the fact that systematic analysis of what is of value independent of agency, including developing an account of value for nonautonomous individuals, can have practical implications because it can have implications for how autonomous individuals ought to treat nonautonomous individuals.

There is a good reason why moral philosophers focus on moral agency: It is the core of the moral life. In the present work, I want to consider the possibility that this claim has gotten conflated with the claim that what we do is relevant to our interests only when we autonomously engage in the action or behavior, or it affects us personally. Roughly, the claim to be pursued here is that the focus on autonomous agents leads to the view that the act of contributing to important projects has value for the contributor only to the extent that the individual autonomously decides to make the contribution, only, as I shall phrase it, the contribution "goes through" the individual's agency. Undoubtedly, this view is correct when understood as a claim about the primary ways in which making a contribution has value for the contributors. But, without further argument, we should not regard this fact as implying that making a contribution to an important project has no value for those who are not autonomous, including young children. That conclusion needs to be argued for, not simply assumed.

I will argue that previous attempts to connect nonbeneficial pediatric research in some way to the participating children's agency fail to provide a compelling justification. The failure to connect the acceptability of pediatric research to some account of the children's agency suggests that we need to accept the fact that children are not autonomous and take on directly the question of the proper treatment of individuals who are not but, if all goes well, will become autonomous adults. When, if ever, is it acceptable to expose these individuals to risks and burdens for the benefit of others? As mentioned, Bartholome suggested, and Ackerman, Ross, and Nelson have pursued, a very different way to answer this question by appeal to the fact that children might derive educational benefit from participating in clinical research. We will try to extend this line of work by considering other ways in which children might benefit from their involvement in nonbeneficial research. In particular, we will consider what implications the fact of making a contribution to a valuable project has for individuals' overall lives and, by implication, their own interests.

One of the problems with focusing too much on moral agency is that doing so ignores the personal relevance of our causal relationships with others and the world. By focusing too much on our agency, we lose sight of our place in the physical world, on the importance of the impact the world has on us, and the impact we have on others and on the world itself. We lose sight of the fact that we are not just agents, we are embodied agents, and the physical interactions we have create connections with and have an impact on various activities, projects, relationships, and ends. These connections can affect our interests, independent of the extent to which they have implications for us as moral agents.

To begin to get a sense for this possibility, consider a tactic sometimes employed in response to procrastinating students. A mechanism is established by which the student is effectively forced to contribute a very small sum of money to a cause, perhaps a political candidate, the student loathes, for every unit of time the student fails to complete the task in question. This approach can be very effective at encouraging students who have previously resisted exhortation, pleading, and threats. When the sums contributed are large, the incentive effects on the procrastinating student are obvious. Most of us at least, do not want to give away large sums of money, especially to causes we loathe, and most of us do not want causes we loathe to receive large sums of money. The incentive effect of this approach is more subtle when the sums of money are negligible. In these cases, the incentive does not trace so much to the amount of money the student loses or the loathed cause gains. Imagine the sums are so low that the monetary impact on both parties is negligible. The student has sufficient reserve funds that the money lost, at least for the first year or so of the arrangement, will have no impact on him. The level of money contributed also will have effectively no impact on the cause. Perhaps the cause is a political candidate whose chances of victory will be unaffected.

Finally, imagine that the student knows all of this ex ante. Nonetheless, the strategy may and, in practice has, influenced students. Why? The explanation in at least some cases, I suggest, has to do with the fact that the contributions establish a connection between the student and the loathed cause. And this connection the student wants to avoid. He wants to avoid contributing to that cause and, thereby, having a connection to it. It is often the desire to avoid making such contributions and having such connections, independent of the monetary consequences, that provides incentive for the student to finish his work. This is just one aspect of our lives in which we recognize that the contributions we make establish connections between us and the projects, causes, relationships to which we contribute. And these connections can have implications for us and our lives.

This line of argument and the present work in general, is informed by a general trend over the past 20 years or so which has begun to question whether the emphasis on autonomy in moral philosophy and bioethics has gone too far, whether this focus, while clarifying the importance of moral agency, has obscured other considerations of importance and value. One of the ways in which we tend to emphasize and promote the things that are of greatest value and significance in our lives is to deemphasize, sometimes to the point of rejection, those things that are of lesser value or significance. In ethics, emphasis on the significance of moral agency has implicitly resulted in the downplaying, to the point of sometimes ignoring, among other things, the importance of emotions and relationships in our lives.[35] In the ethics of clinical research, it has been argued that the focus on autonomy has led to an overemphasis on informed consent and a consequent ignoring of other important considerations, such as the investigator-participant relationship, to the detriment of research participants and the research enterprise itself.

The present work begins with the possibility that the focus on moral agency and autonomy also has resulted in a failure to appreciate the importance of what we do, the physical contributions we make, the causal relationships into which we enter. Deontologists tend to regard what we do as important for us to the extent that it provides evidence regarding our intentions and moral agency, and the extent to which we abide by our obligations and duties. On this view, the relationships into which we enter and the contributions we make that do not go through our agency are of little moral significance. Consequentialist theories regard what we do as morally important to the extent that it has an impact on us and other sentient beings, to the extent that it leads to greater happiness or pleasure or contentment for us and others. This approach runs the risk of incorporating a necessarily subjective element into one's account of a better life for an individual. A better life is one that is experienced in some sense as better by the individual. And both traditions end up eliding, downplaying, or even ignoring those facts of our lives that do not go through our agency or have sufficient impact on our sensory organs. It may be that our agency and experiences largely define how well our lives go. But, they do not exhaust the considerations relevant to how well our lives go, and failure to appreciate this difference has distorted analysis of a number of practical concerns, including the question of whether we can justify nonbeneficial pediatric research.

To consider the possibility that making certain contributions can have value for our lives independent of the extent to which they engage or go through our agency, we first will need to distinguish what is good or valuable for an individual from what is good or valuable for an individual's life. This distinction then presses the question of the extent to which it is in our interests—it is better for us—that our lives go better overall. I shall argue that helping others can be in children's interests, hence, justify some risks in the context of nonbeneficial pediatric research, even for very young children who are not autonomous. Participation in some nonbeneficial pediatric research can be in children's interests because it can make for a better life overall, and this fact can be good *for them*. Here, then, is the primary claim to be defended in what follows: participation in nonbeneficial research can be in the interests of children, even very young children, to the extent that it involves their making a contribution to an important project, and making that contribution does not conflict with any other significant interest. This account implies that nonbeneficial pediatric research can be acceptable when the benefits to the children in this regard justify or compensate for the (net) risks and burdens to which they are exposed. Nonbeneficial pediatric research in which the risks and burdens exceed this level is unacceptable or, at least, stands in need of some other justification.

As the previous paragraph suggests, the present account is intended as a sufficient, not a necessary justification on some nonbeneficial pediatric research. It may be that some other justification could be developed for some nonbeneficial pediatric research that remains unjustified on the present account. For example, I will argue that participation in clinical research offers a certain kind of benefit in most cases. It might be that there is a different kind of benefit that some (or many) children also gain from participation in some or all nonbeneficial pediatric research. That conclusion would provide an independent argument for the ethical acceptability of nonbeneficial pediatric research.

In making the present argument, I often will rely on general phrases such as "having implications" for one's life, and "saying something" about one's life. These phrases are intended to capture, without the need for continual repetition, the fact that the things we do, the actions we perform, the behaviors we engage in, the physical interactions we have with others and the world, often become a part of our biography or life narrative, hence, aspects of our lives overall. In this way, they can influence the extent to which our lives are better or worse overall. A life that includes making contributions to valuable projects is better overall compared to the same life absent these contributions. This claim applies to us all. Its generality leads to questions about its implications for clinical research with groups other than children.

We will consider in some depth the concern that the present analysis implausibly implies that investigators may force competent adults to participate in nonbeneficial research on the grounds that making even forced contributions is in their overall interests. One also might wonder what implications the present analysis has for clinical research with adults who are unable to provide informed consent, such as those with advanced Alzheimer disease. I will have less to say about this question because it involves issues that would take us far from our focus on research with children, including analysis of what is required to show proper respect for individuals who once were, but no longer are competent. To what extent should we treat them on the basis of their competent preferences and values? To what extent should we treat them in light of their current preferences and values, independent of the extent to which this results in treatment that is consistent with the preferences and values they espoused when competent?

An Initial Example

Our lives are defined in large part by the ways in which we are influenced and the ways we, in turn, influence others and the world. Whether a given contribution goes through one's agency, whether the individual understood what was happening, whether he had any control over its occurrence, whether he intentionally performed an action that led to the contribution in question, determines a great deal. It determines, in particular, whether the contribution has implications for the individual as a person or as a moral agent. In contrast, whether a contribution goes through an individual's agency does not determine whether the causal relationship obtained. It also does not determine whether the causal relationship was part of one's life, whether it is in fact one's contribution. The possibility that the things we do can have implications for our lives even when we are not morally responsible for them is a result of the fact that we are embodied beings and is most clearly seen with respect to the contributions we make to unfortunate, negative, or harmful causes or relationships.

On July 10, 2008, Ted Lilly, a pitcher for the Chicago Cubs baseball team, was batting in the second inning when he fouled off a pitch, sending it into the stands.[36] Unknown to Lilly at the time, the ball hit 7-year-old Dominic DiAngi, fracturing his skull. After the game, the Cubs took up a collection of memorabilia, a bat, a glove, and a ball signed by all the players, to give to Dominic. Many players contributed to the gifts; Lilly also planned to call the family and visit the boy in the hospital. Everyone on the team recognized the accident as unfortunate and hoped to compensate the boy for his injuries. Only Lilly felt a personal connection to the injury as a result of the fact that it was a ball that he hit which caused the injury. Lilly, unlike his teammates, was a vital part of the immediate causal chain that resulted in the injury.[37]

Lilly's reaction was typical—a common feature of our lives, reflected by the fact that none of the many news reports of the story expressed surprise that Lilly felt a personal connection in a way the others did not. None of those reporting on the incident wondered why Lilly in particular planned to call the family and visit the boy in the hospital. Although the response to this incident is commonplace, it is worth noting the ways in which it looks puzzling. Most importantly, Lilly is not to blame morally for the boy's injury. He did not in any way attempt to hurt the boy, or hurt anyone. There is no sense in which he intended this outcome and, presumably, he would have done a great deal to avoid injuring the boy. Lilly was no more responsible, qua moral agent, for the injury than any of his teammates. Thus, to the extent that our causal contributions are relevant to us and our lives only to the extent that they go through our agency, it seems puzzling that Lilly responded in a way very different from his other teammates.

Some might be tempted to respond that this outcome, and Lilly's relationship to it, involves a kind of moral luck. Perhaps Lilly made a small mistake in fouling the ball off, and the universe was arranged in just such a way that this minor mistake led to the boy's injury. The problem with this characterization is that fouling off the ball was, independent of the ultimate outcome of hitting the boy, the right thing for Lilly to do in the circumstances. Attempting to hit into fair territory a well-placed pitch often leads to an out. Fouling off such pitches gives the batter the opportunity to see another pitch, one that may well be easier to hit.[38] Fouling off pitches also forces the other team's pitcher to throw more pitches. Doing this early in the game can result in the pitcher tiring and losing his effectiveness as the game continues. Effectively fouling off good pitches is an art, an impressive one for any hitter and especially impressive for pitchers like Lilly (who typically are not good hitters).

Lilly is also not to blame legally. Foul balls are part of the game. Everyone (including Dominic DiAngi's father) knows this, and those who come to the game (and bring their children) accept the very small but real risk of getting hit. So, Lilly is not to blame morally, nor is he to blame legally. He did the right thing, at the right time, and it led to an unfortunate accident. Moral theory offers us little that might help to clarify Lilly's relationship to the injury. In particular, moral theory offers few resources for thinking about how the unfortunate consequences of Lilly's good action should be understood in the narrative of his life. Moral theories that focus too much on agency may end up concluding that the accident says nothing at all about Lilly's life.

Although there is a good deal more work to do on this issue, the conclusion that these accidents say nothing at all about our lives, or about Ted Lilly's life in particular, ignores an important part of our view of ourselves and our relationship to others. As Barbara Herman points out, our causal relationships count, not just because they allow for the possibility of moral agency, but in and of themselves. As Herman puts the point: "We accept causal responsibility" for the outcomes that result from our actions.[39] "I caused that injury" can be true even when I did not intend it and even when I was acting properly. There is a reason why Ted Lilly in particular decided to visit the child in the hospital. Presumably, many others did as well, well-wishers sorry for what happened. But Lilly, in visiting the hospital, was doing much more: He was recognizing that he was causally, even though not morally or legally, an important part of why the boy was in the hospital.

This is not to argue that Lilly's recognition is based only on the fact that he causally was an important part of the injury. It is bad enough to have one's skull fractured by a baseball; it is even worse in standard cases to have this come about as the result of another's intent to do harm. By visiting the boy and emphasizing that it was in no way intentional, Lilly is able to remove that potential insult from the realm of possibility. By expressing genuine regret that the harm occurred, Lilly removes another possible insult, the possibility that he benefited from the injury. *Intentionally* contributing to a negative outcome has negative implications for one as a moral agent and, thereby, has implications for one's overall life. One's life has led to at least that bad outcome, and such a life is worse overall compared to the same life absent the negative contribution. Although the involvement of one's agency is important to our evaluations of the contributions one makes, a contribution going through an individual's agency is not a necessary condition for its having negative valence for one's life. All things being equal, Ted Lilly's life would have been, to a very slight degree, better overall if it had not included being part of the causal process that led to the fracturing of Dominic DiAngi's skull.

This conclusion is supported by strong intuitions regarding our evaluation of our own lives and the lives of others. Undoubtedly, the worst part of the accident was the injury the boy suffered. But the outcome is not all that matters; the way in which it was realized also can have an impact on how we evaluate individuals' lives. It is worse to be harmed as the result of an intentional act of another compared to being injured as the result of an accident of nature. Worse to have your skull fractured as the result of an intentional assault than the result of a tree limb breaking off and striking you in the head. The significance of the way in which goods and evils come about is not limited to those who experience them. We are not indifferent, in some cases at least, to a world in which an injury is caused by an accident of nature versus one in which it is the result of a causal chain that includes us and our actions, even when our actions are not directed toward the resulting harm.

We will pursue this line of reasoning more fully in Chapter 7 when we consider children who contributed to the Nazi cause. The fact that a child was old enough to understand and willingly contribute to the horrors of the Nazi regime says a great deal about one's person and life, all of it negative. Too strict a focus on agency might lead to the conclusion that contributions made for which one is not morally responsible have no implications at all for one's life. Examples that contradict this initially plausible view point to the possibility of making judgments about individuals' lives independent of our judgments about the individuals as persons. A life may go less well without the individual being in any way to blame for it. We will see this when we consider the lives of the very young children who contributed to the Nazi cause without in any way understanding what that cause involved, including a 3-year-old girl we will meet in Chapter 7 who may personally have contributed to helping Hitler. While she is in no way to blame for what happened, her life would have gone better overall if she had not made this contribution (assuming she did). She, better than most, recognized, as she looked back on the episode, that an absence of moral responsibility is not sufficient to entirely eliminate a contribution to a negative cause from one's life narrative, from a complete telling of one's life.

This conclusion has significant implications not only for how we should think about our lives, but for how we should think about—and the extent to which we should care about—social structures and institutions. This is a vital point that I will not be able to do justice in the present work. The physical structure of society and the world can result in our actions having horrible causal consequences, beyond our intention and control. The fact that these consequences have implications for our overall lives provides us with a self-directed reason to care about those structures. It provides us with a reason to insist that social structures help protect individuals from such fates. Baseball players have reason to insist that adequate protection be included in stadiums to minimize the chances that the foul balls they hit harm spectators. There is even more reason to structure society so as to minimize the chances that children are put in a position to contribute innocently to evil causes, thus keeping them from contributing to such causes and, thereby, having a personal relationship with those causes. The fact that the contributions occur at a time when the children are unable to understand what is happening is some comfort, but not enough. In developing structures to protect all of us from inadvertently contributing to harmful outcomes, society is protecting more than the potential victims; society also is protecting potential contributors from becoming part of the cause that leads to others being harmed.

Outline of the Argument

There are several ways to defend the claim that a given contribution or relationship has implications for one's life overall in ways that are relevant to one's own interests, implications for whether it was a better or less good life overall for the individual whose life it was. The first-person perspective asks whether, all things considered, one would prefer that the contribution or relationship in question be a part of one's own life. Presumably, at least most of us would choose a life that, all things considered, involved making no contributions to the Nazi cause. If given a choice between making these contributions as a 20-year-old or a 3-year-old, we likely would choose the latter option, which tarnishes us, as moral agents, not at all, and tarnishes our lives less. But, if given a choice between a life that includes no such contributions versus a life that contributed to the Nazi cause as a 3-year-old, we prefer the former option. Put differently, we are not indifferent between a life in which we contribute to the Nazi cause at age 3, and the same life absent that contribution, even if we assume that the Nazi cause would not have been at all diminished by the absence of our contribution.[40] Lucky are those of us for whom this is only a theoretical question. As we shall see in Chapter 7, many individuals personally faced these very questions. And many of them emphatically preferred a life that did not include contributing to the Nazi cause, even though the contribution occurred when the individuals were too young to know the nature of the cause to which they were contributing. As adults, they both wished that these things had not occurred and independently wished that they had not contributed to them.

We can evaluate these options from a second-person perspective as well. From this perspective, we can ask what we would want for a loved one for his own sake. To take an instance of this approach that has special relevance for the present analysis: What do we want for our children? Stephen Darwall has developed this second-person perspective into a full analysis of what is good for an individual. Darwall argues that an individual's well-being or welfare is determined by what someone who cares for the individual (including possibly the individual herself) would want for the individual for her own sake.[41] What we want for those for whom we care is greatly influenced by, but also often diverges from, what they want for themselves. What we want for ourselves to the extent that we care about ourselves and our welfare also may diverge from what we in fact want. We may not want what is good for us or we may want things that are not good for us, possibly because we do not care for ourselves. An individual also may be mistaken about her own interests and want something, a cigarette perhaps, that is not in her interests.

Naturalistic accounts, of which Darwall's is one example, face the question of whether they can provide a complete account of welfare. For example, if we are not thinking straight, we may want things for those for whom we care that are not in their interests. The possibility of mistakes seems to suggest that what we want for those for whom we care may often track, but does not *determine* what is in their interests. For present purposes, we need not consider this concern because we shall not appeal to the second-person perspective to determine what is good for an individual for their own sake. Rather, this perspective, like the first-person perspective just considered (and the third-person perspective to come), will be employed as a heuristic to evaluate the plausibility of claims regarding what is in our interests, including the question of when participation in nonbeneficial pediatric research is or is not in the interests of individual children. The second-person perspective—what we want for those for whom we care for their own sakes—provides a useful mechanism for evaluating these claims, even if it does not provide a complete and independent account of what is in our interests.

Would you care whether your child contributed to the Nazi cause not at all, as a 3-year-old, as a teenager, or as an adult? The fact that the options get progressively worse reveals that the extent to which contributions go through an individual's agency plays an important role in how we judge him and his life in light of the contribution. In addition, and importantly, we presumably prefer the first option for our children to all the others. We are not indifferent, when thinking about our children for their own sakes, as to whether they never contributed to the Nazi cause or did so as 3-year-olds. This preference further supports the claim that agency is not everything for how well one's life goes. Better that our children not make this contribution at all than make it as infants or 3-year-olds, even though contributions made when very young do not have implications for them, as persons, agents, or as moral beings.

Finally, we will evaluate the implications of a given contribution for an overall life from the third-person perspective. All things being equal, is a life better or worse if it includes a given contribution or relationship than not? Positive contributions, like negative ones, can have implications for a given life, even when the individual makes the contribution as an infant or child, and these implications can be such that it was not simply a better life overall, but a better life for oneself. This is so because one of our interests is an interest in how well our lives go overall. And, to that extent, it can be in infants' and children's interests to contribute to important and valuable causes, including important and valuable clinical research studies, even when they pose some risks to them. Individuals may, as they mature, come to value these contributions and regard them as important. They also may become better people for having made the contributions. These are two crucial ways in which making positive contributions can make for a better life and thereby promote one's interests.

There is a further, more direct, way in which these contributions can have implications for one's life. To see this, consider again the case of contributing to the Nazi cause. Making the contribution to the Nazi cause as a child may have a devastating impact on the individual as an adult. Although that fact contributes to, it does not exhaust the negative implications of the contribution for the individual. Such contributions are a bad thing to have in one's life whether they have a negative impact on one's psychology or future behavior. Similarly, a valuable contribution can have positive implications for one's life even though it never influences one's psychology or future behavior.

Many philosophers have written on the topic of what is in our interests, and there is great debate and disagreement over the present question of whether events or contributions can be relevant to our interests even when they do not go through our agency and do not affect or influence us at all. Hedonistic accounts of our interests deny them any relevance. Such accounts regard things as being in our interests only to the extent that they influence our subjective experiences, only, to take Jeremy Bentham's version of the view, when and to the extent they give us pleasure or pain. One of the standard counterexamples to hedonist accounts of our interests asks us to consider whether it can be contrary to one's interests if one's spouse has an affair, even if one never finds out and the affair never influences one's life or relationship (e.g., the spouse never treats one differently as a result of the affair). The intuition that such an affair can nonetheless be contrary to one's interests supports the claim that our interests are not defined fully by our experiences or even our knowledge.

Preference satisfaction accounts of our interests, another type of subjective account, can explain this conclusion. These accounts hold that our interests are determined by those things about which we care. Presumably, we do not want our spouses to have affairs, whether we know about them or not. We take a further step away from purely subjective accounts of our interests if we agree that there is value for us in being involved in meaningful relationships, activities, and projects that goes beyond our personal goals and interests. Consider, for example, the *Depressed Contributor* who is part of and makes important contributions to a meaningful project. Perhaps he is part of a project that works with war refugees, helping them build new lives. The *Depressed Contributor* is so depressed that he derives no satisfaction from the activity or the project, either from his contributions to the project or his involvement in it, and does not regard it as a valuable aspect of his life. The appropriate response would not be to argue that if he could bring himself to embrace his association with and contribution to this project, and regard it as a valuable part of his life, then it would become part of a more valuable life for him. Rather, the argument is that he should embrace the relationship and his work with the project because in fact it is a valuable contribution, and there is value for individuals in making valuable contributions in many, if not most, cases. It typically is valuable for the person whose life it is to make valuable contributions to worthwhile projects. The value of the *Depressed Contributor*'s work for his life does not entirely depend on his valuing it, nor entirely on his experiencing in some way the results of the finished project. Moreover, it is not his valuing the contribution that makes it his contribution. Whether he was part of the project and made important contributions to it is determined by the causal facts: what did he do and what were the consequences of what he did? And whether the project is valuable depends on the nature of the project itself.

Many commentators in ethics argue that something can be in an individual's interests, often characterized in terms of promoting the individual's welfare or well-being, only if it affects the individual in some way, including possibly promoting or realizing a personal goal. I will argue that, in addition to the influence things have on us, our interests also include how we influence others and the world, independent of the extent to which we are influenced in the process or as a result. The claim that, all things being equal, participation in and contributions to valuable and meaningful projects are part of a better, more meaningful life overall, and that we have an interest in living better lives because such lives are better *for us,* need not deny that individuals' personal preferences, projects, and goals are relevant to whether participation in and contribution to a particular activity or relationship is consistent with and furthers their interests. Contributions and relationships that are in the interests of most of us may be contrary to the interests of some, for example, cloistered monks.

The view one takes of human interests involves an entire framework within which to understand our lives and our place in the world. Because these considerations involve fundamental aspects of our lives, the claim that being part of and making contributions to valuable causes or relationships is in our interests, even as young children, cannot be settled with one example or argument. Instead, defense of this claim and the consequent justification of some nonbeneficial pediatric research will require a fundamental account of how we think about our lives and our interests. Thus, it is only when the entire account is in place that we will be able to evaluate the argument fully. In the end, the question will essentially be one of which account of our lives is more compelling, all things considered.

Three preliminary stages will be required before we will be in a position to evaluate this view. To consider what contributions might be part of a better life overall for an individual, we first will need an account of what constitutes a better life overall. We will then consider to what extent it is better for us that our lives go better overall. This will require a general account of human interests. Second, we will need to consider what conditions must be satisfied for it to be the case that one has been part of and made a contribution to a given project or outcome. We will see that the central issue here is not whether the contribution goes through an individual's agency, but whether one is causally connected in the right way to the project or outcome. Third, we will consider when it is the case that making a given contribution to a valuable project is in an individual's interests as the result of being part of a more worthwhile life overall. We will see that while *the extent* to which a given contribution goes through an individual's agency affects what implications it has for the individual's life, this fact does not determine whether (making) the contribution has implications for the individual's life and for the individual whose life it is.

As has been suggested thus far, and as will be seen in much greater detail in Chapter 5, the present analysis of when nonbeneficial pediatric research is ethically acceptable, and when it is ethically unacceptable, will be based on an account of human interests that includes more objective elements. Specifically, this analysis will be based on the claim that it is objectively in our interests in the sense that the value for a given individual of contributing to valuable projects and relationships does not depend entirely on the particular mental states of the individual in question. The claim that it typically is in our interests to contribute to valuable projects and contrary to our interests to contribute to evil, inappropriate, and harmful projects does not require that one endorse these views personally. Griffin endorses a similar view when he writes "making one's life valuable and not just frittering it away, is valuable for everyone; anyone who fails to recognize it as valuable lacks understanding."[42]

This view recognizes that individuals' own goals, values, preferences, and projects have significant influence on what, as a matter of fact, is in their interests. However, this view also holds that individuals can be mistaken, even wildly so, about what is in their interests. At the same time, any plausible account of what is in our interests includes the fact that, among other things, it is in our interests to pursue our own projects and goals. The relationship between what we care about and what is in our interests becomes complicated to the extent that (some of) what is more objectively in our interests may not be in the interests of specific humans once they have adopted and pursued goals and projects the realization of which are inconsistent with those other aspects of the objectively good life.

This tension can be seen in Bernard Williams's retelling, and perhaps recasting, of the life of Paul Guaguin.[43] Williams's Guaguin is confronted with the terrible choice of continuing to provide for his family, or leaving them behind for distant lands where he can pursue his art. Williams uses this example to support his claims regarding moral luck: "I want to explore and uphold the claim that in such a situation the only thing that will justify his choice will be success itself."[44] If Guaguin suffers an accident on the way that prevents his painting, there will be "nothing in the outcome to set against the other people's loss."[45] In that case, Guaguin will have done something terribly wrong; he will have deserted his family and friends for no (good) reason.

Williams's example is useful for present purposes because it introduces the notion of luck and the extent to which factors outside of the agent's control can influence how the agent's life goes. Since at least the time of Socrates, as Williams points out at the beginning of his essay, philosophers have been trying to immunize to one extent or another how well our lives go—what we say about the quality or value of one's life—from the vagaries of fortune and misfortune. As we shall consider in Chapter 9, some philosophers have held that all that matters for us, or all that seriously matters for us, is within our control. It seems, following a very plausible line of reasoning, positively irrational to value, to hold as relevant to one's well-being, things, events, and people that are outside of one's control.

Very few philosophers are willing to go that far today. It is clear that being born with an intact brain and keeping it relatively intact for an extended period are necessary conditions for a good life; yet the former is fully[46] and the latter largely is outside the individual's control. To borrow and adapt a line from a widely cited article on a different topic, absent a (reliable!) army, one cannot fully control whether one's brain suffers permanent injury.[47] Nonetheless, many contemporary philosophers try to carve out a space of value within our lives that is immune to luck. In particular, many philosophers argue that while the overall value of one's life is subject to luck, the moral value of one's life is fully within one's control. One cannot, by ill fortune, on this view, do something immoral. Many of these philosophers then greatly emphasize those aspects of our lives that are within our control, perhaps unconsciously attempting again to wall off as much of our fortune as possible from luck.

The attempt to insulate ourselves from those things that are outside our control will play a fundamental, if somewhat implicit role in the present work. I will argue for the claim that the contributions one makes have implications for one's overall life, even though we often are not fully in control of what sorts of contributions ultimately are the fruits of our actions. This is not to say, as Williams does, that the outcomes of our actions which are the result of luck have implications for a *moral* evaluation of us and our lives. Rather, the consequences of our actions have implications for the overall preferability of our lives. Although I will not argue for the claim here, I suspect that the failure to distinguish these two possibilities is part of what gives the examples Williams and others use to defend the notion of moral luck much of their force. Without taking on that argument, it will be useful as we proceed to keep in mind the extent to which our desire to remain in control of (the most important aspects of) our lives shapes our views, and how appropriate that shaping is on the significance of the contributions we make for our overall lives.

One can read Guaguin's dilemma as supporting the possibility of a conflict between moral considerations (care for one's children, discharge one's responsibilities to others) and other values, including artistic ones. Williams writes: "While we are sometimes guided by the notion that it would be the best of worlds in which morality were universally respected and all men were of a disposition to affirm it, we have, in fact, deep and persistent reasons to be grateful that that is not the world we have."[48] One can also understand the dilemma as one regarding the nature of our interests. What is in Guaguin's interests in this case? One might argue that his own interests are determined by those things he most cares about. And if that is painting rather than caring for his family, then it would further his overall interests to leave his family to paint. It might be thought that this conclusion is inconsistent with an objective account of interests that presumably will tend to prioritize doing the right thing for others. Yet, one may regard it as an objective fact that it is in individuals' interests to pursue their own goals. Thus, depending on the significance of the different considerations for Guaguin's life, it may turn out, on an objective account, that it is in his interests to leave his family. Of course, this conclusion need not imply that leaving his family is the morally right thing for him to do.

While the present analysis will be based on the claim that it is to some extent objectively, or at least not fully subjectively, in our interests to contribute to valuable projects, the conclusions regarding the acceptability of some and the unacceptability of other nonbeneficial pediatric research studies will not depend on one's accepting an objective account. This argument could be recast using a subjective account. This version of the argument would maintain, roughly, that, as a matter of fact, many individuals do value making contributions to valuable projects and outcomes. And it seems to make sense for parents to want their children to have such preferences and for parents to raise their children both to have such preferences and to structure the children's lives so that they contribute to valuable projects, even as children. Or, one could argue that parents are justified in making decisions for their children based on plausible empirical assumptions regarding the preferences and values their children are likely to develop. To reject on subjectivist grounds the conclusions drawn here regarding nonbeneficial pediatric research, one would have to hold that the good for any individual is fully determined by his own preferences, values, and goals and, furthermore, it is inappropriate for parents to attempt to structure their children's lives or influence the values, preferences, and goals their children develop. We will come to reasons to think that this position is implausible and, for most purposes, self-defeating.

TWO | Background

Scope of the Debate

The studies that evoke the greatest concern, what I will call the paradigm instances of nonbeneficial pediatric research, involve investigators directly interacting with pediatric participants and thereby placing them at some risk for the benefit of others. A paradigmatic nonbeneficial research study might involve an investigator giving pediatric participants a few doses of an experimental medication to see how quickly the concentration of the medication rises and falls in their blood. A paradigmatic nonbeneficial intervention occurs when investigators take a few milliliters of blood purely for research purposes as part of a study that offers a compensating potential for clinical benefit. In addition to these paradigm cases, investigators also sometimes expose children to research risks without directly interacting with them. An example of this type of research occurs when investigators systematically analyze children's medical records in a way that poses some confidentiality risks.

In objecting to nonbeneficial pediatric research, critics do not cite examples in which researchers look through the medical records of children or use children's left-over biological specimens for research purposes. They cite examples in which researchers insert a needle into the veins of children for research purposes. Because the paradigmatic studies are thought to raise the greatest ethical concern, our focus will be on evaluating possible justifications for them: how might it be justified for researchers to insert a needle in a child's vein purely for research purposes. To the extent that nonparadigmatic studies expose children to research risks, these stand in need of justification as well. Thus, although we will spend little time on these studies, a complete justification of nonbeneficial pediatric research should address both the paradigmatic and nonparadigmatic cases.

Our focus will be further limited to nonbeneficial interventions and studies conducted by nonprofit entities and designed to benefit future patients. This focus is intended to bracket the increasing number of clinical research studies conducted by pharmaceutical companies as opposed to governmental agencies and nonprofits: "Impatient with the slow pace of academic bureaucracies, pharmaceutical companies have moved trials to the private sector, where more than 70 percent of them are now conducted."[1] This change raises a number of important ethical issues, central among them how to regulate the inherent financial conflicts of interest that arise when companies are entrusted with testing the safety of medical interventions they will market and from which they hope to profit. This change also has the potential to alter the goal of clinical research, including pediatric research.

The primary ethical question raised by pediatric research is whether it is acceptable to expose children to research risks for the benefit of others. In the standard formulation—the one that will be the focus of the present work—the benefits that others enjoy as the result of pediatric research are medical and health benefits, better treatments for disease, and better methods to prevent disease. Pharmaceutical company-funded research introduces the potential for monetary benefit and, thereby, potentially alters the moral concerns raised by pediatric research. Pharmaceutical companies typically focus on generating profit and increasing stock price and market share. Depending on market conditions, achieving these goals may lead them to pursue new treatments that also have the potential to increase overall health and well-being. Or, they may not. The latter possibility is illustrated by the phenomenon of so-called "me-too" drugs.

A purely me-too drug is one that is identical in all clinically relevant respects to approved drugs already in use for a given condition. Me-too drugs offer in place of the potential to increase overall health and well-being, the potential to redistribute the market so that some consumers who previously purchased the drug of company A will instead purchase the effectively identical drug from company B. There is considerable debate over how many me-too drugs really exist, and what is required for a drug to count as effectively identical. Does a difference between once- versus twice-a-day dosing constitute a clinically relevant difference? Does the fact that a drug need not be taken with meals? We will not engage this debate, except to note that a company may well be interested in a drug that qualifies as a me-too drug on all relevant counts, whatever they turn out to be. Despite the similarities between existing drugs and the newly developed one, the company may be able, by relying on an effective marketing department, to convince physicians to prescribe (and consumers to request) the new drug rather than the existing ones.

The oft-cited claim that a company's primary obligation is to earn a profit and increase stock price seems to imply that pharmaceutical companies are obliged to focus on earnings and to pursue improvements in health and well-being only to the extent that they are sufficiently profitable. It seems to follow that pharmaceutical companies are obligated to pursue me-too drugs when the evidence suggests that they will be sufficiently profitable. This possibility raises the question of whether it can be ethically acceptable to enroll children in nonbeneficial research that has the potential to earn profit for a company, but does not have the potential to improve overall health and well-being. Is it acceptable for a company to enroll children in a nonbeneficial trial that poses risks in order to make a profit? Although the present account will have implications for this question, I will have little to say about it. Instead, I shall focus on the question of whether it is acceptable to enroll children in studies designed to develop medical interventions with the potential *ex ante* to promote and improve health and well being. The normative dilemma here is not trading risks to children against potential profits for others, but trading risks to some children for benefits in health and well-being for others.

Focus on research with the potential to help others medically brings with it a temptation to demand too much of individual studies and then criticize as wanting and perhaps unethical those that fail to satisfy this standard. Many studies are necessary preludes to future treatment studies, and their value is represented by the incremental gain in knowledge that they offer, not by any potential to identify a new treatment. Years of examination and many preliminary studies are required before investigators are even in a position to determine the efficacy of new interventions. In the case of the rotavirus vaccines, scientists first had to determine what causes the gastroenteritis, and then had to develop and test different vaccines and different ways of delivering them to children. The benefit of these preliminary, and typically nonbeneficial studies, was not identification of an effective new vaccine, but collection of information crucial to achieving that result in the future.

The fact that developing new medical treatments for children typically takes many studies and many years places limits on the possible justifications for most nonbeneficial pediatric research. Any justification that appeals to the potential for a given nonbeneficial study to yield improved medical treatments will be unable to justify most pediatric research studies, including the preliminary studies that are necessary precursors to those studies that do offer this potential. It also is important not to assume that the value of a given research program—for example, the years and series of studies that culminated in the identification of effective rotavirus vaccines—resides solely or even largely in the final study that identifies an effective vaccine. For many years, Sandra Day O'Connor was the swing vote for many important cases before the U.S. Supreme Court. There were four fairly reliable liberal votes and four fairly reliable conservative votes, such that the majority in many cases fell on whichever side turned out to be more congenial to her. In these cases, it is easy to assume that hers was the most important vote.

We tend to credit the deciding vote with more value because it defines the point at which we can be confident of the outcome. Although we privilege the conclusive step for the certainty it provides, we should not make the mistake of assuming that the input that makes the outcome certain is also the input that alone determines the outcome. We should not conflate epistemological significance with ontological importance. In a 5–4 court case, the deciding vote influences the outcome no more and no less than the other votes. In the context of clinical research, preliminary studies are just as important, if not nearly as dramatic, as the final study or studies that establish the safety and efficacy of an experimental treatment. Even studies that turn out to be negative typically have some value. As anyone who has attempted to locate a missing item recognizes, it can be very useful to know where the item is not to be found.

Terms of the Debate

Fairly wide agreement exists concerning the necessary conditions for informed consent to clinical research. Individuals must be able to understand, at a minimum, the research in question and their own circumstances. They should understand the risks, potential benefits, and alternatives to a given research study. Individuals also should be competent and in a position to make an autonomous decision whether to enroll. Most children are unable to meet these conditions because they are unable to understand sufficiently the research and their own circumstances.

It is the inability to understand and give informed consent that makes the enrollment of children in nonbeneficial research particularly troubling.[2] This is not to imply that all children are unable to give informed consent to research participation. Human development occurs at a fairly predictable but varying pace. Some children are able to understand and give informed consent early, and most children are able to understand before they reach the age of legal consent. Recognizing these facts, the present work will consider a child to be an individual who is too young to give informed consent. This, in turn, is not to imply that once children are able to give their own informed consent they should be treated in exactly the same way as adults. The fact that children live with and are dependent on their parents raises the distinct question of whether the parents should have a say, even a veto, regarding whether their children, no matter what their level of maturity, participate in clinical research.

The term that one uses to describe the individuals in clinical research itself says something about how one views the ethical concerns it raises and, in some sense, reflects at least preliminary conclusions one has drawn regarding those concerns. Calling these individuals "patients" emphasizes the fact that they often suffer from disease and may be especially vulnerable. This view also runs the risk of confusing the ethical analysis of clinical research with the ethical analysis of clinical care, and does not apply to research with healthy volunteers. The term "subject" seems more apt and emphasizes that the individuals are involved in research and are being subjected, especially in the paradigmatic cases of non-beneficial research, to some risks and burdens for the benefit of others.

For reasons that will become clearer as we proceed, I will use "participant," a term that has gained in popularity more recently and is intended to draw attention to the fact that those enrolled in research are not merely being exposed to risks and burdens. They also are contributing to the research effort, a fact that has important implications independent of the extent to which they face risks and burdens. One may object that even if the term "participant" is appropriate for adults who provide informed consent, it does not apply to children who cannot consent and are enrolled in research based on the permission of their parents or legal guardians. Adequate response to this concern will require full evaluation of the arguments to come. A preliminary response was anticipated by the outline of the argument provided in Chapter 1. Children, even those who are unable to give informed consent *are* participants, although often unwitting ones, in the sense of making an important contribution to the research in question. "Contributor" might be a better term were it not already used to refer to the clinicians who are part of the research team.

The literature uses a number of different terms to refer to research interventions and studies that expose participants to risks for the benefit of others. Previously, this type of research often was labeled "nontherapeutic" research, in contrast to therapeutic research. *Therapeutic research* has been defined in different and sometimes conflicting ways, but typically is thought to involve research that is *intended* or *designed* to benefit participants. This distinction, and these labels, are problematic for the simple reason that investigators often intend, in the same study or even during the same intervention, to both help participants and to gather generalizable knowledge. Similarly, research interventions and studies typically are designed both to collect generalizable information and to benefit participants to the extent possible. In the end, then, essentially all procedures and studies qualify as both therapeutic and nontherapeutic. This is one of the reasons why Robert Levine argues that "every document that relies on a distinction between therapeutic and nontherapeutic research contains errors."[3]

The U.S. regulations avoid these particular errors, referring instead to research that offers the "prospect of direct benefit" to participating children. This terminology represents an improvement, but is unclear regarding whether the research to which it refers offers any chance of benefit, or is limited to research that offers some minimal level of potential benefit. To avoid these terminological debates, I will use the term "nonbeneficial research." The term "nonbeneficial" as a qualifier refers to the fact that the study or intervention in question does not offer a compensating potential for clinical benefit to participants. This term has the potential to mislead to the extent that it might be taken to suggest that the research in question offers no potential for benefit of any kind, even to future patients, in which case it would be puzzling why the research is being conducted at all. Against this possibility, I assume that nonbeneficial pediatric research can be justified, if it can be justified at all, only when it has the potential to gather valuable information with the potential to improve health and well-being.

One might worry that a definition of nonbeneficial research procedures that relies on the notion of a "compensating" potential for clinical benefit commits us to substantive assumptions regarding the extent to which it is possible to compare risks and potential benefits in a single individual. In particular, one might worry that the postulation of research procedures that do not offer a compensating potential for clinical benefit assumes that some single metric exists on which experts, at least in theory, can directly compare risks and potential benefits. Such experts might find that the risks of a given study have a negative value of X, while the potential clinical benefits have a positive value of Y, in which case a nonbeneficial study would be one for which X is greater than Y.

We can avoid this apparent implication, and the resulting debate, by basing the present distinction on the clinical judgment of informed and expert clinicians. Whether a given pediatric research intervention or study offers a compensating potential for clinical benefit can be understood as referring to the recommendations of an informed and expert clinician who is concerned only with furthering the clinical interests of the children in question. Specifically, would such an expert recommend that the child or group of children undergo the intervention or enroll in the study in question? If yes, the research offers a compensating potential for clinical benefit. If no, the research constitutes what I am calling "nonbeneficial" pediatric research.[4]

It may turn out that a range of studies exist for which it is unclear whether enrollment is consistent with an individual child's clinical interests.[5] In that case, the present approach would determine whether these studies should be categorized as offering a compensating potential for clinical benefit by establishing a default of enrolling or not enrolling children. Although I will not pursue the question here, the standard in pediatric research ethics is to default to the side of not enrolling children.[6]

In what follows, I shall argue that participating in nonbeneficial pediatric research can be in children's overall interests to the extent that they have an interest in a better life overall, such a life is better for them, and being in the research makes for a better life overall for them to the extent that it involves their contributing to an important project. This claim may seem to undermine the assumptions on which the argument is based. If nonbeneficial research is defined as research that conflicts with the interests of the participating children, how is it possible that participation in such research might promote their overall interests? This terminological conundrum is resolved by distinguishing different types of benefits to participating children.

Whether an intervention or study qualifies as nonbeneficial depends on whether it offers a compensating potential for clinical or medical benefit. Research interventions that satisfy this standard may, nonetheless, offer children the potential for other sorts of benefits that may justify the risks they face. As mentioned previously, this possibility may first have been considered by William Bartholome, who argued that participation in nonbeneficial research can offer children the potential for educational benefit in the form of moral growth. This example highlights the fact that a research intervention or study that does not offer a compensating potential for clinical benefit, and therefore qualifies as nonbeneficial in the sense used here, may be in children's overall interests because it offers the potential for other types of benefits. The question, then, is whether nonbeneficial pediatric research consistently offers some other type of benefit that is sufficient to justify the risks to which are exposed participating children who cannot consent.

History of Abuses, Early Guidelines

The early history of pediatric research includes far too many examples of abusive research. One account maintains that: "The history of pediatric experimentation is largely one of child abuse."[7] In addition, many of the abuses cited by Henry Beecher in his famous 1966 article listing research abuses at prominent institutions in the United States included children, and a number of these studies focused on children specifically. Pappworth also cites many abusive studies involving children.[8] There is inevitable debate over whether one or another of the cited examples in fact involved abusive research. What options did the children have? How are those options relevant to the appropriateness of the study in question? What impact did the study in fact have on the participating children?

Bracketing these questions, which largely are of historic interest, it is clear that many instances of unethical and abusive studies have occurred in the history of pediatric research. One of the earliest recorded cases of abuse occurred in 1892 when Albert Niesser, a medical professor at Breslau, gave serum taken from syphilis patients to unwitting individuals. Several of the recipients contracted syphilis, leading to public outcry and a government ruling, promulgated in 1900 and codified in the 1931 German guidelines, resulting in perhaps the first systematic regulations governing clinical research.[9] These guidelines explicitly prohibit nonbeneficial research with children, as well as pediatric research that "in any way endangers the child."[10] It is difficult to imagine a research study that does not pose some risks to participating children. Seemingly innocuous surveys of health behavior, for instance, pose some chance of upsetting children. Even widely accepted pediatric research that offers a compensating potential for clinical benefit poses some chance of harm. In practice, then, these guidelines may prohibit essentially all pediatric research.

The German ruling of 1900 is one instance among many in which research guidelines were developed in response to a specific scandal. Most famously, in response to the horrific experiments perpetrated by the Nazis, the Nuremberg Code stipulates that participants' consent is "essential" to ethical research. This approach, even more so than the German guidelines of 1931, appears to prohibit essentially all research with children.[11] There is an obvious and very important virtue to this approach. If children are prohibited from being enrolled in clinical research, it will be difficult for investigators to exploit them in that context.

By the 1960s, increasing sentiment indicated that the Nuremberg Code needed to be modified in several important respects, especially to address the fact that it did not include a requirement that clinical research studies should be reviewed and approved by an independent ethics board. This requirement was included in the Declaration of Helsinki, promulgated by the World Medical Association in 1964, and intended to address the shortcomings in the Nuremberg Code. The Declaration of Helsinki also is based on recognition of the shortcomings of attempting to protect individuals who cannot consent by excluding them from clinical research. This approach protects individuals in the short term but dramatically undermines investigators' ability to identify better medical treatments for these groups. The Declaration of Helsinki attempts to protect individuals who cannot consent without excluding them from the potential benefits of clinical research by allowing them to be enrolled in clinical research based on the permission of an appropriate surrogate. This clause allows the enrollment of children in clinical research based on the permission of a legal guardian, typically the child's parents.

The abuses perpetrated as part of the infamous Tuskegee syphilis study were made public in 1972, 40 years after the study was initiated. The resulting outcry led to the formation of the U.S. National Commission, which was charged with evaluating the ethics of clinical research with humans and developing recommendations regarding appropriate safeguards. As part of its deliberations, the National Commission spent a good deal of time considering whether it can be acceptable to expose children to research risks for the benefit of others. These deliberations resulted in an entire volume dedicated to the ethics of pediatric research, including what are still some of the most important writings on the topic. These deliberations also produced a series of recommendations for the conduct of pediatric research, which became the framework for the existing U.S. regulations for research with children, one more instance in which scandal led to new regulations for clinical research.

Current Regulations

National regulations governing human subjects research are relatively recent. The U.S. federal regulations for clinical research are not yet 30 years old. Many countries, including countries where research is taking place, do not yet have formal research regulations, and others have adopted them in only the last 10 years. For example, the Indian Council of Medical Research (ICMR) guidelines were adopted in 2000.[12] Halpern argues that clinical research communities had informal ethical norms, especially regarding consent, risks, and benefits, in place long before formal codes were developed.[13] Unfortunately, as Halpern notes, there was "tremendous inconsistency in whether and how they [the moral norms and traditions] are implemented."[14] Indeed, these informal codes and protections proved inadequate to protect many pediatric research subjects from abuse.

Unlike the early German regulations and the Nuremberg Code, current research regulations around the world attempt to allow important pediatric research while still protecting pediatric research participants. They try to achieve this balance by mandating specific safeguards, especially safeguards concerning risk level. The National Commission argued, and the framers of the U.S. regulations agreed, that what I am calling nonbeneficial pediatric research can be acceptable provided the risks are sufficiently low and several other safeguards are satisfied, including independent review and approval, and permission of the child's parent or legal guardian.

Current U.S. regulations refer to sufficiently low risks as "minimal" risks and define them in terms of the risks of daily life. Specifically, minimal risk are risks that are "not greater in and of themselves than those ordinarily encountered in daily life or during the performance of routine physical or psychological examinations or tests."[15,16] Many guidelines, including those from Nepal, use this standard.[17] Australia's guidelines categorize research interventions as posing minimal risk when "the probability and magnitude of harm or discomfort anticipated in the research are not greater in and of themselves than those ordinarily encountered in daily life."[18] This standard is also used by guidelines in Canada and Uganda,[19] and a variation of it is used in the South African guidelines.[20] Finally, a few countries, including Kenya[21] and the Indian Council on Medical Research,[22] allow nonbeneficial pediatric research without defining what constitutes sufficiently low risks, leaving this determination to the judgment of the ethics review committees.

There has been significant discussion regarding the proper interpretation of the "risks of daily life" standard, with much of the discussion focusing on whose life should be used as the index case. The risks allowed in nonbeneficial pediatric research would vary significantly if one based this standard on the risks faced by children who live in unsafe or dangerous environments as opposed to children who lead a very sheltered life, children who live in Norway versus children who live in current-day Iraq. To address the possibility of exploiting some children's already unfortunate circumstances, widespread agreement has developed over the past several years that the risks of daily life standard should be interpreted based on the risks faced in daily life by average, healthy children.[23]

The U.S. regulations, unlike most other regulations around the world, allow nonbeneficial pediatric research of greater risk in two circumstances. Review boards can approve nonbeneficial pediatric research when the risks are greater than minimal provided they are no more than a "minor" increase over minimal and several additional safeguards have been satisfied.[24] In addition, the Secretary of the Department of Health and Humans Services (DHHS) may approve research that poses risks too great for review board approval following review by a panel of experts. In principle, if not in practice, these regulations would allow approval of nonbeneficial pediatric research that posed risks substantially higher than those average, healthy children face in daily life. We will discuss the minimal risk standard in more depth, as well as some alternatives to it, in Chapter 3.

Efforts to Increase Pediatric Research

Child health and medicine is enormously better than it was 200, or even 50 years ago. A great deal of this improvement has occurred as the result of public health measures, such as clean water and sanitation.[25] Clinical research also has been central to at least some of the advances. One example has been the dramatic improvements in treating pediatric cancer, many of which are the result of clinical trials. Another is the development of a number of vaccines.

Despite these examples, and explicit regulations allowing nonbeneficial pediatric research, it is estimated that up to 70% of all medications given to children have not been tested for safety and efficacy in children.[26] The relative paucity of pediatric research traces to a number of sources. First, the market for pediatric medical treatments is much smaller than the market for adults for the simple reason that children develop serious illnesses much less often than adults. As a result, pharmaceutical companies are less likely to make a profit on drugs developed for children. Second, concern exists that conducting pediatric research carries with it an increased potential for legal jeopardy. Third, concern exists over the ethical acceptability of pediatric research. Institutions have been reluctant to support, review boards have been reluctant to approve, and clinicians, trained to promote the best interests of individual children, have been reluctant to conduct pediatric research studies.

A number of rules and regulations have been developed to encourage research designed to improve pediatric medical care.[27] In 2000, the International Conference on Harmonization published guidance on the evaluation of medicinal products in children (ICH E-11). The objectives are described as follows: "The number of medicinal products currently labeled for pediatric use is limited. This guidance is intended to encourage and facilitate timely pediatric medicinal product development internationally. The guidance provides an outline of critical issues in pediatric drug development and approaches to the safe, efficient, and ethical study of medicinal products in the pediatric population."[28]

Data that approximately half of all drugs provided to children in Europe represent off-label or unlicensed use has led to calls for more research on medications in children, while the European Forum for Good Clinical Practice has called for legislation in Europe to promote research with children. In 2004, the U.K. Health Minister announced a new initiative to encourage the development of medications for children. In the United States, the National Institutes of Health (NIH) now requires the inclusion of children in a broad range of research,[29] and the Food and Drug Administration Modernization Act[30] passed by Congress in 1997, offered 6 months additional marketing exclusivity to firms that submit data pertaining to the use of tested agents in pediatric populations. In October 2000, the U.S. Congress passed the Children's Health Act, which considers research on childhood illnesses to be a national priority.[31] In 2002, the U.S. Congress passed the Best Pharmaceuticals for Children Act, which extended the marketing exclusivity opportunity for an additional 5 years.[32] And in 2003, the Pediatric Research Equity Act was passed, requiring studies in children on certain drugs and biological products.[33] These regulations, which were scheduled to lapse at the end of 2007, were renewed in September of that year and are now effective until October 1, 2012.[34]

Data suggest that these efforts are leading to increases in the number of pediatric studies. Approximately 45,000 children have been enrolled in studies reviewed by the U.S. FDA in an 8-year period from 1997 to 2005. As of 2007, 125 products have been studied, leading to 128 label changes as of March 2007. These changes include new information on dosing and safety of medications in children. It has been estimated that 1 in 5 to 1 in 3 studies conducted as a result of the Best Pharmaceuticals for Children Act have produced new information regarding dosing, effectiveness, or risks.[35]

New European Union (EU) regulations to encourage research on pediatric medicines were passed in January 2007.[36] These regulations offer incentives to the pharmaceutical industry to test products in children and call for a pediatric committee at the European Agency for the Evaluation of Medicinal Products (EMEA) to oversee and assess investigators' plans for developing medicines for children. The main responsibility of the pediatric committee (PDCO) is to assess whether applicants have an adequate plan for testing in children, including assessment of applications for a full or partial waiver and assessment for deferrals of the requirement to test products in children.[37] Beginning in July 2008, all applicants for marketing approval are required to have a pediatric implementation plan, which includes either a plan to collect pediatric data or the request for a deferral or waiver, reviewed and approved by the pediatric committee. Although it is far too early to assess the impact of this legislation in Europe, it highlights the increase in efforts around the world to encourage and conduct clinical research with children.[38] These efforts in turn underscore the importance of determining whether and under what conditions nonbeneficial pediatric research can be ethical.

The Legal Landscape

The law, at least in the United States, offers little on which to base an analysis of when it is acceptable to enroll children in clinical research. In 1993, Leonard

Glantz pointed out that "perhaps the most notable point concerning the legal aspects of research on children is the small role the law has played in this area."[39] Little has changed since then, although there have been a few notable legal cases, which we will consider in the next section.

The U.S. federal regulations for pediatric research often are regarded as legal statutes. In fact they only establish guidelines for how pediatric research must be conducted to receive federal funding or product approval by the FDA. These regulations do not specify when it is lawful to conduct pediatric research in the United States. Essentially, the existing federal regulations represent agreements that institutions conducting research enter into with the federal government. To receive U.S. federal funds to conduct research and to apply for product approval by the FDA, institutions must agree to abide by the regulations of the DHHS and the FDA. However, the fact that one has followed these regulations does not imply that one necessarily has acted in accord with relevant law. In particular, adhering to the federal regulations on pediatric research may lead researchers to violate the laws of the state in which the research is conducted.

Several attempts have been made in the U.S. Congress to introduce legislation that would create national legal standards for clinical research. None of these efforts has succeeded, in part because of the historic practice of deferring to the individual states in matters of health. Yet, few states have developed laws on pediatric research. In the absence of legal statutes, one looks, in the United States at least, to case law. The earliest relevant cases involve tissue or organ donation in which one child faces risks for the benefit of another child. In these cases, the courts typically appeal to the best-interests standard for the donor, allowing donations to proceed only when the court finds that it offers the donor important potential benefit in the form of helping the recipient, often a close relative.

One of the earliest donation cases, *Madsen v. Harrison* involved 19-year-old twin brothers and took place in 1957, when the age of majority was 21. The court ruled in part that the donor would benefit by avoiding the negative psychological impact of the death of his brother. In the case of *Strunk v. Strunk,* the mother of 27-year-old Jerry Strunk, who had a reported mental age of 6, petitioned the court to allow Jerry to donate a kidney to his 28-year-old brother, who had kidney disease. The court found that the loss of his brother posed a greater risk to Jerry than the surgery and donation, and allowed it. In the 1972 case of *Hart v. Brown* the court allowed a transplant from a 7-year-old to her sister after hearing testimony from a psychiatrist that the procedure would benefit the donor in the form of a happier family.

The *Farinelli* case represents a rare instance in which a court did not rely on the fact that the donation was in the best interests of the donor. This case involved a bone marrow transplant from a 6-year-old girl to her 10-year-old brother with aplastic anemia. The court argued that the transplant was acceptable, not because it would benefit the donor, but on the grounds that it was the "fair and reasonable" course of action. This ruling is significant because it raises the possibility, which we will pursue, of considering whether it is possible to justify on other grounds interventions—research or clinical—that do not promote a child's clinical interests.

The (Few) Legal Cases Involving Pediatric Research

In the early 1970s, James Neilson, a member of the Committee on Human Subjects at the University of California at San Francisco, objected to a proposed longitudinal study of children with allergies.[40] The study planned to use healthy children as a control group and to subject them to nonbeneficial procedures, including blood draws and the administration of pharmaceutical agents. Neilson contended that these nonbeneficial procedures violated the healthy children's constitutional rights. He sought a judgment forbidding parents from enrolling their children in the study on the grounds that it would not benefit them directly. The case received wide attention, but was dismissed on the grounds that Neilson lacked sufficient standing to bring the case.

In 1996, several individuals and organizations challenged regulations of the New York State Office of Mental Health that allowed for the enrollment in greater than minimal risk research of minors and adults who lacked the capacity to give informed consent.[41] The trial court invalidated the regulations on the grounds that the Office of Mental Health lacked statutory authority to adopt them. The next year, the intermediate appellate court in New York agreed with the trial court's conclusion, but added a wide-ranging critique of the regulations, indicating that they violated both constitutional due process rights and the substantive protections granted these research subjects under New York's statutory and common law. The court ruled that parents and guardians "may not consent to have a child submit to painful and/or potentially life-threatening research procedures that hold no prospect of benefit for the child." In *T.D. v. New York State Office of Mental Health,* New York's highest court narrowed the judicial holding to the original decision of the trial court.

The case that most directly involves nonbeneficial pediatric research in the United States is the case of *Grimes v. The Kennedy Krieger Institute*. The *Grimes* case stems from a lead paint abatement study, sponsored by the Kennedy Krieger Institute (KKI) and conducted in Baltimore, Maryland from 1993 to 1995. The study was designed to evaluate whether partial lead paint abatement might protect children from lead poisoning. Viola Hughes and Cantina Higgins, parents of children enrolled in the study, sued KKI on behalf of their children,[42] alleging that the investigators failed to warn them in a timely manner when testing indicated elevated levels of lead dust in the plaintiffs' homes. The lower court dismissed the case, and the plaintiffs appealed to the Court of Appeals, Maryland's highest court.

The Court of Appeals' main ruling attempts to specify the conditions under which children may be enrolled in research. Citing the Nuremberg Code, and legal precedent that parental decisions should be in their children's best interests, the court ruled that, in Maryland, children may not be enrolled in research that poses "any risk of injury." KKI asked the court to reconsider, warning that its ruling could "cripple the pursuit of critical" pediatric research. The request for reconsideration points out that even minimal risk research, as well as research that offers subjects a potential for medical benefit, poses some risks of injury, and thus would be precluded by the court's ruling. The court denied the motion for reconsideration, but issued a clarification stating that it had intended to ban only pediatric research that poses:

> any articulable risk beyond the minimal kind of risk that is inherent in any endeavor. The context of the statement was a nontherapeutic study that promises no medical benefit to the child whatsoever, so that any balance between risk and benefit is necessarily negative.

This attempt at clarification has triggered ongoing debate regarding precisely which categories of pediatric research the court intended to ban. Some have argued that the ruling allows minimal risk research, but prohibits minor increase over minimal risk research. Others have argued that the ruling is consistent with the existing federal regulations, including the category of research that poses a minor increase over minimal risk and does not offer the prospect of direct benefit.[43] The Maryland Court of Appeals sent the case back to the lower court to hear all the relevant facts and make a final decision on that basis. The lower court ultimately dismissed the case with prejudice, and it is closed.[44]

The Maryland Court of Appeal's rejection of pediatric research that poses a "negative" balance between risk and benefit illustrates the degree of suspicion that exists regarding nonbeneficial pediatric research. Following the *Grimes* ruling, the Maryland legislature adopted a statute governing human subjects research modeled on the federal regulations. It allows nonbeneficial pediatric research that poses minimal risk or a minor increase over minimal risk.[45] Despite this, the *Grimes* ruling still applies in the state of Maryland, leaving unclear the legal status of pediatric research that poses risks to children and does not offer them a compensating potential for clinical benefit. A few other state legislatures, including Virginia's, also have passed statutes that govern clinical research, including nonbeneficial pediatric research.[46]

A recent article considers the possibility of regulating pediatric research based on existing standards for child abuse and neglect.[47] The thought is that the lack of clarity in evaluating the risks of pediatric research might be addressed by appeal to the standards developed over years of enforcing abuse statutes. The problem with this claim is that risk standards used in child abuse cases seem no clearer, and the enforcement of these standards by child welfare agencies seems no more consistent, than existing practice with respect to nonbeneficial pediatric research. The same article points out that the courts have historically required direct benefit to children to justify exposing them to risks. This history places some doubt on the legal status of appeals to more indirect benefits, including educational and altruistic benefits, and the types of benefits considered here which involve furthering the child's overall interests. The article goes on to point out that courts may be willing to consider such benefits but worries that at least very young children are not in a position to realize educational benefits.

The *Grimes* case nicely illustrates the range of responses common to nonbeneficial pediatric research. The lower court does not seem to have been concerned at all with the ethics or legality of the research. In contrast, the highest court in Maryland regarded such research as clearly unethical, while the state legislature endorsed the view that such research may be acceptable provided it satisfies the federal standards of not posing greater than minimal or a minor increase over minimal risk. The Maryland Court of Appeals arguments against nonbeneficial pediatric research, like Ramsey's earlier arguments, were never addressed publicly and have yet to be countered. In the law, as in the existing literature, we remain in the situation of allowing some nonbeneficial pediatric research without a satisfactory response to the claim that it is necessarily unethical. The next chapter begins by considering this dilemma. We will then consider, in the remainder of Chapter 3 and in Chapter 4, previous attempts to resolve it.

THREE | Evaluating the Worry

Ramsey's Argument

The standard justification for exposing adults to research risks for the benefit of others cites the fact that they consented to being so treated. In most cases, nonbeneficial research with adults can be acceptable when the participants consent and is unacceptable if they fail to do so. This line of reasoning leads to a general presumption that the ethical acceptability of nonbeneficial research depends on the consent of its participants. It seems to follow that nonbeneficial research with children is necessarily unethical.

This argument has powerful intuitive appeal and has seemed almost self-evident to some. Paul Ramsey has been perhaps its most prominent and eloquent defender. In arguments offered in his book *Patient as Person*[1] and further developed in a series of articles,[2,3] several of which contribute to an iterative debate with Richard McCormick, Ramsey argues from the importance of consent for research with adults to the conclusion that "children, who cannot give a mature and informed consent" should not be made the subjects of medical experimentation unless it "may further the patient's own recovery."[4] Ramsey goes on to argue that "no parent is morally competent to consent that his child shall be submitted to hazardous or other experiments having no diagnostic or therapeutic significance for the child himself."[5]

As these citations suggest, a good deal of Ramsey's argument focuses on the fact that nonbeneficial pediatric research exposes children to research risks without their consent for the benefit of others. Ramsey, perhaps more clearly than any other writer on the subject, recognized that nonbeneficial pediatric research raises an additional ethical concern. Because participation in clinical research involves individuals contributing to the goals of the study in question, nonbeneficial pediatric research, in effect, forces children to contribute to the goals of a project they do not understand. Ramsey argues that, in this way, enrolling children in research without their consent necessarily treats them as a mere means and thereby wrongs them, even when it poses no risk of harm. In his words, children can be "offensively touched without risk of or actual harm"[6] and should be protected from "both the degradation of the body's fortress and from being treated as a means only."[7]

The Value of Consent

Informed consent is often described as being morally transformative.[8] It transforms the moral landscape by making it permissible to do things to and with an individual that would be impermissible in the absence of the individual's informed consent. Obtaining an individual's informed consent can transform a punch in the nose from assault to a sporting event.[9] Similarly, inserting a needle into an individual's arm contrary to his medical interests can constitute assault and battery or appropriate clinical research, depending in part on whether one first obtains the individual's consent.

It is true that clinical investigators typically must obtain parental permission before enrolling children in clinical research. It is also true that, no matter how old children are, their parents often are better judges of their own interests than they are. It follows that the requirement to obtain parental permission could provide an acceptable—indeed, often would provide a preferable—substitute for an individual's own consent to the extent that consent is purely a means for protecting an individual's interests. However, informed consent is not morally transformative because it provides assurance that the action consented to is consistent with the individual's interests. To the contrary, informed consent tends to be most important and is most clearly transformative when the action in question is not (at least otherwise) in the individual's interests. It is when we choose against our own interests that the fact of our having made the choice ourselves carries the most weight.

Informed consent is not the only way to overcome the general prohibition against intentionally exposing others to risks of harm. A second way is to appeal to the individual's own interests. The importance of protecting an individual's life and limb can justify exposing him to risks when it is impossible to obtain his consent. It is just this line of reasoning that justifies the very ordinary activity of pediatric medical care, exposing to risks of harm on a daily basis individuals who cannot provide informed consent. By definition, nonbeneficial pediatric research does not offer participants a compensating potential for clinical benefit. As a result, investigators who conduct nonbeneficial pediatric research cannot appeal to participants' clinical interests, nor can they appeal to participants' informed consent, to justify violating the general presumption against intentionally exposing them to risks of harm.

Parental permission does not offer a substitute for individuals deciding for themselves the causes to which they will contribute. This view is reflected in the legal principle, affirmed by the U.S. Supreme Court, that: "Parents may be free to become martyrs themselves. But it does not follow they are free, in identical circumstances, to make martyrs of their children before they have reached the age of full legal discretion when they can make that choice for themselves."[10] This brings us to the standard articulation of the ethical concern posed by nonbeneficial pediatric research. Nonbeneficial pediatric research is ethically concerning because it involves exposing children to risks for the benefit of others and also involves having children contribute to the goals of the research without their consent and often without their knowledge and understanding.

When Is Consent Necessary?

Ramsey's argument against nonbeneficial pediatric research is based on a very common way of analyzing research with children. If a given treatment of an adult would be unethical if that adult does not consent to it, then the same treatment is unethical for children who are unable to consent. Since it would be unethical, at least in most cases, to insert a needle, without informed consent, in a competent adult's arm for research purposes, then it is unethical to do so with respect to children who cannot give informed consent. Put in this way, it becomes clear that, even if we grant Ramsey's claim regarding nonbeneficial research without the consent of competent adults, he needs to show that the norms that govern our treatment of adults in this regard also govern our treatment of children who cannot consent. The question, in effect, is whether unconsented treatment (i.e., treatment of a competent adult who could consent but does not) raises the same ethical concerns as nonconsented treatment (treatment of an individual who is unable to provide consent).

The distinction between unconsented and nonconsented treatment raises the question, roughly, of whether the necessity of obtaining consent before enrolling adults in nonbeneficial research traces to the nature of the individuals in question or the nature of the research. Ramsey assumes the latter view. He assumes that nonbeneficial research procedures require consent because they involve exposing individuals to risky procedures that are not in their medical interests and, thereby, involve individuals contributing to the project of helping others. In the absence of consent, the first involves contradicting participants' medical interests without their consent; the second involves effectively forcing them to contribute to a given project, thus contradicting the individuals' rights to determine for themselves the course of their own lives, including the projects to which they contribute. The fact that the project is for a good cause, assuming that it is, does not remove the taint of using individuals as means. It implies only that they are being used as a means for a valuable project. In Ramsey's view, this fact may provide solace to investigators and others, but it does not make our treatment of the participants acceptable.

To clarify the distinction I have in mind here, consider again the example of inserting a needle into a research participant's arm to obtain a blood sample for research purposes. Ramsey's argument appeals to the intuition that, in standard cases, when researchers do this with adults, they first should obtain the adult's informed consent and that failure to do so undermines the ethical acceptability of this nonbeneficial research procedure. Although this seems right, there are at least two explanations for the need to obtain consent in this case. One possible explanation is that the nature of the situation is such that one needs the individual's consent (no matter who the individual is). For all individuals, one must not insert a needle in their arm for research purposes without first obtaining their informed consent. An alternative explanation is available, however, for the same intuition. One must not do this *to competent adults* without their consent. This principle, unlike the first, is silent on the proper treatment of children in the same context. Defense of Ramsey's position requires some reason to endorse the first principle over the second.

Why Is Consent Valuable?

Some actions or ways of treating others are unacceptable unless they provide their informed consent. In these cases, the requirement to obtain informed derives from the nature of the act itself. Put differently, informed consent is morally transformative in these cases by making acceptable an action that otherwise would be unacceptable.[11] Punching someone in the nose, at least in standard cases, seems to be an instance of this kind of action or treatment.

In general, the act of punching another person in the nose is unethical. But, if you first obtain that individual's sufficiently informed consent, punching them in the nose can be ethically acceptable, as the (presumed) acceptability of boxing shows us. In these kinds of cases, informed consent is vital because it is required to make an action ethical; without informed consent, the action is unethical.

In other cases, the importance of consent attaches not to the act itself, but to specific individuals or, better, to the conjunction of this action with this (type of) individual. Feeding another person is an instance in this class of actions or behaviors. Feeding competent adults without their consent would be unethical. Assuming they are in a position to decide for themselves, appropriate respect for them as autonomous individuals implies that we should get their informed consent first; they should control whether they eat what we have to offer. The strength of this principle is supported by common practice regarding the possible force-feeding of individuals, such as hunger strikers. Most guidelines allow adults to be force-fed only under very strict conditions, typically including a determination that the individual is at that time incompetent to decide for himself.

Granting the necessity of obtaining the consent of competent adults before one feeds them, it would be a mistake to conclude that informed consent is a necessary condition for feeding others in all cases. Put differently, it is not the case that, for all individuals, one must obtain their informed consent before feeding them (ethically). It is acceptable for parents to feed their infants, despite the fact that the infants do not give their informed consent. Ramsey's argument that nonbeneficial pediatric research is necessarily unethical assumes that it falls into the first category; it is more like punching someone in the nose than feeding them. One way to support his view would be to show that exposing individuals to risks without their informed consent for the benefit of others always involves unethically using those individuals as means, no matter who the individuals happen to be. Ramsey may have assumed that this claim was almost self-evident. It turns out to be false.

Consider an example. While on a hike, your young daughter falls down an abandoned well. You cannot reach her, do not have any rope or other way to pull her out, and there is no means of available communication to summon assistance. Nearby, fortunately, is another person, a very tall, thin (read light) person. This person's legs are sufficiently long that if you grasp his wrists and dangle him into the well, your daughter could grab hold of his feet and climb out of the well. Further imagine that, given the size and weight of your daughter, there is compelling reason to believe that this could be accomplished at extremely low risk to all parties involved. Imagine that there is no chance of the thin man being serious injured. Perhaps the most significant risk is a very low chance that you will sprain one of his wrists in the process of dangling him into the well.

Presumably, you should ask for the thin man's consent and, if you obtain it, it would be acceptable to use him as a human ladder in this way.[12] Because we will return to related cases, it is worth noting several features of this example. It is acceptable to ask the thin man to contribute to the goal of saving your daughter. And, if he consents, it is acceptable to carry out the rescue mission. Notice that this conclusion does not depend on knowing to what extent the thin man embraces the goal of saving your daughter. It would be nice if he endorsed the project, but it would not be unethical to use him as a ladder if he did not. Imagine the thin man responds to your request by saying "Yes, I will consent, but I do not care a straw for you or your daughter." The conclusion that it can nonetheless be acceptable to use the thin man provides the first hint to which we shall return that individuals need not always embrace the goals of the projects to which they contribute at some risk to themselves for it to be acceptable to rely on their efforts to achieve those goals.

Second, using the thin man in this way, with his consent, seems acceptable despite the fact that it involves asking him to contribute in a very passive way. As we are imagining the case, the thin man is supposed to make himself into a ladder, the more passive and motionless the better, and simply allow your daughter to clamber over him and out of the well. The thin man is not asked to do anything in particular, and certainly is not asked to provide a service that requires anything nearing what we would regard as skill. In an important sense, you are appealing to him purely for some physical properties he happens to possess—his length and weight—independent of his will and autonomy. The more he resembles an inanimate ladder, the better. Despite the passivity of the role, this all seems acceptable when you have his consent.

This conclusion underscores a point that will be important for our analysis of nonbeneficial pediatric research. Often our analysis of the ethics of particular cases depends on the alternatives available to the individuals in the example. Cases in which one individual is passive and is used by another to benefit some third party frequently are ones in which the individual need not have been passive. Indeed, they often involve cases in which it would have been better if the individual had not been passive. The conclusion, in these cases, that there is something troubling in the individual's passivity is sometimes thought to imply a concern with passivity in general when in fact it reflects concern regarding passivity in cases where there are other and better options. This example also highlights the fact that passivity can involve the will or the body. The present version of the example involves a physically passive, but willing thin man. The next version involves one who is passive in both senses.

Before we consider that version of the example notice, in the present version, that after it is over we will say that the thin man provided a crucial contribution to saving your daughter. The thin man makes an important contribution despite the fact that he does not actively contribute to the goal of saving your daughter and may not even endorse that goal. His only contribution involves the willing provision of the very passive means for your daughter to climb out of the well. Moreover, while the thin man makes this contribution, his contribution is only one of many necessary contributions. Without your holding the thin man's wrists, your daughter would not be able to escape, hence, the thin man would not be able to contribute to her escape.

One might conclude from the importance of obtaining the thin man's consent that it is unethical to treat others as passive human ladders without their consent. This argument follows Ramsey's line of reasoning that the need to obtain the consent of competent individuals for nonbeneficial research implies that consent is necessary to enroll all individuals in such research. To evaluate this view, we can revise the example to one in which the thin man is unconscious and you are not able to awaken him in time. While it might be a bit odd to dangle an unconscious person into a well, it seems ethically acceptable if it is the only option available for saving your daughter's life. The ethical acceptability of treating the thin man in this way seems especially clear if we again assume that you have compelling reason to believe that the risks to him are extremely low. Dangling an unconscious thin man seems acceptable despite the fact that you are engaged in unconsented touching and using an individual as a passive (in both senses) means to helping another. The fact that you are using the thin man as a means does not imply, in this case at least, that you are using him in an ethically objectionable sense.

This conclusion seems especially compelling if we imagine a case in which the parent declines to use the unconscious thin man as a human ladder on the grounds that doing so would involve a failure to respect his autonomy. There are many responses appropriate to such a parent. None of them involves congratulating him for understanding correctly the ethics of the situation. One might grant this conclusion, but argue that using the thin man in this way is acceptable because we can assume that he would consent if he were in a position to do so. In Chapter 4, we will evaluate several arguments that attempt to justify nonbeneficial pediatric research based on presumed consent. This analysis will suggest that presumed consent cannot do the ethical work required of it here. Until then, imagine that the facts of the case do not support an argument from presumed consent. Imagine that you have no information on which to predict the likelihood that this particular individual would consent if he were conscious. Perhaps you are in a foreign country and are unaware of the relevant views of the locals. In this case, you (a foreigner) have no reason to think the (native) thin man would consent and no reason to assume that he shares the goal of saving your daughter. Nonetheless, assuming the risks to the thin man are very low, it seems acceptable to use him as a human ladder while he is unconscious.

This example suggests that, in at least some instances, whether one must obtain consent prior to exposing individuals to risks for the benefit of others depends on whether the individuals in question are able to consent. You should obtain the consent of the conscious thin man, but ethically you are allowed to dangle the unconscious thin man, despite the fact that you do not obtain his consent. To bring this example back to nonbeneficial pediatric research, imagine that the very tall individual is a child rather than an unconscious adult. You cannot, by hypothesis, obtain his informed consent. He is too young to understand, perhaps he does not understand death or sprained wrists, and cannot give his own consent. Would that render it unethical to dangle him into the well? It would be ethically acceptable to use the child as a ladder, again assuming that you have very good reason to believe that the risks to him are extremely low (including reason to believe that the child will not be terrified by the experience) and very good reason to believe that the benefits to your daughter will be substantial. Finally, imagine that although the thin child is too young to understand what you propose, he does not object to being used in this way, to the extent that he understands it. Indeed, imagine that the child assents to your proposal. Here, too, this seems a matter of acceptable using, as opposed to inappropriately using a child as a mere means, despite the fact that the child is too young to understand and is not able to consent to contribute to the project in question.[13]

Ramsey assumes that the case of competent adults establishes what rights or interests individuals have and what they need to consent to. Since competent adults typically should not be touched, at least intentionally, without their consent, he concludes that there is a right against unwanted touching for all individuals, or at least all human beings.[14] What Ramsey fails to consider is the possibility that competence not only gives individuals the ability to consent, it also affects what rights or interests they have. The problem with touching without consent an individual who can consent, or getting him to contribute to some project without his consent, is that you thereby fail to respect his ability to determine what happens to him and the projects to which he contributes. This is not an interest or a right that you can contravene with respect to children. And the conclusion that it can be acceptable to dangle the child into the well, especially when there is compelling reason to believe that the risks to the child are very low, the benefit very great, and the child does not object, suggests that exposing children to risks for the benefit of others without their informed consent does not always constitute treating them unethically.

We have concluded that exposing children to some risks for the benefit of others is not always unethical. This is a long way from establishing that it is ethically acceptable to enroll children in nonbeneficial research. But it does establish that we cannot simply conclude that nonbeneficial pediatric research is necessarily unethical on the grounds that it involves exposing children to risks for the benefit of others. We will need a more nuanced argument, one which clarifies when it is acceptable and when it is unacceptable to expose children to risks for the benefit of others. Analysis of Ramsey's argument effectively leaves us back where we started. We can dispense with the argument that nonbeneficial pediatric research is necessarily unethical simply on the grounds that children cannot consent, but we still are in need of an argument to justify exposing them to risks that conflict with their clinical or medical interests. Examination of Ramsey's arguments further reveals that a complete account should consider when it can be acceptable to have children contribute to the goals of projects to which they cannot consent.

Clarifying the Worry

It is a common feature of daily life that we expose children to risks without their consent. Typically, the activities in question are in the children's interests, but not always. Parents often expose their children to risks for the benefit of other family members. Similarly, parents might instruct their children to help an infirm neighbor by mowing their lawn or shoveling their sidewalk, even though they recognize that doing so involves the child facing some risks for the benefit of others. One might respond that the beneficiaries of these activities, unlike most instances of nonbeneficial pediatric research, are individuals to whom the child has a close relationship, such as a sibling or close neighbor. However, children also are frequent and appropriate contributors to charitable activities in which they are exposed to risks for the benefit of unidentified others.[15] Going door to door to collect charitable donations exposes children to some risks, washing cars likely exposes them to even greater risks.

One might argue that these activities are acceptable because they are part of a complete education for children. These activities teach children the value of helping others. We will consider this argument later, when we consider this as a possible justification for nonbeneficial pediatric research. At this point, it is sufficient to note that this possibility, while important to the extent it is present, does not seem necessary to justify charitable activities for children. This is suggested by current practice. We do not know whether allowing and even instructing children to perform charitable activities teaches them valuable lessons, yet we endorse them. Imagine if future research on cognitive development reveals that children are unable to learn valuable lessons from helping others during some periods of their development. Imagine that a child is in a position to provide an important benefit to an infirm neighbor while in one of these phases of development. Does it necessarily follow that it would be unethical to instruct the child to assist the neighbor? The fact that the child will not benefit personally seems relevant, but not determinative. Asking or even insisting that the child assist the neighbor seems acceptable, assuming the risks are sufficiently low, the benefit is important and, perhaps, the benefit cannot be provided readily by someone else (e.g., a child who would gain educational benefit).

Those skeptical of nonbeneficial pediatric research may regard the analogy with charitable activities for children as reason to question their acceptance of the latter, rather than reason to endorse the former. While I think this is a mistake, it will take the arguments to come to explain why. Others may be sufficiently convinced by the analogy to conclude that ethical concern over nonbeneficial pediatric research must be mistaken. To the extent that nonbeneficial pediatric research involves exposing children to risks for the benefit of others, it is no different than widely accepted charitable activities of daily life. One might conclude from this comparison that we do not need a justification for nonbeneficial pediatric research, so much as we need an account for why some consider it to be so problematic and in need of special justification.

I suspect that ordinary instances of exposing children to risks for the benefit of others are widely accepted because they are so ordinary. The acceptance thus traces to the fact that we tend to effectively ignore the risks of ordinary activities as we go about our daily lives. We do not, for instance, calculate the risks of crossing the road each time we have reason to do so and evaluate carefully whether the potential benefits of reaching the other side justify the risks. Instead, we carry on with our lives, allowing these risks to fade to the background unless something unfamiliar or noteworthy brings them back to our attention—someone is killed crossing the road in our neighborhood or an eight-lane highway is built in front of our house.

Some of our casual acceptance of ordinary charitable activities for children likely traces to this attitude regarding the risks of daily life. We essentially ignore the risks of ordinary crossings of the street, thus ignoring the risks to children of selling cookies or soliciting donations door to door. To this extent, our intuitive acceptance of these activities traces to a failure to recognize the risks, not to a considered judgment that it is acceptable to expose children to risks for the benefit of others. To this extent, there remains good reason to evaluate the acceptability of exposing children to risks for the benefit of others. Moreover, a fundamental difference exists between charitable activities and nonbeneficial pediatric research in terms of the process by which the children are exposed to risks. The harms children experience in the case of charitable activities are largely outside of the control of the responsible adults and typically are the result of the child's own actions. While going door to door to collect money for charity, a child might twist an ankle on the curb; while planting crops or washing cars the child might cut a finger. Contrast this with the role that investigators play in the conduct of nonbeneficial pediatric research. In this case, the investigators give a child potentially toxic medication, insert a needle into the child's arm, or place the child in an MRI machine. Of course, the investigators take many steps to minimize the consequent risks to the participating child, such as using sterile needles and testing the medications extensively first in the laboratory and in animals. Still, it is the investigator who is directly exposing the child to risks and, if the child is harmed, the investigator who is the direct or proximate cause of the harm.[16]

To appreciate this difference, imagine that some parents proposed to help an infirm neighbor by having a nurse come over and stick needles in their child's arm for the neighbor's amusement. Presumably, we would be horrified by a neighbor who found this behavior entertaining. In addition, it seems that this means of helping the neighbor would be unacceptable on the grounds that the nurse is doing something unacceptable, even when the risks to the child are the same or less than the risks the child would face from shoveling snow from the neighbor's sidewalk. The difference between the shoveling the walk case and the entertaining the neighbor case suggests that it is not just the level of risks to which children are exposed, and the benefits that others might derive, that determine our normative evaluation of these cases. It matters how the risks are realized, by what process they are introduced into the children's lives. Do the adults introduce the risks or, put differently, are they the proximate causes of any harms the children experience?

I suspect that a good deal of the ethical concern surrounding nonbeneficial pediatric research traces to this role of the investigators, that they are introducing risks in the name of all of us. This concern is evident in a good deal of the writings of critics of nonbeneficial pediatric research, which tend to focus not specifically on the risks the children face, but on the role the investigators play in posing the risks to the children. It is said that the investigators invade the children's bodies or force them to take potentially toxic medications. It would take a good deal of analysis to evaluate fully the ethical significance of this difference. In particular, there is a great deal of disagreement regarding the extent to which the means by which one brings about a particular result are morally relevant. Do the means matter when other ethically relevant factors—the risks, potential benefits, intentions—are the same? Is it more problematic to help others by inserting a needle into a child's arm than by asking the child to dig a hole or shovel a sidewalk, even if we assume that both activities offer the potential for important benefit, the risks are equivalent, and there is no less risky way to bring about the benefit in question?

Two comments about this concern. First, the assumption that the means by which the end in question is brought about sometimes matter is consistent with the widely endorsed active/passive distinction. This distinction holds that it is morally worse to actively cause harm as opposed to allowing the same harm to occur. One way to think about this distinction is in terms of a difference in responsibility. In paradigm cases of causing harm, one is more responsible for the resulting harm compared to cases in which one merely allows a harm to occur.[17] While a good deal more would need to be said to develop this into a complete account, the level of responsibility may be thought to be different in clinical research cases compared to charity cases. The fact that the investigator is the proximate cause of the risks faced by pediatric research participants implies that the investigator bears a greater level of responsibility for the risks and any resulting harms. This difference in the level of responsibility in the two cases may explain a good deal of the intuition that nonbeneficial pediatric research is ethically more troubling.

We need not settle this issue for present purposes. Either way, we need a justification for nonbeneficial pediatric research. It may turn out that exposing children to risks when conducting (the paradigm cases of) nonbeneficial pediatric research is morally problematic in a way that allowing children to be exposed to risks in charitable activities is not. If this is right, we clearly need a justification for (the paradigm cases of) nonbeneficial pediatric research. Alternatively, it might be that exposing a child to risks for the benefit of others in general raises concern to the extent that it violates the principle of promoting a child's best interests. In this case, we will need a justification for nonbeneficial pediatric research and for charitable activities involving children.[18]

McCormick's Response

Richard McCormick offered a number of arguments in response to Ramsey's claim that nonbeneficial pediatric research is necessarily unethical.[19] While his arguments fit with the arguments considered in the next chapter, I include them here because they were offered in direct response to Ramsey. McCormick points out that even Ramsey does not restrict allowable touching to instances in which the individual gives consent. This view would have the absurd conclusion that emergency room physicians must wait for car accident victims to regain consciousness before they can be resuscitated. McCormick argues that we do not wait for accident victims to regain consciousness because we have compelling reason to believe that they would consent to our resuscitation efforts if they were able to consent.

If this is right, it suggests that touching another is acceptable either when they consent to it or when we have reason to believe that they would consent to our doing so, if they were able to consent. McCormick then argues that parents' decision to enroll their children in nonbeneficial research is acceptable provided there is good reason to think that the child would have consented, if the child had been able to consent. McCormick argues that enrolling children in nonbeneficial research is a reasonable presumption of what they would want because it is the right thing to do; in effect, we can assume that the child would consent because there are good reasons to do so.[20]

On one reading, McCormick's argument involves an empirical generalization based on the behavior of individuals who are able to consent. The argument is that individuals who have the ability to consent predictably consent to helping others when the risks and burdens to themselves are minimal. Thus, we can assume that children, if they were able, would consent to nonbeneficial research, at least when it offers the potential to gather valuable knowledge and poses minimal risks. The problem is that it is not clear how strong the empirical evidence is for this claim. Certainly, there are many times when individuals in a position to help others at some risk to themselves choose to do so. There also are many instances in which competent adults choose not to provide assistance. On purely empirical grounds, then, there is reason to question the strength of McCormick's position.

An alternative reading is not that individuals predictably will consent to minimal risk, nonbeneficial research, but that there are good reasons why they ought to do so. Here McCormick's argument is more that children have good reason to consent, thus we can enroll them on the assumption that they would consent if they were able to appreciate these reasons. To evaluate this argument, we need to consider more carefully the claim that a child would consent to enrollment in a given study if the child were able to consent. In the case of the accident victim, the claim that the individual would consent if he could consent seems to mean roughly that the counterfactual "this individual would consent to medical treatment provided he was able to consent" is true. Notice that we cannot evaluate the truth of this counterfactual simply by imagining that the person is able to consent because he did not suffer an accident. In that case, a person likely would not consent to treatment for the simple reason that he would not need it.

One way to evaluate the truth of a counterfactual is to determine whether it is true in what philosophers refer to as the "nearest possible world." Roughly, we consider whether it would be true in a world that is as similar to the present world as possible, including holding the individual's injuries constant, with the exception that the individual is able to consent. The relevant world to consider in the resuscitation case is the one in which the individual needs the treatment and has the same values and preferences, but is conscious rather than unconscious. What decision would the individual make in that world, or that case? Since the individual in that world has the same basic identity—including interests, values, and preferences—as the individual in front of us, it seems reasonable to conclude that the individual would consent to the resuscitation efforts if he could consent (assuming this was an individual who typically sought out or at least accepted needed medical care).[21]

Now imagine running the same thought experiment on infants. In this case, it will not do simply to give them the ability to make a decision. Who knows what, if any, decision would be made by an infant who has the ability to make decisions, but who possesses no values, preferences, goals, dreams, hopes, or view of the world and beliefs about medical research, doctors, and people who have the disease under study.To address these concerns, we need to determine what values and preferences the (competent) infant will have. Our answer thus depends on the interests, values, and preferences we ascribe to him. We previously saw that looking to competent adults for the appropriate preferences and values yields an indeterminate answer. Moreover, it is not clear on what grounds we attribute to hypothetically competent infants the preferences and values of (some) adults. Why think that infants, if competent, would be like competent adults? This is the first of several instances in which the attempt to justify nonbeneficial pediatric research by appeal to some version of consent forces us to treat infants like competent adults. This move thereby ignores, rather than answers, the challenge we face.

To take a different tack, we might try to predict not what decision infants would make now if competent. Instead, we determine what decision they would make by imagining that now they have the preferences and values they will develop as adults. Obviously, it is difficult to imagine what preferences and values a given infant will develop as an adult, especially with respect to issues on which competent adults have divergent views. Moreover, even if we get this right, even if it turns out that the individual becomes the person we predict, it is not clear why that is relevant to the index case. The index case is one of how to treat individuals who are unable to consent. Turning the individual in question into a competent adult does not provide an answer so much as it changes the question. Even if it were true that most individuals who could consent would consent when given the chance, the fact is that children, at least young children, cannot consent. And it is precisely their inability to consent that raises the ethical concern in the first place.

Finally, one might try to base McCormick's argument on the mere fact that there is good reason for the child to enroll in research. The argument is not that children would consent given that there is a good reason to do so. Rather, the argument is that we are justified in enrolling the child since there is a good reason to do so.[22] The difficulty with this argument is that moral reasons per se do not seem to provide sufficient reason to treat individuals according to those reasons. Rather, moral reasons provide a basis on which competent individuals might or should decide to pursue the action in question. The fact that it would be good of you to help your mother might provide reason for me to encourage you to help her. But, it does not provide good reason, much less a determinative reason, for me to force you to do so. The finding that moral reasons in general do not provide definitive reason to force someone else to engage in the project in question is underscored by considering how we might balance the moral claim to enroll children in nonbeneficial pediatric research against the children's best interests. How should we decide whether the moral reason to enroll children outweighs the fact that participation in nonbeneficial pediatric research is not consistent with their clinical interests?

McCormick's argument starts with a child, imagines effectively turning the child into an adult, and uses the presumed consent of that individual to justify nonbeneficial pediatric research. This argument, like many arguments of its type, fails for the simple reason that it fails to take seriously the fact that children are children and not able to give their own consent. Ramsey puts this point nicely in rejecting McCormick's defense of nonbeneficial pediatric research: "To attempt to consent for a child to be made an experimental subject is to treat a child as not a child. It is to treat him as an adult person who has consented."[23] This seems right and suggests we need an account of the way that we ought to treat children, taking seriously their status as individuals who currently are not but if all goes well, will become competent adults.

McCormick offered a second defense of nonbeneficial pediatric research according to which children are viewed as part of the moral community and have a general obligation to contribute to the general welfare when doing so poses little or no risk to them. On this argument, it is not so much that children would consent if they could, but that children are obligated to participate in efforts to help others in the community. Presumably, this includes nonbeneficial research when the risks are sufficiently low, when, in McCormick's words, the research poses "no discernible risk" and offers an important potential to benefit others.[24, 25] One might try to argue for such an obligation from the fact that children have enjoyed the benefits of prior nonbeneficial pediatric research. We will consider this argument below.

Before leaving Ramsey and McCormick, it is worth anticipating the argument to come by noting that McCormick had available to him a different understanding of how we should treat individuals who cannot consent. McCormick argues that we can treat emergency room victims because we have good reason to think that they would consent if they could. An alternative explanation exists for why it is acceptable to perform emergency medicine. Physicians in this situation do not attempt to determine what the individual would consent to if the individual could consent. Sometimes even competent individuals make bad decisions and decline medical treatment that is in their interests. To appropriately conduct emergency medicine, physicians need not ask themselves how common this is and whether the individual in question might be such an individual: Were they in a particularly sour mood before the accident? Was their marriage in trouble? Rather, the reason why it is acceptable to resuscitate an accident victim is that there is reason to believe that doing so promotes the individual's interests and no clear evidence suggests, as in the case of a living will, for example, that doing so contradicts the individual's preferences and values. While the difference here is a subtle one it has important implications for the present analysis. It is a mistake to try to run all claims of appropriate interaction with individuals through consent, whether actual or not. Instead, the question of the individual's interests is primary here, and the question of what they might consent to, rather than a necessary element in the argument, is seen as a perhaps useful heuristic for assessing the individual's interests (based on the assumption that individuals would consent to those actions which are in their interests).

The Negligible Risks Threshold

Those who do not make the mistake of pretending that children are competent often try to justify nonbeneficial pediatric research when it poses sufficiently low risks. One version of this argument claims that nonbeneficial pediatric research does not raise serious ethical concern provided the risks are negligible, in the sense of posing only low burdens to the children, with no chance of serious harm. For the most part, we think of childhood as a kind of preparation for adulthood. In particular, parental and societal obligations to children are based largely on the importance of protecting children from harm and nurturing their potential to become autonomous and thriving adults. Parents and society more broadly are obligated to ensure children receive the necessary tools for adulthood, including a basic education, and to feed, clothe, house, and protect them from physical and psychological insults. On this view, exposing children to risks without their consent raises special ethical concern only when it threatens their ability to acquire the capacities needed for a flourishing adulthood.

Exposing children to minor burdens and a risk of slight harm does not threaten their long-term potential to lead an autonomous life as an adult. This explains in part why we allow parents to further their own interests, even when doing so conflicts slightly with the interests of the child or children in question. It is permissible to have a child miss school for one day so that an adult might pursue an important interest of her own. Presumably, parents also may decide to have their child face burdens of this sort for the benefit of strangers, perhaps sitting in a waiting room for several hours while a parent attends a stranger in distress. This possibility suggests that nonbeneficial clinical studies that meet this negligible risk standard similarly raise no serious ethical concern. Thomas Murray, an advocate of this approach, writes: "parents act within the bounds of good parenting when they consent to a wide range of research protocols for their children, including research likely to benefit their child but also research that might benefit others without being unduly risky to their children."[26] The central idea here is that nonbeneficial pediatric research is acceptable when the research poses no worse than some burdens and some risks of minor harms. In that case, parents are not violating their duties to protect their children from serious harm and are not violating their duty to prepare the child to live an autonomous life as an adult.

Imagine a study to establish norms for height and weight of children of different ages. For this study, a randomly selected group of children are measured and weighed each year, from birth until they reach 18 years. Participation in this study, we can presume, does not pose any risks of serious harm to the children and involves relatively minimal burdens. Assuming participation does not involve any major opportunity costs for the children (e.g., coming to the clinic does not force the children to miss an important educational opportunity), enrollment in the study does not conflict with their basic needs or with the parental and societal obligation to prepare them for adulthood. This finding suggests the study is ethically acceptable, despite the fact that it offers no potential benefits to compensate for the minor burdens involved and, as such, constitutes nonbeneficial pediatric research in the sense used here.

A number of guidelines and commentators agree with Murray. The Council of Europe and the U.K. Medical Research Council allow what I am calling "nonbeneficial" pediatric research when "it is to be expected that [the research] will result, at the most, in a very slight and temporary negative impact on the health of the person concerned."[27,28] Similarly, Curran and Beecher allow nonbeneficial pediatric research when the risks are negligible,[29] and Bartholome allows it if there is "no discernible risk or significant discomfort" to the participating children.[30] Fried endorses this, or a very similar position, arguing that nonbeneficial research is acceptable for younger children provided it does not involve "undue" risk or it is only "marginally" risky.[31]

These arguments for nonbeneficial pediatric research can be read in either of two ways, depending on whether the reference to "negligible" risks is intended to modify the *probability* that children participating in the research will be harmed or intended to modify the *magnitude* of the possible harms the children might experience. On the former reading, this justification would allow nonbeneficial pediatric research that poses risks of serious harm, even death, provided their probabilities are sufficiently low.[32] Because this reading is very similar to the minimal risk view, I will postpone consideration of it until the next section, when we take up the minimal risk standard.

An alternative reading of the "negligible" risks justification holds that children may be enrolled in nonbeneficial research only when no chance exists that the children will experience serious harm. This seems to be the view endorsed by Murray. On this reading, the clause in the British regulations that "it is to be expected that [the research] will result, at the most, in a very slight and temporary negative impact" is to be understood in a very strong sense, mandating that there must be no chance of any harm beyond slight and temporary bumps, bruises, and boredom.

Risk standards for clinical research typically refer to the presence or absence of some level of risk. In the process of reviewing actual research studies, these standards inevitably, and often implicitly, are translated into epistemological standards. What does the evidence suggest regarding the risks of the study or procedure in question? With respect to the negligible risk standard, does the available evidence suggest that the study or procedure poses any risk of serious harm or harms?

Requiring absolute certainty in this regard is to require too much. It is difficult to imagine any intervention for which we can be certain that it poses no chance of any harms beyond very slight ones. More plausibly, the standard might require compelling evidence, or confidence on the part of the review committee. Is there compelling evidence that the procedure poses no risk of serious harm? Almost no research procedures satisfy even this somewhat relaxed version of the standard. The examples of measuring height and weight considered previously are almost unique in this regard.[33] There are at least three reasons for this. First, risks are a function of the magnitude of the possible harm and the probability that undergoing the intervention in question will result in that harm. To be confident that a given procedure does not pose even a very low—say 1 in 200,000—chance of serious harm, one must have a great deal of experience with the procedure. Even a finding that a procedure has caused no serious harm in thousands of patients does not preclude the possibility that it leads to serious harms in a very small percentage of cases.

Second, especially when it comes to children, the possibility of experiencing harm from some research procedure may not be manifest for decades. Thus, one needs data not just in a large number of cases, but the data must cover a good deal of the children's lives. A finding of no allergic reactions or other acute toxicities is not sufficient to establish that an experimental medication does not cause serious harm. One would need to follow the children over time to see whether their participation in the research leads to harms later in life, whether they develop cancer later in life, or increased rheumatoid arthritis, or peripheral neuropathies. We have no data of this extent for any research procedures, and we may never have it.

Third, even if investigators could determine for a particular group of children that a procedure poses no risks, the possibility remains of idiosyncratic reactions. Prospectively, it is typically impossible to be certain that a given child does not have any characteristics implying that, for her, the procedure in question poses some chance of serious harm. The 150,000th child may experience an allergic reaction not seen in any previous child. These considerations reveal that, in almost all cases, one cannot, be certain that a given research intervention will not lead to serious harm in a given child. It follows that the negligible risk standard is able to justify at most an extremely narrow range of nonbeneficial pediatric research, leaving us with the task of determining whether it is possible to justify the vast majority of the nonbeneficial pediatric research that is needed to improve children's health and well-being.

The Risks of Daily Life Threshold

Many commentators and guidelines allow nonbeneficial pediatric research when the risks are "minimal," often defined as risks that do not exceed the risks children face in daily life or during the performance of routine examinations. In my experience, many of those involved in pediatric research implicitly adopt the view that this standard is essentially equivalent to the no serious harms standard. That is, when evaluating nonbeneficial pediatric studies they assume that minimal risk studies are acceptable because they pose no chance of serious harm.

As an attitude regarding the risks we face in daily life, this view makes sense. We could not get through our daily lives if we were conscious of all the risks we face. Sitting down to lunch poses more risks than one can catalog, much less process over the course of an hour-long lunch break: the floor may be insecure, the chair flimsy, the chandelier loose, the soup poisoned, the meat rancid, the waiter psychotic, the water tainted, the table placed in the line of fire from a dispute on the street. Assuming these risks are sufficiently low, psychologically healthy individuals place them in the background so to speak, ignoring them unless circumstances provide reason for special concern (e.g., the person at the next table starting to gag might bring the risk of food poisoning to one's awarenes). The minimal risk standard gains a good deal of its normative support not from the ethical acceptability of the risks thus allowed, but by appealing to comparator risks that we tend to ignore.

Paul Ramsey, commenting on the extensive deliberations by the National Commission on the ethics of nonbeneficial pediatric research, notes that members often used the terms "minimal" and "negligible" risks in a way that seemed to imply that these standards precluded the possibility of serious harm. The members then went on to argue that an additional ethical requirement for pediatric research would be that there must be a guarantee of compensation for any research injuries. Ramsey writes: "To think of compensation shows that the net of protection thrown around uncomprehending subjects (by stipulating minimal risks) is exactly that: a net with holes in it, however small or few, through which slips actual harms."[34]

The members might have been consistent if they were assuming compensation was needed only for the minor harms that children might experience, but it seems doubtful they would then be so adamant about its importance as an ethical requirement. It seems doubtful that the members were troubled by the possibility that children might not receive compensation for a small scratch or bump. Rather, the Commission's intuitive response to minimal risk pediatric research seems to highlight nicely the different attitudes we take toward risks, especially the risks of daily life. We go about our daily lives as though risks of very low probability are not going to occur.[35] But this is an attitude that one adopts as one goes about one's daily life; it does not imply that one thinks there are no risks in daily life. The implicit assumption that one's house will be there at the end of the day does not prevent one from buying fire insurance.

Although our attitude toward the risks of everyday life makes sense psychologically, it does not provide an ethical justification for exposing children to the same level of risks. First, the extent to which we ignore the risks of daily life is not a fully rational process. In many cases, our attitude regarding risks has to do with features of the situation that are not correlated directly with risk level, such as our perceived level of control and our familiarity with the activity.[36] We are aware typically of the possibility of getting mugged when walking down a city street at night, but not aware of the risk of getting in car accident, even though that risk may be higher. We also tend to be more worried when driving on unfamiliar streets or walking in new neighborhoods compared to being on familiar ground. Recognizing the different factors that influence our perception of risks undercuts the attempt to ascribe moral significance to the threshold for which risks we attend to.

Next, to the extent that the process of ignoring some risks is rational, it involves a rough cost/benefit analysis. If we get it right, the question is basically which risks are worth our paying attention to. Some risks are so low that they are not worth paying attention to. That is, paying attention to these risks would be more harmful (would cost us more) than the expected value of being aware of them in the first place. The fact that the costs to an individual of paying attention to a given risk in daily life are greater than the benefits to that individual does not seem to have any relevance for what risks we may expose children to for the benefit of others.

Bracketing what impact this attitude has during the review and conduct of nonbeneficial pediatric research, it seems clear that this attitude does not provide an argument for the conclusion that the practices thus allowed are ethically acceptable. Before we countenance this attitude in practice, we must determine that it is in fact acceptable to approve and conduct research that poses risks of this level.

Data on the risks children face in daily life reinforce the point that meeting the risks of daily life standard does not ensure that pediatric research participants will not suffer serious harm. In the United States, children face up to a 1 in approximately 300,000 chance of death from riding in a car and a 1 in 5,000 chance of permanent disability from playing sports. These data reveal that the "risks of daily life" standard does not preclude the chance of some children experiencing serious harm. Indeed, one could put the point in a much stronger way. Probabilities being what they are, these data reveal that under the risks of daily life standard, enrollment of a sufficient number of children in minimal risk research eventually will result in a few children dying and scores being disabled. This is not to say that these harms will be the result of mistakes or negligence. Rather, the harms may be a result of the simple fact that in a sufficiently large series of events, it is expected that even very-low-probability outcomes will occur. The challenge, then, is to justify nonbeneficial pediatric research that meets the minimal risk standard, recognizing that it allows some very low chance of serious harm to participating children.

To make this challenge somewhat more concrete, imagine a nonbeneficial pediatric study that poses a 1 in 500,000 chance of death, a 1 in 50,000 chance of serious harm, such kidney dysfunction, and a 1 in 5,000 chance of relatively minor injury along the lines of a bone fracture. Although exact data on the risks of nonbeneficial pediatric studies are almost nonexistent, these levels of risk likely provide a fairly accurate picture of many current studies. The negligible risk standard considered in the previous section either ignores these risks or, given that they exceed negligible burdens, implies that all such research is unethical. The 'risks of daily life' standard implies that these studies can be appropriate because the level of risk likely does not exceed the level of risks that average, healthy children face in daily life. The present question is why that fact provides a reason to think that such research is appropriate.

One possible response would be to defend nonbeneficial pediatric research that poses risks no greater than those children face in daily life on the grounds that it does not *increase* the risks to which children are exposed. It seems plausible to assume that at any given time a child will either be participating in research or involved in the activities of daily life. But, by assumption, the risks of the two activities are essentially equivalent, implying that enrollment in the study, as opposed to allowing the child to continue to participate in activities of daily life, does not increase the risks to which the child is exposed.

The problem with this argument is that the risks of research often add to rather than replace the risks children face in daily life. For example, a study may require that the child rides in a car to the clinic for a research visit. The present defense works if this trip in the car replaces a trip the child would have taken or an otherwise similarly risky activity in which the child would have been involved. In practice, this often is not the case. The parent instead may simply put off the trip to the mall until after the research study. In that case, the child's risk of serious injury from a car trip would double as a result of his participation in research. This additive effect often will be the result of the approach taken by many researchers of trying to disrupt the child's daily life as little as possible. The attempt often is to time research procedures so they do not displace activities of daily life. Although this approach seems respectful of the children, it undermines the proposed justification.

The second problem is that many of the activities of daily life offer children the potential for direct benefit. Thus, even when research participation displaces the activities of children's daily lives and thus does not increase the risks they face (as when children come to the clinic rather than playing basketball), it often will thereby eliminate the potential benefit that the child might have gained from the daily life activity in question. Research participation eliminates the potential to enjoy playing a game during that time. This problem faces another prominent defense of the risks of daily life standard.

It has been argued that the 'risks of daily life' standard provides an appropriate threshold for assessing the risks of nonbeneficial pediatric research because the risks of daily life are themselves considered acceptable. In one of the most prominent articles in pediatric research ethics, Freedman and colleagues argue that the "concept of 'risks of everyday life' has normative as well as descriptive force, reflecting a level of risk that is not simply accepted, but is deemed socially acceptable."[37] On this view, we allow children to face the risks of daily life because we judge those risks to be acceptable. If we did not find them acceptable, we would either change them or prevent individuals from facing them. Unfortunately, we do not exercise the level of control over the risks of daily life assumed by this view. Healthy normal children face many risks in their daily lives—risks of violent crime to humiliating teasing, for example—not because we deem them acceptable, but because we have not yet learned how to eliminate them from children's lives.

Furthermore, as mentioned, many risks in daily life are accepted only because they are linked to activities that offer a prospect of direct benefit. Parents do not allow their children to hike, ski, and play basketball because they deem the risks of these activities inherently acceptable. They accept the risks because they assume the activities to which they attach offer a compensating potential for benefit. In the absence of this potential benefit, the risks would be unacceptable. Imagine a parent who allowed her child to go snow skiing and face the attendant risks even though the parent believed that the child would not enjoy the experience and would not benefit from it in any way.

The Routine Examinations Threshold

The U.S. federal regulations define minimal risks using two clauses, the first referring to risks that are "not greater in and of themselves than those ordinarily encountered in daily life," the second to risks ordinarily encountered "during the performance of routine physical or psychological examinations or tests." Some have hoped to sidestep the problems we have been considering that face the minimal risk standard by dropping reference to the risks of daily life and limiting the definition of minimal risk to the second clause. The Council for International Organizations of Medical Sciences stipulates that children may undergo research procedures that will provide no direct benefit only when the risks do not exceed those "associated with routine medical and psychological examinations of such persons."[38]

The risks of "routine examinations" are justified when the examinations can benefit the recipients and are unacceptable otherwise. Clinicians who expose children to routine examinations when those children cannot possibly benefit from the examinations are guilty of medical malpractice. This suggests that the routine examinations standard, understood as a justification for nonbeneficial pediatric research, suffers from a flaw similar to that faced by the risks of daily life standard. The fact that we accept some risks in the context of a potentially beneficial activity does not imply that those risks are acceptable in the absence of that potential for benefit.

Next, in practice, routine examinations for normal, healthy individuals in most higher-income countries pose essentially no risks. The Bright Futures health guidelines, endorsed by the American Academy of Pediatrics (AAP), recommend that healthy children be assessed for height, weight, head circumference, vision, and hearing.[39] The only invasive examinations typically recommended for healthy children are a single heel stick at birth to screen for metabolic disorders and a blood draw to screen for genetic diseases. In practice, then, the routine examinations standard would be extremely restrictive, categorizing all procedures beyond a blood draw or two as greater than minimal risk. Finally, this standard is vulnerable to advances in standard medical care in a counterintuitive way. Development of a noninvasive test for metabolic and genetic disorders in the clinical setting would imply, under the routine examinations standard, that children could no longer be exposed to even this level of risk in the context of nonbeneficial research. It is not obvious why improvements in clinical medicine should render unethical research that was acceptable prior to those improvements.

Appeal to Long-term Benefits

Improving pediatric clinical care requires the conduct of pediatric clinical research, including nonbeneficial research. This necessity provides an important reason for adopting a social policy that allows pediatric research and for conducting pediatric research itself. Some commentators go further, seeing this necessity as a justification for enrolling children in nonbeneficial research. It is, of course, a justification for conducting pediatric research. If it were not in some sense necessary to enroll children in research, if pediatric medical care could be improved without pediatric research, for example by doing computer simulations, there would be little justification for enrolling children. But, the fact that pediatric research offers important benefits does not seem sufficient justification for enrolling specific children.

One possibility would be to argue that, since X is a child, studies to benefit children as a class will also benefit members of the class, including X. The first version of this argument holds that studies likely to benefit children as a class are likely to offer future medical benefit to the individual children who participate in them. The nonbeneficial research blood draws experienced by children in the placebo arms of the rotavirus vaccine studies can be justified, on this view, by the possibility that a successful trial will yield an effective vaccine which these children may then receive.

There are two problems with this argument as a general justification for nonbeneficial pediatric research. First, even if the children who undergo nonbeneficial research procedures will have access to any treatments proven effective by the study, it does not follow that this potential benefit justifies enrolling a particular child. The potential to realize this benefit establishes only that the research needs to enroll some children, not that it is in a given child's interests to be in the study. On the assumption that proven medications are not restricted to those who participated in the studies which established them, children's clinical interests are better served by having others face the risks of the research process, allowing one's child to reap the benefits without facing the risks.

Of course, one might argue that this approach would be unfair and simply involves allowing one child to act as a free-rider, benefiting from the sacrifices of other children. Although this concern does not establish that it is in a given child's clinical interests to participate in nonbeneficial research, it does raise the possibility that failing to participate may be unjust. We will consider this possibility in the next chapter when we consider the claim that receiving the benefits of clinical research obliges one to participate in it.

The second problem with the present justification is that a generational gap typically exists between those who participate in nonbeneficial pediatric research and those who benefit from it. The time from first identification of a medication to its availability in the market takes approximately 10 to 15 years on average.[40] Current early-phase studies likely will take a decade or more, if ever, to yield new medications. By that time, the children who participated in the study often will no longer be eligible for the treatments, which will benefit the next cohort of children. For example, rotavirus is a serious threat to children younger than 5 years of age. By the time the rotavirus vaccines were approved for clinical use, the children who participated in the final studies were over age 5, and the children who participated in the earlier (nonbeneficial) phase studies were teenagers and no longer candidates for the vaccine.

Helping Children as a Group

A modified version of the previous argument claims not that participating children ultimately will benefit in the long run from the results of nonbeneficial studies in which they participate, but simply that a good deal of nonbeneficial research intended to benefit children must be conducted on children. The U.S. National Commission emphasized this fact as reason for allowing some nonbeneficial pediatric research.[41] The need to enroll children in some research often is turned into a protection for pediatric research subjects by stipulating that children may be enrolled in nonbeneficial research only when it will provide important information regarding treatment of children and there is no way to obtain the information without enrolling children.

It is important to distinguish justifications for enrolling children in nonbeneficial research from safeguards. Restricting enrollment of children to nonbeneficial studies that poses no greater than minimal risk (or perhaps a minor increase over minimal risk) and that must enroll children to answer the scientific question at hand offers an important safeguard. If implemented appropriately, it keeps children from being enrolled in research that poses very high risks, as well as all of the research that can be conducted with adults. Yet, there remains the need to justify the class of studies thus allowed. As long as we allow some nonbeneficial studies, the question remains how we can justify enrolling children who cannot consent in those studies. It is not obvious at first how the fact that we have to enroll some children in order to achieve an important end provides justification for doing so. One has to assume that adopting this approach to achieve that end is acceptable, and that is precisely the issue.

One possible justification is based on the fact that nonbeneficial pediatric research will help other children, along with the assumption that children have an interest in helping other children. A number of commentators suggest this kind of argument. Charles Fried argues that research with very young children can be acceptable provided there is a "much closer connection between that child and the benefit he or she is producing," as there would be when the research is likely to benefit "a close relative or perhaps those suffering from a disease this child is also suffering from. For there the community of interests is tightly drawn."[42]

There seem to be two closely related ways to run this argument. One might argue that individuals tend to identify with other individuals who share important characteristics with them. As a result, individuals tend to be more willing to help other individuals who share these characteristics. This fact suggests a kind of substituted judgment justification for enrolling children in nonbeneficial research. Basically, the assumption here is that the children would agree to the research if they were in a position to do so. If they could make the decision to enroll, they would enroll because the study is designed to help others who share important characteristics with them. Previously, we considered the shortcomings of justifications based on substituted judgment. In essence, they fail to take seriously the fact that children cannot consent and thereby elide the central ethical concern. The fact that an individual who could understand likely would agree to enroll does not provide an adequate justification for enrolling individuals who cannot understand.

A slightly different version of this argument moves not from the fact that the individuals enrolled share important characteristics with those who will benefit—in this case, age—to the conclusion that the individuals would consent to enroll assuming they were able to do so. Instead, the argument moves from the fact that the individuals enrolled share important characteristics with those who will benefit to the conclusion that participating in the research is in the interests of the individuals enrolled. Notice that this line of argument also provides a possible response to Ramsey's charge that nonbeneficial pediatric research involves recruiting individuals for causes the goals of which they do not understand or embrace. Contributing to those goals, helping children, is in the interests, it is assumed, of the children we enroll. We will return in the next chapter to the possibility of justifying nonbeneficial research on the basis of the interests of the children enrolled. Here I want to focus on a common thread between this and the previous version of the present argument.

Both versions of this argument assume that the question we are faced with in justifying enrolling individuals who cannot consent because of their age is to justify the enrollment of individuals who are of that age. This way of describing the requirement is useful because it highlights the fact that it is one instance of a general class of requirements that many commentators place on research with individuals who are not able to provide informed consent, sometimes referred to as the "subjects' condition" requirement. In the words of the U.S. Office for the Protection from Research Risks (now OHRP): "it is widely accepted that research involving persons whose autonomy is compromised... should bear some direct relationship to their condition or circumstances."[43] The U.S. Federal regulations stipulate that IRBs may approve nonbeneficial pediatric research that poses more than minimal risks only when it is likely to yield generalizable knowledge about the subjects' disorder or condition (45CFR46, subpart D). Similarly, the Belmont Report states that individuals who cannot consent should be enrolled in nonbeneficial research only when the "research is directly related to the specific conditions of the class involved."[44]

Hans Jonas claims that individuals with the condition under study are more likely to identify with the goals of the research, compared to unaffected individuals. For instance, one might assume that adults with Alzheimer disease are more likely than adults with Down syndrome to have the goals of supporting research on Alzheimer disease. If this were the case, individuals' own goals would offer a reason to prefer the enrollment of affected individuals. However, much of the plausibility of this view derives from the way in which the options are framed. Proponents ask whether an individual with disease X is more likely to support research on disease X, compared with an individual who does not have disease X. Framed in this way, the only information we are given is that the individual shares a characteristic with those who might benefit from the research, namely, the disease in question. A complete description of those individuals who do not have the disease under study would reveal that many of them share other characteristics with those who will benefit. Indeed, it may be that some individuals without the disease share a greater number of characteristics with those who will benefit than many individuals who have the disease, but have little else in common with them. Individuals' allegiances and willingness to help others may equally well track these other characteristics, leaving little reason to think that those with the disease will be more likely than those without the disease to endorse helping individuals who have the disease.

This possibility is supported by the few data collected to date. These data reveal that individuals are not more willing to participate in nonbeneficial research on conditions from which they suffer. In one study, respondents were asked how willing they would be to give advance consent to participate in a nonbeneficial, minor increase over minimal risk study in the future when they had lost the ability to consent.[45] There was essentially no difference in individuals' willingness to participate in research on their own condition (98%), compared to research on other conditions (97%). The fact that these individuals were equally willing to participate in research on other conditions may be explained by the fact that adults develop numerous allegiances during their lifetimes. Hence, what kinds of research one assumes these individuals will be likely to support depends, in large part, on which of their allegiances one focuses on. Identifying individuals who cannot consent based on their medical conditions suggests that they will support research on those conditions. Identifying them based on their age suggests they will support research to benefit individuals of the same age. Indeed, the Council of Europe allows investigators to enroll individuals who cannot consent in nonbeneficial research when the research concerns a condition the individuals have, or the research has the potential to benefit "other persons in the same age category."[46]

But why stop there? There is no a priori reason to think patients will be more likely to support research to help others with the same condition, than research to help others of the same age, religion, culture, or birthplace. Given these possibilities, no nonarbitrary way seems to exist to limit the enrollment of individuals who cannot consent to research on their own conditions, compared to research on conditions that affect their friends, grandchildren, or members of their church. This analysis supports the prior suggestion that the present argument has intuitive appeal because it is framed in a somewhat tendentious way. We ask in what research it would be acceptable to enroll children, and the intuitive answer is that they would support research to benefit other children. But the intuitive appeal of this response seems largely an artifact of our description of the individuals in question as children. Describing individuals as children is pertinent when one considers the importance of competence and informed consent. It is less pertinent when the issue is the causes or goals with which the individuals identify.

We assume implicitly that children will identify with other children because, in essence, that is how we classified them for the purposes of the analysis. But the individuals in question could be identified in myriad ways, to the extent that it seems we could allow them to be enrolled to help just about anyone—individuals from New Jersey, tall people, Methodists. To make an argument for or against one or more of these groups, we would need to know with whom the children identify; we cannot assume that these individuals will identify with, in the sense of wanting to benefit, those with whom we group them based on characteristics relevant to medical research, especially the disease they have and the fact that they cannot consent.[47] Moreover, infants do not preferentially identify with any group, to the extent that they identify with others at all. In the end, the present justification offers a reason why we should choose to enroll some individuals rather than others, not a justification for why it is acceptable to expose those individuals we so choose to risks for the benefit of others.

FOUR | Proposed Justifications

The Argument Thus Far

The previous chapter considered arguments that attempt to determine whether nonbeneficial pediatric research is acceptable, in effect, by analyzing the nature of the research itself and the standard guidelines under which it is conducted. We considered arguments that such research is necessarily unethical because it violates children's autonomy, exposing those who cannot consent to risky procedures that are not in their medical interests, and also involves forcing them to contribute to the goals of projects they do not understand, much less embrace. The problem with this approach is that it ignores the possibility that children's inability to give consent does not merely alter their ability to decide the course of their lives; it transforms what constitutes appropriate treatment of them. Although this negative conclusion removes certain arguments against nonbeneficial pediatric research, it does not provide a positive argument regarding whether it can be acceptable to expose children to research risks for the benefit of others.

McCormick's attempt to justify nonbeneficial pediatric research on the grounds that children would consent to it if they could consent fails to take seriously the fact that children are not autonomous. Next, we bracketed for consideration in the present chapter McCormick's claim that children are obligated to participate in nonbeneficial research when the risks are sufficiently low. Finally, we considered the claim that nonbeneficial pediatric research does not raise serious ethical concern when the risks are negligible or low. Understood as allowing research that poses no risk of serious harm, this approach fails to address the majority of nonbeneficial pediatric research or, alternatively, implies that the majority of nonbeneficial pediatric research that is being conducted, and has been conducted under existing regulations is unethical.

Proposed justifications of the first type are unsatisfactory because they do not take seriously the fact that children are children. Those in the second set do not take seriously the fact that nonbeneficial pediatric research often poses some risk of serious harm to participating children. This is not to say that such research is necessarily unethical, only that proposed justifications should be consistent with this fact. One way to think about this point is in terms of the function of the existing risk standards. These standards allow nonbeneficial pediatric research when the level of risks does not exceed some threshold, most notably, the level of risks average children ordinarily face in daily life. The present claim is that research which satisfies this standard may well be ethically acceptable. That standard may provide approximately the correct threshold for the level of risks to which children may be exposed in this context. The problem comes when we regard this standard as providing not simply a metric for which risks are acceptable, but also a *justification* for studies that satisfy the endorsed metric: nonbeneficial pediatric research that meets this standard is acceptable because the risks are no greater than the risks average children ordinarily encounter in daily life.

As we have seen, the risks of daily life tend to be accepted in most cases because they attach to activities that are thought to offer the participating children a compensating potential for personal benefit. Because nonbeneficial pediatric research does not offer participating children a compensating potential for clinical benefit that justification appears lost when we apply the standard to nonbeneficial pediatric research. An alternative justification cites the fact that we tend to ignore the (familiar) risks of daily life when going about our lives. The problem with this justification is that this attitude toward the risks of daily life is either itself unjustified, or it depends on a kind of rough cost/benefit calculation regarding which risks are worth paying attention to.

The fact that it might not be worth parents' time to pay attention to very low risks to their children does not provide a justification for society to support and clinical investigators to engage in an activity which exposes children to those risks for the benefit of others. We saw this point with respect to the comparison between the risks of nonbeneficial pediatric research and the risks of charitable activities for children. The fact that it is widely regarded as appropriate to expose children to some risks for the benefit of others in the context of charitable activities provides reason to think that exposing (nonconsenting) children to risks for the benefit of others is not necessarily unethical, as Ramsey claims. The problem, of course, is that this comparison begs the question of whether in fact it is acceptable to expose children to risks in the context of charitable activities, and why. A further problem arises from the fact that clinical investigators actively expose children to risks, giving them medications, inserting needles into their veins.

The thought that charitable activities for children can be appropriate because it is good for the children to participate in them begins to suggest one way to try to justify exposing children to risks for the benefit of others. This suggestion brings us to the work of Ramsey, Bartholome, and others who argue that it might be possible to justify nonbeneficial pediatric research by appeal to the fact that it can promote the nonmedical interests of pediatric participants. We will pursue this suggestion further in the following chapter. For the present, it is sufficient to note that this approach also may offer a justification for the active role that investigators play in the context of pediatric research. It is one thing to insert a needle in a nonconsenting child's arm for the benefit of others. This is the perspective from which Ramsey and other critics argue that nonbeneficial pediatric research is necessarily unethical. It is a very different thing to insert a needle in a child's arm for the benefit of others, in a context in which the child stands to benefit in some way. To set the stage for that consideration, the present chapter first considers prominent attempts to justify nonbeneficial pediatric research which take seriously the fact that it exposes children to risks, including some risks of serious harm, but do not appeal to the possibility that the participating children themselves stand to benefit.

Utilitarianism as an Epithet

The puzzle offered by (the paradigm instances of) nonbeneficial pediatric research is to justify directly exposing some children to risks for the benefit of unrelated others, and thereby having them contribute to ends they do not understand and do not positively endorse. Utilitarianism provides a possible solution to this puzzle by largely ignoring the distribution of benefits and burdens that arise from a given policy or practice. A Utilitarian justification would focus on whether a given nonbeneficial intervention or study is expected to produce on balance positive benefits to the extent that the net benefits are greater than what could be realized by pursuing available alternatives.

On this argument, it is acceptable to expose children to research risks when the study offers the potential for benefit that outweighs the risks and burdens the participants face (and the burdens and costs of conducting the research), independent of the extent to which the participants themselves will benefit.

Although Utilitarianism offers a straightforward argument, this view, at least in the simplistic form assayed here, is rarely endorsed by supporters of nonbeneficial pediatric research. It is more often cited by opponents who oppose current regulations on the grounds that they are thought to justify nonbeneficial pediatric research on purely Utilitarian grounds. These arguments are regarded as criticisms because it is assumed that purely Utilitarian justifications are inadequate. Nonetheless, evaluation of the possibility of developing a straightforward Utilitarian argument will be useful because it reveals the extent to which current regulations for nonbeneficial pediatric research are not consistent with a Utilitarian calculus and also provides important insights into what a successful justification might look like.

One virtue of the Utilitarian approach is that it connects any possible justification of nonbeneficial pediatric research and its value in what seems like the right way. Intuitively, one assumes that any justification for nonbeneficial pediatric research will cite in some way its social value. It is after all the potential for benefit that is the reason for doing the research in the first place. And, yet, since the benefits do not accrue to those who face the risks, it is hard to see how to connect the justification for exposing subjects to risks to the benefits it offers to others. Indeed, while the value seems central to the justification of nonbeneficial pediatric research, it similarly raises concerns about exploitation or unfair use of children for the benefit of others. The accounts we have considered thus far, and several we will consider in the present chapter, address this dilemma by providing a justification for doing the research in the first place, and then a distinct justification for enrolling children in the research. The research is justified by its potential to gather information of significant social value. Enrolling specific children is justified on independent grounds; for example, on the grounds that the children would consent to it if they could.

This is not to say that these justifications ignore the social value of the research. The claim that individuals would consent is based, at least in part, on the assumption that the research has sufficient value. It is assumed that reasonable individuals would consent because the research is valuable (and presumably not excessively risky or burdensome). Although such justifications cite the value of the research, the fact that the studies have value is not, in theory, necessary for them. One could argue that individuals would consent to participate on other grounds, perhaps to satisfy a desire to confront risks or to assist one's colleagues in an endeavor that is important to them. In this sense, the value of the research is not necessary for the proposed ethical justification. It is, instead, just one reason to draw a conclusion that one might arrive at for other reasons.

I will argue that none of the existing justifications for enrolling children succeeds in the sense of providing a justification for the range of research that seems intuitively acceptable. This conclusion will provide impetus to consider attempts that justify the enrollment of children by citing more directly the social value of the research. This approach will have a second virtue. By focusing the justification for enrolling children on the social value of the research, it will emphasize the importance of ensuring the research is valuable. Accounts that attempt to justify nonbeneficial pediatric research by citing the low risks involved tend to focus almost exclusively on the risk level, losing sight of the importance of ensuring the research is valuable.

Similarly, nonbeneficial pediatric research is thought to provide a paradigm case of exploitation because it involves the use of some (without their consent) for the benefit of others. If the research offered no social value, enrolling children might be wrong on other grounds, but it would not involve possible exploitation of the enrolled children (since it would not benefit others). The social value of the research thus seems to represent at best an embarrassment, at worst an ethical affront and the source of the primary ethical concern posed by the research.

Many of those who are involved in nonbeneficial pediatric research tend to ignore the fact that the interventions are designed to benefit others when considering the acceptability of enrolling specific children. They do not emphasize to themselves, the children, or their parents the fact that the interventions are designed to benefit others because doing so raises the concern that the participating children are thereby being exploited. They instead focus on the requirement for low risks and try to convince themselves that this precludes the possibility of serious harm. Or, they focus on the possibility, sometimes extremely remote, that the child might derive some kind of clinical benefit, perhaps as the result of an incidental finding of the type that we considered in the first chapter, or in the long term as the result of new medications identified by the series of studies of which the present study is a part. An approach that connects the justification for enrolling specific children to the social value of the research might offer the pragmatic benefit of reassuring those involved in nonbeneficial pediatric research and possibly making more transparent the nature of the research itself. That is, it might clarify the ways in which the social value (i.e., the potential to benefit others), far from being an affront and the possible basis for a charge of exploitation, provides the basis for a justification for enrolling some children in some nonbeneficial research.

What we might think of as a simple-minded Utilitarian justification connects the social value of nonbeneficial pediatric research and the justification for enrolling children by dropping the requirement that those who face the risks must stand to benefit, and instead evaluating the overall balance of risks and benefits independent of the actors to whom they attach. A Utilitarian account can explain why it is acceptable to expose children to risks, provided the expected risk–benefit profile of enrolling them is more favorable overall than other available options. Indeed, when these condition are satisfied, one might argue that doing otherwise than enrolling children in the research would be unethical since the other options, by hypothesis, are expected ex ante to yield lower benefits overall. It follows that it would be acceptable for parents to enroll their children, and it would be acceptable for investigators and society at large to involve themselves in such efforts. Doing so is the ethical thing to do.

This same aspect of Utilitarianism famously explains why almost no one regards it as an acceptable ethical justification. By splitting apart the burdened from the benefited, it allows for the possibility of increasing, essentially without limit, the risks and burdens to which some are exposed provided doing so brings with it a compensating potential for benefit somewhere in the system. The implication for nonbeneficial pediatric research would be that it would be acceptable to expose children to essentially any level of risks provided the study offers sufficient potential for social benefit.

The costs of exposing children to risks in a given nonbeneficial research study is, at least on this first pass, a relatively fixed sum: the risks or the harms and burdens caused by the study to the children who are enrolled in it. Of course, most interventions require a series of studies, not a single one. Thus, we need not assume that just one cohort of children will face the risks of research participation. Nonetheless, the harm is fixed to a relatively small set of children. The potential benefit, in contrast, can be thought of as an ever-increasing sum in real time. Improved medical treatments benefit all children who are helped by them. If the disease in question affects many children, the number benefited could be enormous. And, if the disease remains active for generation after generation, each treated cohort would add to the sum of total benefits realized. Or, if the research produces a cure, the beneficiaries would be all future children who thereby avoid the disease. The rotavirus vaccine studies considered in the first chapter have the potential (again, assuming funding is made available to provide it to children in lower-income countries) to benefit hundreds of thousands of children each year, possibly for decades to come.

This potential benefit underscores another common concern with straightforward Utilitarian approaches, namely: a relatively minor benefit to the members of a sufficiently large group can justify very serious harms to a small number. At some point, we could justify serious harms, even deaths, to children in a study of a new treatment for acne, since the new treatment could benefit so many children. To take a frightening, but potentially actual example, testing of HIV vaccines takes many years, not to mention the fact that the studies cost a great deal. Essentially, investigators must give the putative vaccine to one group and a placebo vaccine to another group and then wait many years to see whether there is a significant difference in the rate at which individuals in the two groups acquire HIV. Because the risk of acquiring HIV for a given individual tends to be low, these studies must enroll very large numbers of individuals in both groups, typically in the thousands, and must wait a long time to get a result, up to 10 years. This approach to testing vaccines is extremely inefficient. In addition, while we wait 10, 20, perhaps 50 years for an effective vaccine to be identified, millions more will become HIV infected.

To address this concern, HIV vaccine studies often are conducted in groups at higher risk for acquiring HIV, such as intravenous drug users and prostitutes. Although possibly decreasing the time to a significant finding, this approach raises a host of additional ethical concerns linked to the focus on vulnerable populations. From the perspective of overall benefit, independent of who benefits and who is harmed, a more efficient approach would be to do injection studies in which you give a few individuals the vaccine and then inject them with HIV virus. Clearly problematic studies of this type could be justified on a strictly Utilitarian approach. The fact that existing regulations would not allow these studies in children, or even allow an injection study of a vaccine for a disease that was significantly less risky, say hepatitis A, reveals that these regulations are not, as critics have argued, based on a Utilitarian justification alone.[1]

There are various ways in which one might try to develop a more nuanced and plausible Utilitarian justification for nonbeneficial pediatric research. One might argue on rule Utilitarian grounds that we need to consider not only the consequences of a given study, but also the consequences of adopting a policy which permits that type of study. It might turn out that a policy of allowing what we regard as excessively risky nonbeneficial pediatric research studies would have worse consequences in the long run. This possibility could be made even more plausible by citing our intuitions that such studies are wrong.

The fact that this is a fairly deeply ingrained intuition—assuming that it is—would suggest that the implications of adopting a policy that contradicts the intuition need be considered as well, and might tip the balance of risks and benefits against a policy of allowing such studies.

One likely could come up with a Utilitarian story that roughly matched our intuitions. The final account might not match our existing intuitions exactly. But, that result in itself is not a knock-down objection. Our intuitions in this regard are relatively rough and ready, and reasonable people can disagree about where to draw the line on acceptable risks. However, as a justification, the present approach would remain problematic because it explains why some nonbeneficial pediatric research is acceptable based on the fact that we think it is acceptable, and explains why riskier research is unacceptable based on the fact that we think it is unacceptable. But, the intuitions regarding where to draw the risk threshold for nonbeneficial pediatric research are not supposed to be the explanation for why the line should be drawn at that point. Rather, the explanation is supposed to provide some story that is independent of and makes sense of our intuitions. Moreover, if this account were correct, it would provide what seems a very unstable defense of present regulations.

The claim here is that extremely risky pediatric research studies should be prohibited because a policy that allows them would be traumatic, an offense to our feelings on the matter. This argument provides a defense of current regulations only to the extent that we continue to find extremely risky studies troubling. As such, this line of reasoning provides a reason to change our views on these studies, if that can be done in a relatively cost effective way. It suggests that a better world would be one in which we conduct such research and find it unproblematic. The intuition that this would not be a better world ethically undermines this approach.

To consider one final version of the Utilitarian argument, one might attempt to develop a justification that allows nonbeneficial pediatric research on consequentialist grounds, subject to plausible side constraints. One version of this approach would argue that nonbeneficial pediatric research is acceptable provided the research is valuable, the risks are low, and the child's parents give their permission. Although this framework seems reasonable and mirrors many existing regulations on pediatric research, it does not provide a justification for allowing children to be exposed to some risks, nor does it offer a justification for the side constraints on the pursuit of social benefit. With respect to the former aspect, this account does not offer a response to Ramsey's claim that exposing children to risks for the benefit of others is unethical. One might respond that the side constraints minimize the extent to which children are exposed to risks for the benefit of others. That response, however, effectively grants Ramsey his central claim and then tries to minimize the ethical damage.

Second, this approach provides no justification for placing a threshold on nonbeneficial pediatric research. If some risks are allowed for an important study, significantly greater risks seem acceptable for even more important studies. Arbitrary side constraints on the level of allowable risks do not provide a very reassuring safeguard against incremental increases in the risks to which children may be exposed in the context of nonbeneficial research. A more effective response to this concern would provide a framework that not only insists on a particular risk threshold, but justifies the choice and explains why greater risks in nonbeneficial pediatric research are unethical, even if the research thus precluded offers the potential for enormous social benefit.

The Scope of Parental Authority

Most attempts to justify nonbeneficial pediatric research focus first on the children and the impact the research has on them. The hope is to show that, on the proposed analysis, this impact is of such a nature that parents can enroll their children in nonbeneficial pediatric research and investigators can conduct it. A different approach effectively reverses the priority of these considerations, arguing that a proper analysis of parents' authority to make decisions for their children implies that they may enroll their children in at least some nonbeneficial clinical research. The level of risk to which children may be exposed in nonbeneficial clinical research is determined, using this approach, not directly based on what it is acceptable for investigators to do in research, but on the scope of parental authority, on the level of risks to which parents may expose their children.[2]

One of the most prominent proponents of this view is Lainie Ross. She begins with a general analysis of the scope of parental decision making in a liberal society, and then systematically applies the resulting account to decision making for clinical care and clinical research.[3] Ross points out that the two primary standards for health care decision making for individuals who are unable to make their own decisions are the best interests and substituted judgment standards.[4] The latter directs surrogate decision makers to try to make the decision the patient would have made in the circumstances, given the patient's competent preferences and values. Although important to decision making for adults who have lost the ability to make their own decisions, for instance, those who fall into a coma as the result of head injury, this standard does not apply to children, at least not to younger children who have yet to develop competent preferences and values.

This conclusion seems to imply, and many commentators and courts agree, that decisions for children should be governed by the best interests standard. Ross points out that endorsement of a strict best interests standard ignores the fact that children typically are reared in the context of a family, often with other children who have needs, preferences, and values of their own. The fact that siblings' concerns and interests can conflict implies that parents cannot adopt the best interests standard all the time, at least not with respect to all their children. Attending the school play of one child can necessitate leaving a younger child with a baby sitter. This can be an acceptable choice to make even though it often is not in the best interests of the child left temporarily behind. Strict adoption of a best interests standard also would require parents, implausibly enough, to "disregard all personal interests in order to fulfill the children's needs, interests, and wants. That parents are individuals with needs, interests, and rights is ignored."[5]

Ross argues that, in liberal societies, parents should have wide latitude to make decisions for their children, what she calls a model of "constrained parental autonomy." In this model, parental authority to make decisions for their children is constrained only by a negative and positive obligation. The negative obligation specifies that parents may not abuse, neglect, or exploit their children, whereas the positive obligation requires parents to respect their children as developing persons and provide them with the means to live an autonomous life.[6] Some have argued that parents' obligation to provide their children with the means to live an autonomous life places very strict demands on parental decision making. Specifically, it has been argued that the ability to lead an autonomous life requires that individuals have a sufficiently rich range of life choices from which to choose.

Joseph Raz argues that realization of personal autonomy presupposes that individuals "have available to them many forms and styles of life" thus providing them with an "adequate range of options" for their lives from which to choose (not to mention the mental capacities to make this choice and lead the life thus chosen).[7] Similarly, Joel Feinberg argues that, in the absence of wide agreement on what constitutes the best life, parents have the obligation to provide their children with an "open future," one sufficiently rich in possible life plans from which the future adult can choose.[8]

Ross does not see the proper relationship between parents and their children in a liberal society in the same way. To a certain extent, she prioritizes parental autonomy over the developing autonomy of the child. She regards the absence of any "consensus on what the good life entails" as implying that "parents in a liberal society must be free to choose whether to expose their child to a wide or narrow array of coherent life plans."[9] On this view, parents have the right to mold their children as they see fit, provided the children are given the means to live a viable adult life. Ross gives the example of parents who may choose to not motivate, or even to discourage their children from developing an interest or talent in sports that would conflict with the religious life the parents envision for their children.

Parents, of course, may make mistakes in deciding which type of life to prepare their children for. But as long as they provide for the child's basic needs and prepare them for some viable form of life, the state must respect the parents' decisions.[10] Applying this view of the family and parental decision making authority to clinical research, Ross argues that as long as the risks of the research are sufficiently low, enrolling children in research is one of the things that parents can do free of state intervention: "Parental authorization or prohibition of their child's participation in minimal-risk research is not abusive or neglectful, even if the child is forced to participate against his will."[11] She also allows minor increase over minimal risk pediatric research, provided the investigators obtain parental permission and the assent of children who are capable of providing it. The child's assent in this case "signifies that his participation promotes goals that he identifies as consonant with his ends (without seriously threatening his future well-being)."[12] Ross argues that nonbeneficial pediatric research that poses more than a minor increase over minimal risk "is always immoral and must be prohibited" on the grounds that enrolling children in such research conflicts with parents' obligation to protect the child's "self-regarding interests and developing personhood."[13]

Ross supports the claim that parents have the authority to enroll their children in nonbeneficial research that poses minimal risk or a minor increase over minimal risk on the grounds that parents have the right to help shape their children's values and the type of adults they will become. Within the scope of appropriate parental authority is the right for parents "to steer their child's development into a socially responsible adult." The parents may not succeed, but "it is reasonable for them to try to guide his development in this way."[14] Ross repeats this stance in her more recent book. Referring back to her earlier work she writes:

> In brief, I have argued that parental autonomy should be respected unless their decision is disrespectful of the child's developing personhood. Parents who value participation in social projects like advancing science may try to inculcate similar values into their child.

Even if the child never shares in these goals, they are goals which responsible parents may try to inculcate.[15]

Two slightly different ways to read this view differ in terms of how strict one sees the constraints on parents' authority to make decisions for their children. On the first reading, parents have the right to enroll their children in research that does not offer a prospect of direct benefit, provided the risks do not exceed a minor increase over minimal. This simply is within the purview of parents' decision making authority, and the state has no claim to intervene. This argument captures one version of the parental authority assumption; namely, that parents are allowed, that it is within the scope of parental authority, to make this decision for their children.

With respect to the example of choosing between different life plans (or more accurately deciding what range of life plans their children will be prepared to pursue), it seems plausible to argue that parents can choose in a way that is not in their children's best interests, and yet still in a way that is consistent with the children's basic needs and developing autonomy. Of course, there may be disagreement regarding the extent of the range of life plans that should be open to one's children. Some argue for a wider range, others might argue for the acceptability of a narrower range, perhaps even preparing one's child for only one viable form of life. Bracketing that debate, Ross's view seems plausible in the case of life plans because it seems clear that children's basic needs can be satisfied within a wide range of more and less optimal ways of life, or ranges of life options.

Parents faced with the possibility of enrolling a child in nonbeneficial research face a different sort of decision in an important respect. Here, the question is what decisions are consistent with the parents' obligation to protect the child's basic needs. Under this authority, parents may enroll their children in research that offers a compensating potential for clinical benefit. Parents also, presumably, may enroll their children in nonbeneficial research when it poses absolutely no risk of serious harm, and there may be, as we have seen previously, research like this. Survey research may provide some examples. But, most minimal risk research poses some risk of serious harm. The research qualifies as minimal risk because the chances of those harms occurring are very low. It is not clear how enrolling children in such research can be consistent with the obligation to protect their basic interests. In the absence of any chance for clinical benefit, how does one determine how great the likelihood of harm has to be before the decision to enroll one's child conflicts with one's obligation to protect her basic interests?

In theory, it seems plausible to assume that a complete analysis would show that the costs and burdens of state intervention, not simply on the state, but on the children themselves, would imply that they are better off without it. Here, in theory, the threshold of risks to which parents may expose their children free from state intervention would depend largely on the costs of state intervention. There are costs to allowing the state to prohibit parents from making these decisions, and that level of costs could be used to set the level of risks to which parents may expose their children in the context of nonbeneficial research.

In some cases, state intervention can have enormous costs on the children it is trying to protect. It is not in children's interests for their parents to fail to compliment them, and one might think that the state should force parents to do so. In addition to dramatically curtailing the ways in which parents may raise their children, enforcement of this requirement would involve enormous intrusion into family life that likely would be contrary to the interests of many children. Prohibition of nonbeneficial pediatric research, in contrast, likely would not place a high burden on the children themselves. It would not require children to be taken from their parents, or even require the state to enter the home and chastise the parents. Instead, the state could prevent parents from making these decisions by directly prohibiting such research. On the assumption that few parents are likely to conduct research on their children, this approach would protect children from research risks without requiring direct intervention into the home or family life.

More importantly, Ross focuses on the decisions that parents can make free of state intervention. She concludes that we allow parents to make certain decisions. Although this argument is important for present purposes, it is not sufficient to justify pediatric research. To that end we need to answer the further question of whether it is ethically appropriate for parents to make these decisions for their children. Specifically, what level of risks, if any, is it ethically appropriate for parents to expose their children to in the context of nonbeneficial research? This question is not directly germane to Ross's task of developing an account of the proper scope of family decision making, but it is crucial for determining whether and when it is acceptable for parents to enroll children in nonbeneficial research, and when it is acceptable for investigators to conduct and society to sponsor and benefit from it.

To consider a specific instance of this difficulty, it clearly is within parental authority to at least occasionally curse at their children free of state interference. Unless the behavior rises to the level of abuse, the state does not have sufficient reason to intervene, not because we think that cursing at one's children is ethically acceptable, but because we place great value on a protected family sphere in which parents get to decide, free from state and other intervention. The serious costs attendant on state intervention imply that states should intervene only at the point at which the cursing becomes abusive.[16]

Nonbeneficial pediatric research poses a different dilemma. Here, it is not simply a question of whether the state should decline to prohibit parents from making certain decisions for their children or treating their children in specific ways. Rather, the question is whether society may establish the system in the first place, encourage, and even participate in it. It would be as if someone concluded from the fact that parents have the authority to mistreat their children slightly that it would be acceptable for society to establish programs, staffed by physicians and nurses, which provide parents with this opportunity free from state intrusion. In this case, it would be feckless to enquire of such programs precisely how much the parents could mistreat their children. It is wrong to set up programs for this purpose, even though parents may do it in their own homes.

Investigators and society do not, unlike parents, have the authority to simply expose children to risks. For these individuals to be engaged in the activity, as is often true for third-party actions in general, there needs to be an independent reason to think that the practice is appropriate. As mentioned previously, a number of other authors, including Ross, offer an independent argument by citing the possibility that enrolling children in research offers one possible way to teach them to become responsible adults. This line of argument offers a possible response to Ramsey's challenge that pediatric research can be acceptable only when it is in the interests of the participating children, and the next section turns to it.

Teaching Children to Be Moral

The process of raising a child to become a mature, responsible, autonomous adult is a long and arduous one. To be successful, parents cannot simply protect their children and provide for their basic needs. The best way of doing that presumably would be to keep the children warm, well fed, and locked in a protective bubble in the attic until age 18, to be unleashed and sent forth. This overprotective approach to raising children, taking the view that one's duty as a parent is to protect one's children from harm, while psychologically understandable, is counterproductive. It has negative effects on the child and also denies him valuable experiences that he can have only when he is a child, and many of the experiences he needs to become a mature and responsible adult. Protecting children from too many risks poses its own serious risks.

This point is crucial for the present analysis. To promote the interests of one's child, parents cannot merely adopt an approach of protecting the child from risks. The parent must be willing to take risks with and for the child. Mature and responsible adults are able to interact with and care about others, and to navigate through the environment. They must have some confidence in themselves, and enjoy some activities, projects, or hobbies. Children are not born with these abilities; they need to learn them. Many things cannot be learned second-hand or by example. Children must do to learn. Many lessons should be learned during childhood, and others must be learned during childhood, if they are to be learned at all.

There are several reasons for this. One is the nature of human development. Parents cannot wait until children reach age 18 to expose them to language for the first time and expect them to become effective users of language. The nature of brain development is such that children need to begin this learning process while relatively young. A second reason is timing. Arguably, it is in children's interests to meet Gandhi, but this opportunity might arise only when the child is young. Third, some experiences are important ones only if they occur when individuals are children. Meeting Mickey Mouse may be an experience like this. A fourth reason has to do with socialization. To lead a flourishing adult life, one must learn to live with and interact with others, to develop and maintain deep and important relationships. And to have a flourishing adult life, one must have a reasonably flourishing childhood, which itself requires the right kinds of interactions with others outside of a protective bubble.

By choosing particular experiences for one's children as a means of helping them to develop the skills necessary for a successful adult life, parents inevitably influence the kind of person the child is and becomes, her character, personality, values, and preferences. As a result, the parents' choices will necessarily slant their children toward certain lives and away from others. To be in a position to earn a music scholarship for college, children must learn to play an instrument and practice a great deal while they are children. A girl who does not hold a tennis racket until age 18 has almost no chance of becoming a world-class tennis player. A child who is never exposed to others will have less chance of hearing mean things said to and of them, but also will have significantly less chance of developing good relationships as an adult.

In many cases, parents cannot determine which experiences to provide their children and which paths to steer them toward by appealing to the values and preferences the child has or will ultimately develop. Often parents need to make these decisions before children have developed the relevant preferences and values, and the decisions the parents make will influence the preferences and values the children ultimately develop.[17] This fact reinforces the point made earlier that parents get considerable latitude in deciding how to raise their children. It is not just that parents are allowed to influence their children based on the parents' own preferences and values. In many cases, these are the only preferences and values extant in the family upon which the parents might base their child-rearing decisions.

In the process of rearing their children, parents certainly have the latitude and, arguably, have an obligation to teach their children to be altruistic, moral, and decent members of a community. A number of commentators have argued that one way of imparting this lesson is to enroll children in nonbeneficial research.[18] Bartholome argues with respect to children that "What warrants our intervention into their lives is not our thesis about what they would or should want. What warrants our involvement is that they stand in need of our help, our care."[19] One way to respond to a child's need is to help her learn to be a responsible adult through participation in nonbeneficial research, when it poses no discernible risk. He argues that this is not obligatory, but the "child and parents might select this activity as one that could enhance the moral development of the child"[20]. Dan Brock offers a nice summary of this argument: "when parents teach their children that they should be willing to participate in medical research designed to benefit others, this is a small, though not inconsequential, respect in which they are helped to become moral beings, with a concern for the well-being of others besides themselves and their close relations and friends."[21]

This argument provides an important lesson for evaluating the different ways in which one might justify nonbeneficial pediatric research. The fact that nonbeneficial research offers no compensating potential for clinical benefit does not necessarily imply that there is no chance for children to benefit in other ways that might justify the risks to which they are exposed. Educational benefits, especially in learning to be moral individuals, but also perhaps in learning about science, medicine, and the research enterprise, are some of the possible benefits children may realize from participating in nonbeneficial research. Notice that the ethical concern posed by nonbeneficial pediatric research, the fact of exposing some children to research risks for the benefit of others, in effect becomes a virtue on this argument. The fact that the research is designed to help others presumably becomes central to its potential to teach children lessons regarding altruism and the importance of helping others.

Learning to be altruistic is an important and valuable lesson. However, to use this as a justification for enrolling children in nonbeneficial pediatric research, one must be clear on why it is in children's interests to learn these lessons. Presumably, we all think that it is a good thing for people in general to be willing to help others. This makes for a better society overall. But this is not sufficient in the present context to justify nonbeneficial pediatric research. We have acknowledged that nonbeneficial pediatric research has the potential to benefit society by improving overall health and well-being. Justifying the enrollment of children in nonbeneficial research on the grounds that it makes the participants better members of society only increases the puzzle, it does not answer it.

What we need is an argument that becoming an adult who is (more) likely to help others is good for the children themselves in some way or other that justifies the risks to which they are exposed.[22] Other kinds of education are more clearly in the child's benefit, such as learning how to read and write. These are to the advantage of the child on most life plans in most (current) cultures. However, without further argument, a skeptic might claim that helping others is a benefit for the child himself only if the child values doing so. Therefore, guiding the child to help others cannot be justified on the grounds that it will benefit the child.

The empirical possibility that enrolling children in nonbeneficial pediatric research may teach them to be moral, and further teach them to value being moral, is both the strength of this view and also its downfall to a certain extent. Whether it provides a justification for nonbeneficial pediatric research depends on the empirical facts. Thus, pending further empirical research, it is unclear whether and to what extent it justifies nonbeneficial pediatric research. The facts may turn out in the right way to allow only the research and the levels of risks that we do allow. That is possible. And some data suggest that participation in charitable activities may provide children indirect psychological benefits.[23–26] However, the existing data are not that strong, and the facts may turn out in ways less congenial to this justification.

Bracketing the question of how these data might turn out with respect to older children, it seems extremely unlikely that enrolling very young children in research before they can understand it has any chance of teaching them to be moral. In this way, the present argument will not offer a justification for nonbeneficial research using infants and very young children. Furthermore, the existing data on pro-social behavior, while relatively scant, suggest that children do not develop the concepts necessary to understand that there are moral reasons to help others until approximately age 10, or older.[27] Before that age, they help others when they think that they have to, or they assume that they will be punished if they do not. Relying on those notions to teach children to help others might be an effective way to get them to act in accord with morality, but it does not seem an effective mechanism for teaching children to be moral; that is, getting them to do the right thing for the right reason.

Next, many nonbeneficial research studies seem particularly ill suited for teaching children to be moral. The principal problem is that the children often experience only the burdens and pain of the procedures required, for instance, undergoing a needle stick. Undergoing this experience seems an unlikely way to teach children to be moral. Moreover, the benefits of any given research study often are not realized for many years afterward and require a good deal of sophisticated understanding to appreciate. The process by which someone else eventually benefits as the result of an investigator inserting a needle into a child's arm, taking blood, looking at that blood in a laboratory, comparing it to the blood taken from other children, and developing, testing, and marketing a new treatment is less than a perspicuous one. One who hopes to teach children a sense of altruism likely would do better to focus on contexts in which the connection between the effort and the benefit is clearer and closer.

Learning to be moral is certainly a benefit of participation in nonbeneficial pediatric research to the extent that it occurs. However, this justification applies to only some research for only some children. It follows that if educational benefit is necessary to justify nonbeneficial pediatric research, a good deal of it could not be justified. In addition, pending further empirical study it remains unclear whether any research participation is justified on this view. Given the alternative of trying to teach children these lessons in safer contexts, reliance on this approach would put nonbeneficial pediatric research in jeopardy. This conclusion is problematic if one relies solely on the educational benefit argument. Yet, there are good reasons to think that this argument does not offer the only justification for nonbeneficial pediatric research.

Imagine if future research on neurological development reveals that children are unable to learn to be altruistic between the ages of, say, 12 and 14. What would we conclude from this research? It seems unlikely that we would conclude that it is always unethical to enroll 13-year-olds in nonbeneficial research. We might conclude that it is better to engage older children who can learn from the experience. But, when the risks are low, the benefit important, and particularly when children of this age are the only suitable participants, it seems we would be willing to expose them to some research risks for the benefit of others. This suggests that the potential for educational benefits is supplementary in some cases, not the primary justification for enrolling children in nonbeneficial research. One possibility is that children should sometimes at least act in ways that help others, even at some risk to themselves. It is hoped that they will learn from these experiences, but that is not the justification for having the children act in this way. This suggests a slightly different argument, according to which we allow children to be enrolled, not because it necessarily will teach them to be moral, but in some cases at least because we think that children should do the moral thing. This line of reasoning recalls a widely cited passage in the literature on nonbeneficial pediatric research.

Willard Gaylin quotes a father who orders his son to give a small amount of blood for research purposes after the son has refused to do so on the grounds that the needle stick will hurt. In the father's words: "I'll be damned if I was going to allow my child, because of some idiotic concept of children's rights, to assume that he was entitled to be a selfish, narcissistic little bastard."[28] This passage is quoted frequently by individuals who endorse the argument that enrolling children in nonbeneficial research can teach them to become altruistic and unselfish members of the community. However, from the passage, it is not clear that this is what the father is saying. The father is concerned that the child not *act* selfishly. That is, the father wants the child to do the right thing, now. One assumes that even if this father learned that the child was not of the proper age to learn to be altruistic he would still want his child *to do* the right thing.

The difficulties with the educational benefit argument are underscored by the competing analyses offered of this example. Bartholome argues that the father was teaching the child that physical force wins.[29] Diekema states that the father was "teaching the child that if you want something from someone else, it is okay to try to get it without asking permission first."[30] In Ross's view, the father was teaching the child that others may veto the child's participation, despite the fact that the father endorsed it. This, she argues, "teaches the child that strangers can restrain his parents' authority, even when it is not abusive or neglectful."[31] Which of the interpretations is correct depends on what, in fact, children learn in these contexts. And answering that question will require future research into the very complex process of learning. Future research may turn out to support one view or another, but that is not certain at the beginning and, thus, does not provide much support for the claim that nonbeneficial pediatric research is acceptable.

Granting the limitations of this argument for the purposes of providing a justification for nonbeneficial pediatric research, recognition that children can benefit from participation in clinical research in nonclinical ways suggests the possibility of considering (which we will pursue) whether children might benefit in other ways from participation in nonbeneficial research.

Children's Moral Obligations

A number of commentators argue that nonbeneficial pediatric research can be acceptable, not because it teaches children valuable lessons, but because children have an obligation to contribute to the common good, to helping others. Robert Veatch argues that "if the individual is seen as a member of a social community, then certain obligations to the common welfare may be presupposed even in cases where consent is not obtained."[32] Veatch's argument suggests that children have this obligation as the result of enjoying the benefits of living in a community. Or, more specific to clinical research, children have gained tremendous benefits as a result of the conduct and completion of previous clinical research, and from those individuals who faced the attendant research risks for the benefit of others, including, in effect, if not specifically in intent, the present child.

The enjoyment of benefits typically does not impose obligations on recipients who have no choice but to accept them. You are not obligated to reciprocate if I offer you a gift you literally cannot refuse. Organizations often mail random individuals small gifts, calendars, and greeting cards. These organizations rely on some individuals wanting or perhaps even feeling obligated to reciprocate by donating money to the organization. While this may be a laudable response, individuals who receive these gifts unsolicited are not obligated to donate to the contributing organizations, even if they retain the gifts and benefit from them.

Children likewise do not have the opportunity, at least at a young age, to decline the benefits of past research. Future children who receive the rotavirus vaccine will have benefited greatly from the efforts of those children who participated in the studies to develop the vaccines in the 1980s and 1990s. However, in many cases, the children have this benefit forced on them. Most children, at least at the time they receive the vaccines, try their best to avoid the benefit. The children do not reject the vaccine under the description of the benefit it conveys, because they cannot understand that description at the time they receive the vaccine. But they often do their best to avoid the injection that delivers the vaccine, and certainly are not accepting the benefit in a context in which they meaningfully could have declined it. Similarly, younger children cannot give informed consent to being enrolled in clinical research because they cannot understand sufficiently the potential benefits and risks of the research, including the potential benefits and risks of the studied treatments. It follows that they cannot understand information that would be essential to their being able to agree to participate in future research in exchange for present medical benefits.

One might argue that at least one instance exists in which enjoying a benefit does confer obligations, even though the recipients did not understand the nature of the benefit and did not voluntarily accept it in a context in which they could have declined. Specifically, children might have an obligation once they become adults to care for their parents in the parents' old age. The children benefited enormously from their parents efforts in rearing them. The parents, let us assume, worked hard and sacrificed for 18 years, attending to the children's needs and providing them with the environment to develop the skills and capacities for a valuable adult life. This effort represents enormous expenditure on the parents' part and the receipt of enormous benefits on the children's side, benefits that the children did not understand for many years and may well have never voluntarily accepted.

It does not seem completely implausible to argue that, in these cases, children have a moral obligation to care for their parents. For present purposes, the important point is not to settle this issue, but to note a key aspect of it. Whether this view ultimately succeeds, it is based on the plausible assumption that, if nonvoluntary and even unknowing receipt of a benefit ever can obligate one to help others, the obligation is owed to those who bestowed the benefit. The plausibility of the example of children having an obligation to assist their parents traces to the extent of the parents' efforts for their children. One wants to say that an individual has to help in a time of need or incapacity someone who did so much for them when they were in a time of need and incapacity. The obligation is owed to those who bestowed the benefit, and denying it would be ungrateful, possibly to the point of being unethical.

This line of argument is not being made in the case of nonbeneficial pediatric research and, in effect, this argument cannot be made. Research intended to develop medical treatments for adults must be conducted with adults because they differ from children in terms of their metabolism, physiology, immune systems, and the like. For the same reasons, medical interventions for children must be tested on children. Moreover, as we have seen, the process of testing medical interventions typically takes many years, yielding a generational gap between participants and beneficiaries. This gap is especially extended for pediatric research that does not offer a compensating potential for clinical benefit because such research typically involves the earlier phases of a research project, the phases of identifying possible medications and determining appropriate dose levels and toxicities. These phases occur even before the tests to evaluate the possible efficacy of the treatment in question, and long before possible approval and marketing of the new treatment.

Children who participate in early-phase nonbeneficial clinical trials tend to benefit other children 10-15 years after their participation. At that point, the children who were enrolled in the trials are now teenagers or more typically adults, assuming their diseases were not fatal. As such, the participants no longer need medical interventions designed for young children. In this way, those children who will benefit from the research involvement of this generation are not in a position to repay these same individuals, at least not by participating in clinical research themselves. The research efforts of one generation benefit subsequent, not previous generations. If current children owe a debt that goes beyond gratitude to those who participated in previous research, they will have to discharge it in some way other than participating themselves in nonbeneficial research.

Finally, if the justification for enrolling children in nonbeneficial pediatric research is that these children benefited, however unwittingly and possibly unwillingly, from the research efforts of previous children, it is unclear how one establishes the system in the first place. If the justification for enrolling children in nonbeneficial pediatric research is based on the benefits they have enjoyed from previous research, how does one justify the original nonbeneficial pediatric research studies? By assumption, the children who participated in the earliest clinical trials did not benefit from the research efforts of previous generations of children because there were no previous clinical trials. Thus, either the enrollment of children in the initial studies was unethical or there exists some other justification for enrolling children in nonbeneficial research that does not depend upon their having enjoyed its benefits.

Two authors have developed accounts of an obligation to participate in clinical research that avoid the present concerns. Arthur Caplan considers individuals who receive care in teaching hospitals that pursue research and, it is assumed, provide better care in the process.[33] He argues that at least some of the individuals who repeatedly return to teaching hospitals for their medical care could have instead gone to nonteaching hospitals. These individuals are repeatedly accepting the benefits of past clinical research in a context in which they could have declined them. Caplan argues that in this context: "Fair play requires that those who knowingly and willingly seek out and accept the benefits of better care, closer attention, and the higher levels of medical skill that are often available in a teaching hospital incur a general obligation to serve" as subjects of medical teaching and as subjects of clinical research.[34]

By focusing on individuals who continue to enjoy the benefits of past research over time, and who could have declined to enjoy those benefits, Caplan tries to develop an argument for an obligation to participate in future research in contexts that fall short of one formally agreeing to do so. Whether this argument works for competent adults who have the option of seeking care elsewhere, it does not apply to children who are brought to the hospital by their parents. As with the proposed justifications based on consent, the present argument succeeds only to the extent that one ignores the premise on which the dilemma is based; namely, that children cannot understand and consent, whether it is to receiving the benefits of health care or being enrolled in clinical research.

John Harris claims that the argument from fair play does apply to children.[35] He argues that our duty to help others and the notion of fair play yield an obligation on the part of those who have enjoyed the benefits of previous clinical research studies to participate in future clinical research studies which have the potential to improve health and well-being for others. As he points out, at least everyone living in higher-income countries has benefited from the results of clinical research. Harris is not arguing for an enforceable obligation. He is not arguing that individuals who have realized these benefits can be *forced* to participate in future research studies. Rather, he is arguing that our duty to help others and the notion of fair play provide strong reasons for each of us to participate in important research. And this reason, he claims, applies to children as well:

> If children are moral agents, and most of them, except very young infants are, then they have both obligations and rights; and it will be difficult to find any obligations that are more basic than the obligation to help others in need. There is therefore little doubt that children share the obligation argued for in this paper, to participate in medical research. A parent or guardian is accordingly obliged to take this obligation into account when deciding on behalf of her child and is justified in assuming that the person they are making decisions for is or would wish to be, a moral person who wants to or is in any event obliged to discharge his or her moral duties. If anything is presumed about what children would have wished to do in such circumstances the presumption should surely be that they would have wished to behave decently and would not have wished to be free riders.[36]

This passage suggests three related but distinct arguments. First, children may have an obligation to participate in research simply by virtue of having received and benefited from previous research efforts. This argument we have considered and rejected. A second argument is that in deciding whether to enroll children in research parents should ask what it would be reasonable to assume the child would decide, if the child were able to make her own autonomous decisions. On this view, declining to enroll the child in research is "to impute moral turpitude as a default."[37]

It is not clear when making other decisions for their children that parents ask or should ask what decision the child would make in the circumstances.

This certainly is not the common approach used to determine whether to enroll children in school or music lessons. For younger children, it is not even clear, as we saw previously, that it makes sense to ask what decision they would make if they were able to make a decision. To answer that question, one must first imagine that the children are competent adults. And that supposition eliminates from the children the very characteristics which press the problem in the first place.

A third approach would be to argue that the obligation to participate in nonbeneficial research traces to an obligation to support and participate in the social structure or system of which nonbeneficial pediatric research is a part. On this view, the obligation does not trace to benefits the individuals in fact received from the efforts of previous research participants. Rather, the obligation is to the overall social system of which clinical research is a part. This argument has the potential to avoid the present concerns. In particular, it may offer the possibility of justifying the first nonbeneficial pediatric research interventions and studies, and it does not necessarily imply that those who enjoy the benefits of the system are obligated to help those specific individuals who faced burdens and risks in the studies from which these benefits were derived. The next section considers perhaps the most prominent way to argue for such an obligation.

The View from Behind the Veil of Ignorance

In the previous section we considered the possibility that children are obligated to participate in nonbeneficial research given the medical benefits they enjoy as the result of the research-specific efforts of previous children. Here it is believed that the obligation traces to the fact that a particular child enjoyed specific benefits that were the result of trials conducted previously. The failure of this argument suggests the potential for a more general one. Rather than the obligation following from the receipt of particular benefits, one might argue that the obligation follows from the more general benefits children receive as the result of being raised in the context of a cooperative scheme or society. Children are obligated to do their part for the scheme because of the many benefits they enjoy as a result of their good fortune of being born within it.

Initially, the same challenge arises here of explaining why children have certain obligations as the result of receiving benefits unknowingly and often involuntarily. One way to justify the obligations that arise out of a cooperative social scheme is on contractualist grounds. However, contract theories have difficulties with precisely those groups, such as children, who do not accept in any meaningful way the benefits of the social system under which they are living. It has difficulty with those who are not able to meaningfully enter into a contract.

One might try, in a Rawlsian vein, to establish children's obligation to participate in nonbeneficial pediatric research based on the choices individuals would make regarding the structure of society from a position of ignorance regarding their own place within the society, from behind a veil of ignorance. To make this argument, one will have to modify the Rawlsian argument in several respects. The knowledge that one is an adult could well bias one's decision regarding nonbeneficial pediatric research from behind a veil of ignorance in favor of more, and perhaps more risky, pediatric research. After all, those who know they are adults at the time the decision is being made are no longer in danger of being exposed to the risks of nonbeneficial pediatric research. They may thus be inclined to regard the overall benefits to be worth serious risks to a few children. Conversely, the knowledge that one exists without knowing one's age may well bias one in favor of very limited or even no pediatric research. This information implies that one is in a position to benefit from the research efforts of previous generations. Any further benefits to be realized from the conduct of more nonbeneficial pediatric research are unlikely to be realized during one's childhood, when they would be of interest to oneself.[38]

Dan Brock argues that, to avoid these biases, the "veil of ignorance has to be stretched so that one does not know to which generation one belongs—past, present, or future—when one decides whether to accept and to participate in a practice in which children, though unable to give or withhold consent, participate in research potentially beneficial to other children."[39] He argues that individuals under this stretched veil of ignorance presumably would agree to pediatric research as long as the benefits of the practice exceed its overall burdens. On this basis, one could argue that justice as fairness gives all individuals, even children, an obligation to participate in clinical research when their turn comes.

This approach seems to have the advantage of explaining why we can expose children to some risks for the benefit of others, and why parents can give permission for their children to participate in such research.[40] This approach has the added virtue of avoiding concerns raised by the substituted judgment version considered previously. It does not require us to imagine what decisions a particular child would make, if he were competent. The individuals behind the veil of ignorance are not the specific individuals being enrolled in a given study. Instead, we are to imagine what choices reasonable and competent persons would make in that situation.

Rawls argued from the original position to the basic structure of society; that is, to a fair arrangement of the basic institutions in the society. If the structure of society meets these basic conditions, members of the society cannot argue that the resulting distribution of benefits and burdens is unfair. Thus, in considering what the argument would imply for more specific questions, such as our policy regarding nonbeneficial pediatric research, we are taking the argument beyond the areas in which Rawls used it. This is not to claim that such uses are inappropriate, only that they should be recognized as extensions of the Rawlsian approach.

The conclusion, on Rawlsian grounds, that the structure of society meets the conditions for fairness, does not imply that individuals are obligated to participate in the society so structured. Competent adults can decide to leave a society that meets these conditions (whether they have any better places to go is another question). The right of exit suggests that the fairness of the system does not generate an obligation to participate in it, but instead defends the system against those who would argue that it is unfair to some of the participants over others. At most, then, the present argument can show that it is not unfair to enroll a given child in a research study, that this is a reasonable thing for all children. But the fact that the system is fair in this sense does not provide a compelling reason for enrolling children in nonbeneficial research. Put differently, a system may expose individuals to risks for the benefit of others in a fair way without implying that it is acceptable to expose individuals to those risks in the absence of their consent.

A second concern relates to whether hypothetical contract arguments provide an independent or noneliminable reason for a particular program or policy. To see this, consider why rational individuals behind the veil of ignorance would select one policy over another. The answer presumably is that there are good reasons to select that option, that on balance the relevant reasons support its selection. But, on this explanation, it appears that one does not need to appeal to the hypothetical contract at all. One could simply ask which option the relevant reasons on balance support.[41] To put the same point in a negative frame numerous commentators who have systematically analyzed the ethical appropriateness of nonbeneficial pediatric research have been unable to agree on the appropriate policy governing it. In this context, it is not clear how we might make progress by imagining, say, these same individuals being challenged to select the most reasonable approach from behind a veil of ignorance. The difficulty we have had developing a consensus does not trace to the kind of biases that Rawls attempts to avoid. Rather, the lack of consensus traces to the fact that it is not clear what the right approach or policy is.

Third, it is important to consider the factors to which individuals behind the veil of ignorance can appeal in making their choices. In particular, are these choices constrained or guided by moral considerations? An obvious response is to think that the decisions would be so constrained. After all, we are asking what is the ethical approach or policy with regard to nonbeneficial pediatric research. The problem, then, is that what answer we get in this case may depend significantly on which ethical constraints we build into the system, making the whole approach question-begging. If we include Ramsey's constraint that it is unethical to expose those who cannot consent to research risks for the benefit of others, the reasonable policy to choose from behind the veil of ignorance would be one that prohibits nonbeneficial pediatric research.

Proponents might avoid this dilemma by assuming that individuals behind the veil of ignorance will make decisions based purely on self-interest, unconstrained by moral limits or considerations. Brock considers this approach and points out that, under those conditions, rational and self-interested individuals presumably would agree to any system that on balance produces more benefits than harms overall. Presumably, many different systems would satisfy this requirement. In particular, the system that produces the greatest amount of benefits overall may well be one that we regard as unethical. This possibility raises concern that the present version of the Rawlsian approach is ill-suited to identifying the morally appropriate approach, leaving aside the extent to which it might identify which approach would be reasonable for such individuals or which approach they have reason to endorse.

Consider the example of the HIV injection studies mentioned previously as a (presumably unethical) means to developing a vaccine for HIV. Here, the risks are a high chance of acquiring HIV for a few individuals in the context of research studies until an effective vaccine is developed. Assuming an effective vaccine is identified, the ultimate benefit of this approach will be that of saving tens of millions and, if one stretches the benefit into future generations, hundreds of millions of people from becoming infected with HIV. Redescribing this choice set as one that faces a single individual who makes the decision on self-interested cost–benefit grounds yields the question of whether such an individual would accept the risk of being one of the individuals enrolled in these studies for the benefit of otherwise avoiding HIV infection. If we assume the studies can be completed in a generation or two (assume for this purpose the existence of a sufficient number of potential vaccines), several hundred of the approximately 10 or so billion (assuming current world population figures) people who are alive in the world during that period of time will need to be enrolled. Because the vaccine protects future generations as well, the number of those who benefit is a multiple of those alive during the time the vaccine studies are conducted. Assuming this approach would speed identification of an effective vaccine by even a few generations suggests that enrolling 500 people in vaccine challenge studies might benefit 50 billion people. The choice facing individuals behind the veil of ignorance, then, is: Would a reasonable person accept the risk of approximately a 1 in 100 million chance of being injected with the HIV virus after being given a potential vaccine in order to gain the benefit of otherwise being protected from the virus?[42]

The veil of ignorance filters out facts that would allow individuals to determine their personal chances of acquiring HIV. They do not know if they will be rich or poor, male or female, live in Sweden or Zimbabwe, a priest or addicted to intravenous drugs. Presumably, on the present application of the original position, all they know is the chances that they will become HIV infected based on the probabilities that an average person will become so infected. Under these conditions, it seems likely that the self-interested individual would choose to allow the HIV injection studies for the simple reason that the gamble will likely be a positive one. Specifically, the background average chance of acquiring HIV infection is likely to be significantly greater than the risk of acquiring HIV as a result of being enrolled in one of these studies. It follows that a self-interested individual would allow the studies, a result which we have agreed is unethical.[43]

The problem is that a purely self-interested individual trying to maximize expected benefits from behind a veil of ignorance makes a decision based on overall benefits and burdens, independent of where those benefits and burdens happen to fall. More precisely, the individual wants the benefits to be sufficiently distributed to provide a sufficient chance that he will enjoy them. The problem is that the individual is likely to prefer the option that places all of the burdens on a few individuals so that the chances of his experiencing them approaches zero. For this reason, the individual ends up making a decision on grounds similar to a Utilitarian approach in the sense of not caring about a fair distribution of risks and benefits, nor caring about the way in which the risks and burdens are realized (with the difference that the individual makes the decision based on an averaging of the risks and benefits rather than on the overall risks and benefits).

Rawls famously avoids this concern when he uses the original position to determine the basic structure of society by arguing that individuals behind the veil of ignorance will choose the greatest overall benefits tempered by the so-called maximin strategy. That is, Rawls assumes that individuals behind the veil of ignorance will be conservative in the choices they make in a particular way. They will choose the option that works to the benefit of those who are least well off in the society. For example, Rawls claims that reasonable individuals would not select a world in which the bottom tier of the population lives in misery, even if this allows everyone else to live in opulence. To avoid the chance of having a life of misery, reasonable individuals would instead choose a world in which everyone lives a comfortable middle-class existence.

In the *Theory of Justice* Rawls acknowledges that the maximin principle "is not, in general, a suitable guide for choices under uncertainty."[44] He argues that it becomes plausible in situations, like the original position, that have certain special features.[45] It becomes less clear whether these features are part of the original position when one applies it beyond the question of the basic structure of society, as is being considered here. Leaving aside the question of the extent to which the present argument retains key features of the original position as Rawls envisioned it, it is not clear that appeal to the maximin strategy will save the present version of the Rawlsian argument. The question here is not whether a reasonable person would choose to make the poor even worse off in order to elevate the status of those more privileged. Rather, both options involve some individuals being in very unfortunate circumstances (i.e., infected with HIV). The difference is that the one option involves many more individuals becoming infected over time, whereas the other option involves significantly fewer individuals being infected, but some as the result of being injected with HIV in the process of identifying an effective vaccine. Since the less-preferable option (being infected with HIV) is the same in both cases, the reasonable choice, even if one accepts the maximin strategy, seems to be whichever option reduces the number of individuals who occupy that position. As we have seen, this may well be the world in which the injection studies are allowed.

Finally, the present defense of nonbeneficial research seems to misconstrue the relevance of consent to exposing someone to risks for the benefit of others. The problem comes when one tries to apply the hypothetical contract model not to the basic social structure of society as Rawls did, but to the specifics of the way in which individuals will be treated. It appears that a rational person behind the veil of ignorance, unencumbered by ethical principles, would accept the HIV injection studies. And that conclusion can be avoided only if the background or average rate of acquiring HIV is low enough that the chances of acquiring it are less than the chances of acquiring it in a world in which the injection studies are allowed. This suggests that the current argument will be relatively unstable. Whether it justifies nonbeneficial research studies of different kinds will depend upon empirical facts that may well change over time. That seems problematic in itself, but hides a deeper concern.

If the probabilities turned out that the reasonable person would not agree to allow the studies, we would conclude, as seems correct, that these studies are unethical. But, notice what the argument is for their being unethical. It is that allowing the studies is not something to which a reasonable person would agree behind a veil of ignorance stretched across generations. That explanation seems to misconstrue the primary ethical issue raised by nonbeneficial pediatric research. The concern with enrolling children in such studies is not, at least in the first place, a matter of whether competent and reasonable persons would agree to allow these studies and risk being enrolled in them. The concern is that children are not competent and reasonable, hence, cannot consent to their being so treated. The present approach misses the ethical work done by actual consent, as opposed to hypothetical consent. The very act of consent changes the normative conditions relevant to a situation. In the present case, it seems that very high risks might be acceptable, if they can be acceptable at all, only if the individuals so exposed in fact give their full and voluntary consent. Exposing children to such risks is worrisome because they cannot consent. Their inability in this regard is not remedied by imagining what choices a competent and reasonable individual would make from behind the veil of ignorance. In effect, then, the present concerns echo the problems we have seen with Ramsey's and McCormick's arguments, namely, a failure to take seriously the fact that children are unable to consent.

FIVE | Human Interests and Human Causes

Brief Recapitulation

In the previous two chapters, we considered arguments that nonbeneficial pediatric research is always unethical, as well as attempts to justify at least some instances of it. Although the accounts considered all have virtues, none seems to establish that nonbeneficial pediatric research is unacceptable, or that it is acceptable and the conditions under which it is acceptable. U.S. case law offers little guidance for finding our way, particularly because so few legal cases have involved pediatric research in general, much less nonbeneficial pediatric research. The case law that does exist, especially the *T.D.* and *Grimes* cases, finds courts inclined to regard nonbeneficial pediatric research with suspicion at best.

The need for an account to support or resolve this suspicion was reinforced by our analysis of Paul Ramsey's arguments. This analysis revealed that the ethical unacceptability of nonbeneficial pediatric research does not follow immediately from the fact that it involves individuals who cannot consent. This fact does, however, raise the question of how such research might be justified, given that it is inconsistent with children's clinical interests. The third chapter revealed that allowing children to be enrolled in nonbeneficial pediatric research only when it poses low risks reduces the ethical concerns thus posed, but does not eliminate nor fully address them. Even limiting the risks of nonbeneficial pediatric research to the level of risks that average children ordinarily face in daily life leaves the question of why the level of risks to which we expose children in the context of those activities that offer some potential for benefit should be regarded as an appropriate standard for research that does not offer the potential for clinical benefit. This concern seems especially acute once we recognize that, even when the risks of research are minimal, there often remains some very low chance that the participating children will experience serious harm. This point was characterized in the previous chapter in terms of the claim that the risks of daily life standard may provide an appropriate and approximate metric for the level of risks to which children may be exposed in nonbeneficial research. Nonetheless, this standard does not provide a justification for exposing children to that level of risk in this context.

McCormick's arguments and the hypothetical consent arguments suggested that accounts that attempt to somehow go through the consent of the subjects, agents in general, or idealized agents, will not yield a justification for nonbeneficial pediatric research. These accounts ignore rather than address the fact that children are unable to give informed consent. It seems, then, that any justification for nonbeneficial pediatric research will have to take seriously the fact that the individuals in question cannot consent, and not attempt to connect the justification for nonbeneficial pediatric research to an account of consent or what decision would be right or appropriate for competent individuals who found themselves in the children's situation.

The argument from parental autonomy recognizes that children cannot consent and instead appeals to the decisions that parents are allowed to make for their children. Parents in a liberal state are allowed, without state interference, to expose their children to low risks, even when doing so is not in the child's interests. Yet, the fact that enrolling children in nonbeneficial pediatric research can be within the protected sphere of parental choice in a liberal state does not establish that such research is ethically appropriate. This latter claim is essential to develop a justification for nonbeneficial pediatric research and provide an argument for the involvement of third parties, such as clinicians and state actors, especially when, as in the paradigmatic cases, the clinicians introduce the risks the children face.

Finally, we considered accounts that attempt to justify nonbeneficial pediatric research on the grounds that it is in the child's interests to participate. The most common version of this argument traces children's presumed interest to the possibility of their deriving educational benefit. By participating in nonbeneficial research, children might learn the value of helping others and the value of being part of a community; they can learn to be altruistic. This line of argument provides a justification for, at best, a very narrow range of nonbeneficial pediatric research. It fails to justify, for example, any research with very young children, no matter how important the research is and how low the risks might be. This is not to say that this argument is necessarily defective. It may be the best and perhaps the only justification available for nonbeneficial pediatric research. If so, we will have to accept that a good deal, perhaps most nonbeneficial pediatric research is unethical and consider what implications this conclusion has for our ability to improve medical care for children.

In the next three chapters, we will consider whether it is possible to extend the arguments from educational benefit by taking into account other possible ways in which children might benefit from participation in nonbeneficial clinical research. This approach, in effect, accepts Ramsey's claim that nonbeneficial pediatric research can be justified only when it is in the interests of the participating children. It then assesses whether we can build on the work of previous authors who have examined the potential for educational benefit by considering other ways in which children might benefit from participation in nonbeneficial research. For this purpose, we will pursue the hint developed previously that a more complete analysis of the ethics of nonbeneficial pediatric research should consider to what extent the social value of a given study is relevant to whether participation promotes children's interests.

Because nonbeneficial pediatric research must have social value to be ethically acceptable, this approach offers the possibility of developing a general justification for at least some research. Conversely, a finding that the social value of the research does not justify enrolling children would provide strong evidence that arguments based on children's interests cannot justify a good deal of nonbeneficial pediatric research. We would be left with attempts to develop justifications that do not depend on the consent nor the interests of those affected.

Three Conditions on an Acceptable Account

Theoretical debate continues over whether it is ethically acceptable to enroll children in nonbeneficial research at all, and a number of commentators and courts have argued that such research is necessarily unethical. Recognizing this theoretical debate and bracketing it for a moment, existing regulations suggest a fairly wide if not necessarily deep consensus regarding the conditions that need to be satisfied for investigators to appropriately enroll children in nonbeneficial research. These conditions provide a useful initial target for proposed justifications. This is not to claim that existing practice is justified. That is the question, and subsequent analysis may show that it is not. But the fact that general practice over the past 30 years, across dozens of countries around the world, has led to some agreement on the conditions under which nonbeneficial pediatric research might be acceptable provides reason, although not definitive reason, to think that the agreed-upon practice represents the most justifiable instances of nonbeneficial pediatric research. As such, this practice provides a reasonable focus for attempts to determine whether conditions exist under which nonbeneficial pediatric research is ethically justified.

These regulations and practices suggest at least three conditions for acceptable nonbeneficial pediatric research.[1]

1. *Net risk allowance.* Guidelines around the world allow nonbeneficial pediatric research that poses some risks to participating children. Of course, the very allowance of such research is at question, and cannot be assumed without argument. But, it is worth noting that at least certain examples of such research are widely accepted and seem consistent with our moral intuitions. Imagine, for example, that taking a few extra milliliters of blood from several children could yield information important to finding a cure for a disease that kills thousands of children every year. Further imagine that obtaining this blood requires only a single needle stick, performed with a topical anesthetic so that the children experience almost no pain from the procedure. In that case, the only risks to the children would be the extremely low risk of infection, the transient anxiety from the invasive procedure, and the risk that taking a few extra milliliters of blood might reduce the children's blood levels to the point where they became anemic.

   Assuming that children for whom the anxiety would be very high are excluded and the chances that participating children will require a transfusion is very low, and children with anemia are excluded and participants are monitored closely, this nonbeneficial research procedure seems ethically acceptable, even though it poses risks, including a very low risk of serious harm (e.g., transfusions pose some risk of serious harm). Again, although the claim that even this instance of nonbeneficial pediatric research is acceptable may be one that we end up rejecting, it seems a reasonable place to begin. Indeed, the intuitive plausibility of such examples provides some justification for current practice in response to the claim that, in the absence of a complete analysis of why such research might be ethically acceptable, we should err on the side of caution and prohibit all nonbeneficial pediatric research.

2. *Risk threshold.* Although guidelines around the world allow children to face some research risks for the benefit of others, wide agreement also suggests that the net risks to which children are exposed must be low. This is not to insist on an unvarying risk threshold for all studies, nor for all children. It may be that the level of risks can be slightly higher in some contexts and, perhaps, should be even lower in others. Yet, no project, no matter how great its social value, can justify exposing children to net risks of high likelihood and grave magnitude. One way to characterize this condition is in terms of a significant discount rate on the research risks to which children may be exposed relative to the increasing social value of a given study. Although a very valuable study may be able to justify greater risks, any successful analysis must accommodate this possibility in a way that does not allow extremely valuable studies to justify the exposure of children to high risks. That is, any account that justifies nonbeneficial pediatric research by connecting children's interests to the social value of individual studies should, nonetheless, avoid the Utilitarian commitment of allowing very high risks in the presence of an extremely valuable study. The 'risks of daily life' standard provides one starting point for the kinds of risks that might be acceptable. In particular, the suggestion is that nonbeneficial pediatric research may be acceptable even when it poses a risk of death and serious injury, provided the likelihood of those harms being realized is not significantly greater than the likelihood of their occurring during widely-accepted activities for children in daily life.
3. *Compelling justification.* All things being equal, it is better to enroll adults who can consent rather than children who cannot consent in nonbeneficial research. This condition implies, in effect, that any successful justification for nonbeneficial pediatric research should not be too strong. It should not imply, on final analysis, that enrolling children raises no greater ethical concern than enrolling adults who consent. Such accounts are inconsistent with the need for a compelling justification to enroll children. Instead, any successful account should provide reason why it can be acceptable to enroll children in nonbeneficial research while still maintaining that, all else being equal, it is preferable to enroll competent adults.

Once again, it is important to emphasize that these conditions offer a starting point, not a final conclusion. The process of reflective equilibrium—evaluating these conditions in light of our judgment of specific cases, and then reconsidering our views on specific cases given the principles we adopt—may ultimately lead us to reject one or more of these assumptions.[2] Finally, I claimed previously that, ideally, any proposed justification of nonbeneficial pediatric research would provide insight into the powerful intuition that such research is unethical. Obviously, a justification for nonbeneficial pediatric research cannot be consistent with and support this intuition. At the same time, this intuition is a strong and widely held one. A finding that this intuition is simply mistaken, with no possible support, would be surprising. A final, albeit not necessary, condition on any successful analysis, then, would be that it does not imply that this contrary view is patently false and, even better, that it provides some insight into its appeal.

Brief (and Prospective) Summary

To evaluate the extent to which participation in nonbeneficial research might be in children's interests and whether such an analysis might yield a justification that satisfies the three conditions on an acceptable justification for nonbeneficial pediatric research, we will need to have in place some understanding of what constitutes human interests in general and the interests of children more specifically. We will need an account sufficiently rich to evaluate whether participation in valuable but nonbeneficial pediatric research studies can be in children's interests, and whether the answer to this question depends on the maturity of the children in question, how much they understand of the study, and whether they are able to make their own decision to participate.

I will regard human interests very broadly as those aspects of a better life for a given individual. If earning more money would make for a better overall life for you, then making more money is in your interests. I will argue for an account of human interests situated in the conceptual space between fully subjective accounts, according to which one's interests are fully determined by or dependent in some strong sense on one's individual mental states, and thorough going objective accounts, according to which our interests are facts, or are determined by facts, that are completely independent of not only our individual mental states but independent of the kind of beings we happen to be. Our interests in many cases are influenced by, but are not determined fully by our preferences, by what we want and desire. We may want more than anything else in the world to make more money and, yet, making more money may not be in our interests. Indeed, it is possible that one's desire to make more money is stronger than any other desire one has, yet making more money is positively contrary to one's interests. A fairly common and unfortunate feature of the human condition is that we often are wrong about what is in our interests.

As will be explained shortly, the present account of human interests is consistent with the possibility of mistakes by including elements that are objective in the sense that they are not determined fully by one's individual mental states. Even informed and autonomous individuals, to use a phrase we will encounter again, sometimes have goals and preferences the satisfaction of which are not in their best interests. At the same time, this account of interests is not objective in the sense of holding that what is in our interests is fully independent of the kinds of beings we are and the kinds of minds we have. To take a specific example, I will argue that having a better life overall is in the interests of the person whose life it is, and one way to make a life better, all things considered, is for the individual to contribute to and be involved in or part of meaningful and valuable relationships, activities, or projects. Our lives are better when we are part of and contribute to valuable projects compared to the same life absent those contributions. This claim has a subjective basis to the extent that it follows from our nature, from the kinds of beings that we happen to be. The claim, put roughly, is not that it is in the interests of all beings, no matter their nature, to contribute to valuable projects. Rather, it is in our interests, given the kinds of beings we happen to be.

We considered this possibility in the first chapter with respect to the Depressed Contributor. We saw that the fact he does not embrace or value his contribution to a valuable project does not imply that the contribution was not valuable for his life. Rather, we argued that he should overcome his depression and embrace the contribution because it was valuable, it was his contribution, and it is in the interests of individuals like us to make such contributions. This does not imply that making such contributions is necessarily in the interests of all beings. It may not, for all we know, be in the interests of Martians to make such contributions. We cannot answer that question without knowing a good deal about Martians and what makes for a better life for them. In this sense, the present account is not fully objective.

The conclusion that contributing to valuable projects is in our interests even when we do not embrace them (but possibly not when we reject them) is important because it creates room for the possibility that contributing to valuable research projects may be in children's interests even when they do not understand the research in question, hence, do not have the goal of contributing to the research. This very brief summary is intended to give the reader some sense of the direction of the argument to come. Readers who are not interested in exploring its philosophical details, and who find sufficiently plausible the claim that contributing to valuable projects is one of the many things that is in our interests, may want to quickly skim the present chapter and return to it only as the need for clarification arises.

Three Questions Regarding Our Interests

Numerous accounts of our interests have been proposed. These accounts can be distinguished based on the extent to which they focus on one or more of three central questions and how they answer these questions: 1) What is an interest; 2) What determines what is in an individual's interests (what is the basis of one's interests); and 3) What in fact is in a given individual's interests. Although proposed answers to each of these questions have implications for the others, the entailment typically is not a strict one. Two commentators might agree, in answering the first question, that an interest is an aspect of the "profound" life, yet one may regard the profound life as involving living according to the dictates of self-denial, while the other may regard it as the fully artistic life. Similarly, commentators who answer the second question in the same way may nonetheless disagree over the third, over the specific content of a profoundly aesthetic or ascetic life.

For present purposes, we need not develop a complete analysis for any one, much less all three questions. Not only would that task be unnecessary, but the controversy surrounding these questions is such that relying on any particular analysis would effectively end at the beginning our consideration of whether it is possible to develop a justification for nonbeneficial pediatric research that satisfies the three conditions on acceptable justifications. To the extent possible, the goal here is to develop an analysis of whether and when nonbeneficial pediatric research can be justified that does not rely on more controversial claims that will be found plausible by few readers. Moreover, for reasons we will consider in a moment, I doubt whether we will ever develop a complete theory of human interests, in the sense of a single or unified account that specifies precisely what our interests are, what is in our interests (question 3), and why (question 2).

The attempt to develop a complete account of human interests finds its impetus more in the professional optimism of philosophers than in the feasibility of the task. It is simply unlikely that such a unifying account will exist for individuals as complex as we are. Scanlon offers a similar sentiment, expressing his doubt that we will ever "find a theory of well-being."[3] The present task will be to consider these three questions only to the extent necessary to address our challenge, making assumptions to the extent that they are necessary to proceed, and relying on claims of sufficient plausibility that they (hopefully) will be consistent with any viable, complete analysis of human interests. The point is to develop an account of human interests that is sufficiently rich to evaluate and possibly determine the moral status of non-beneficial pediatric research.

With respect to the first question, I will use the term "interest" in a very broad and general way to refer to the aspects or features of a good life for the individual whose life it is. If it would be better overall *for* X if a given state of affairs were to obtain, then the realization of that state of affairs is in X's interests. So, assuming that a better life for X is one that includes deep and close friendships, then having (some) deep and close friendships is in X's interests. To avoid begging the questions we hope to answer, it will be important that any claims made here about what is or is not in an individual's interests are justified and argued for. Because this terrain has been covered countless times, one runs the risk of appearing to make substantive assumptions merely as the result of one's choice of terminology. To my ear, the concept of a flourishing life for X captures nicely what we are after. In Harmon's view:

> To flourish is to lead the sort of life it is good to lead, by which is meant the sort of life you want your children to lead, as well as the sort of life you want to lead yourself. Such a life is not just good in the sense that it is good that someone should lead such a life—it may be good that someone leads a life of self-sacrifice without that person's life being the sort of life it is good to lead in the relevant sense, good for him or her.[4]

For others, the concept of a flourishing life often and perhaps irretrievably invokes a virtue ethics orientation to human interests. Thus, by adopting the term, one ineluctably begins to make, or at least appears to make substantive assumptions to the effect that a better life necessarily involves something like the better use of one's (distinctive) capacities. Those readers who can divorce the concept of a flourishing life from these particular virtue ethics assumptions can safely replace my usage of "a better life overall for X" with "a more flourishing life for X."

The concept of a better life for an individual is related to a valuable life for that individual and is similar to Scanlon's concept of a choiceworthy life.[5]

I prefer the term "better" life primarily because it is consistent with the possibility that even among valuable or choiceworthy or worthwhile lives, some lives are more valuable or more choiceworthy or more worthwhile than others. That way of putting it, however, tends to imply a somewhat off-putting sense of the moral worth of some individuals over others as assessed from some purely independent perspective. What we are after here is the concept of a better life for the individual in question. Typically, even individuals who have good lives can imagine, or we can imagine for them, ways in which their lives could be even better for them, more satisfying, more productive, more engaged, more enjoyable. The concept of a better life overall for an individual is a vague one, inevitably raising questions of better in what sense, or in what way. It is for precisely this reason that the term serves our purposes, leaving open to the extent possible without substantive theoretical commitments what makes a life better overall for the individual whose life it is. Any conclusions we draw regarding the extent to which participation in nonbeneficial pediatric research might be in the interests of individual children should follow from substantive arguments, not from assumptions smuggled in as part of our particular account of human interests.

One can think of an individual's interests as being grounded in or following from an analysis of that being's well-being or welfare. A theory of well-being understood very generally would provide an account of the good life for an individual whose well-being is in question, an account of the different aspects of the good life, and an account of why these are aspects of the good life for him. Rawls' concept of primary goods involves those things which are part of the good life, or are aspects of well-being for all human lives. Primary goods are, in Rawls words, prerequisites for carrying out one's plan of life: "things that every rational man is presumed to want. These goods normally have a use whatever a person's rational plan of life."[6]

Rawls distinguishes between social and natural primary goods. Rights, liberties, and opportunities are social primary goods, things that are under the control of society and that all rational individuals want in order to pursue their own life plan. Natural primary goods—health, imagination, and vigor—are influenced by the basic structure of society but are less within the control of society. Rawls sometimes writes as though it is always better to have more of the primary goods than less: "Other things equal, they [rational individuals] prefer a wider to a narrower liberty and opportunity, and a greater rather than a smaller share of wealth and income."[7] At least several of the examples Rawls uses here are almost surely mistaken. This seems particularly clear with respect to choices and options. At some point, increasing an individual's opportunities merely adds to his stress, transactional costs, and opportunities for regret, without increasing his actual or felt sense of liberty. This view is supported by empirical studies, which find that increasing the number of choices or options available to individuals also increases the chances that they will make a bad choice.

The problem here is not simply a function of the fact that a greater number of options decreases the chances that an individual will pick any given option, including those options that would be better for her. The characteristics of the different options also influence the choices we make.[8] For example, one study showed that, when given a number of options, individuals tend to choose the more distinct option in the group.[9] These data suggest that increasing an individual's range of opportunity by offering additional, similar options, any one of which would be good for the individual, may lead them to choose a less preferable but more distinctive option. This example provides a very important lesson for present purposes by reminding us that a priori analysis can take us only so far in developing an account of our interests. It is one thing for some consideration to fit nicely into an elegant and clear philosophical analysis of our interests; it is quite another thing for it to be in our interests, for our lives to go better for us, if that consideration is realized.

The primary goods in the Rawlsian sense are part of, but do not exhaust individual's interests as I am using the term here. In effect, the primary goods are those things that allow individuals to pursue their interests and, for that reason at least, are themselves in individuals' interests. Good health is in our interests largely because it allows us to pursue the projects, activities, and relationships that make for a better life. However, our interests extend beyond securing primary goods. As Scanlon argues: "Well-being is what an individual has reason to want for him- or herself leaving aside concern for others."[10] Roughly, an individual's interests are those aspects of the good life (for that individual) or those things that will help him realize those aspects. This approximates the account offered by Joseph Raz: "Well-being signifies the good life, the life which is good for the person whose life it is.[11] Well-being includes what Scanlon calls the "experiential quality" of a life, what it is like for the individual who lives the life in question.[12] Well-being includes having positive experiences and avoiding negative ones. Having such experiences is in our interests.

To avoid smuggling in substantive conclusions when introducing terminology, it will be important not to make any assumptions regarding the extent to which other directed actions or behaviors, including moral actions or accomplishments, are in an individual's own interests. It begs the important questions at hand to assume that helping others or acting according to the dictates of morality is in, or is contrary to, an individual's own interests. Doing the morally right thing is in an individual's interests insofar as doing the morally right thing is part of a better life overall *for that individual.*

One concern with even entertaining the possibility that doing the morally right thing can be in an individual's interests is that it may seem to rule out the possibility of sacrificing one's interests for the interests of others. Since such sacrifices seem possible and even, at least occasionally, occur, this implication would count against the claim that doing things for others is in the interests of the contributor. This concern arises if one takes the view that *every* instance of doing something good for someone else counts toward a better overall life for the individual, compared to the other options available to that individual. One can hold that helping others promotes the interests of the contributor in some cases and that doing so can make for a better overall life for her. This can be stated without committing to the claim that, in every case in which one has the option of either helping others or doing something for oneself, helping others always is to a greater extent in one's overall interests, in the sense that the life path that includes that option will lead to a better overall life for the individual than will the alternative(s).[13] To see the plausibility of this view, note that we rarely make the same mistake with respect to other things that are in our interests. Having relationships with others is in our interests. But, at some point, pursuing and maintaining an increasing number of relationships becomes one too many.

Coming to the second question of what makes it the case that some states of affairs, but not others, are in an individual's interests, existing accounts often are distinguished based on the assumed or postulated relationship between an individual's interests (or well-being) and the individual's mental states, such as the individual's hopes, goals, preferences, and values. For fully objective theories, no necessary relationship exists between whether a given state of affairs is in an individual's interests and that individual's mental states broadly construed. Certain states of affairs may be in one's interests even though one does not want, desire, hope, or prefer that these states of affairs be realized. On this view, whether a state of affairs is part of a better overall life is a question of fact in the same way that the laws of physics are facts of the universe, independent of what anyone or any group of individuals happens to think about them. Here, the question of why some things are on the list of what is in our interests is essentially tantamount to asking why it is the case that the list of the laws of physics includes some laws but not others.

The most straightforward objective accounts are what Derek Parfit has termed "objective list" accounts. According to these accounts, there is in effect a list of things—states of affair, accomplishments, experiences—that are in our interests, and our lives go better to the extent that they include things on this list: "On the objective list theory, certain things are good or bad for us, even if we would not want to have the good things or avoid the bad things."[14] Objective accounts have the virtue of explaining the apparently commonplace fact that we often are mistaken about what is in our interests. We often badly want things that are not in our interests. On objective accounts, this is possible because it is an open question of whether we want or care about the things that as a matter of fact are in our interests (the things on the list). The challenge for objective accounts is that it is not clear why we should care about what is postulated by these theories to be in our interests. Without some reason for us to care about the items on the list, without some explanation for why they should matter to us, one's theory of human interests seems too far divorced from those humans over which one is theorizing.

Subjective accounts address this concern by positing a necessary relationship between an individual's mental states and those things that are in the individual's interest. On these views, what is in an individual's interests depends in some sense on what that individual thinks, wants, desires, or prefers, perhaps under some idealized circumstances. If an individual does not value, and never would value a given state of affairs, it cannot be of value for that individual; it cannot be in that individual's interests. The standard concern with which subjective theorists grapple is to make conceptual space for the possibility of error: that a given individual might be wrong about what is good for him, and that we might be wrong about what is in general good for us. As we will consider briefly later, some subjective accounts (e.g., preference satisfaction accounts) also must address the problem of scope, the fact that we are interested in many things—the plight of the capybara perhaps—that are not necessarily relevant to our interests, to how well our lives go for us. A rich literature is devoted to whether subjective accounts can satisfactorily address these concerns.[15]

Objective accounts readily address the possibility of even systematic and intractable error by divorcing, to the extent considered previously, what is in our interests from our mental states, from what we think and from what we think is in our interests. The problem is that, in divorcing what is in our interests from the content of our mental states, objective theories face two concerns. First, it becomes unclear why a given individual should care to realize the states of affairs postulated to be in her interests. Depending on the account, one might also face the epistemological problem of determining which states of affairs are in our interests. Any potential for motivational force seems to drain out of the theory as it becomes more fully an objective one. The second problem concerns the foundations of the theory. Why is it the case that these things are in our interests and other things are not? What makes this the case? Depending on one's view, fully objective accounts either fail to answer this question or present us with a metaphysical mystery claiming that what is in our interests is simply a matter of fact.

The present analysis can be understood as one that either rejects the distinction between objective and subjective accounts of interests, or one that embraces elements of both accounts. R.M. Hare argues for the former approach with respect to moral judgment.[16] James Griffin endorses the latter with respect to accounts of well-being, arguing that, if pressed to choose whether his informed desire account is objective or subjective, he would answer "Both."[17] On the present view, what we want for ourselves and others for whom we care takes into account, but is not fully determined by what those individuals want for themselves.[18] If a child loathes science and loves art, we take that into account when asking what career would be best for him. We also think that our children, even as adults, can be mistaken about what is in their interests. They might think they would be hopelessly lost forever if they do not marry a particular individual. But we might think they are mistaken, and we might be right, despite their preferences and views of the matter. In this way, accounts that include some objective elements need not and typically are not committed to the implausible claim that what is in an individual's interests is completely insensitive to the individual's mental states.

Whether one would be better off living the life of an ascetic monk or a movie star depends in good measure on what the individual wants, what he hopes for, and the kinds of things he enjoys. Which option is in the individual's interests may even depend to some extent on which of the two options the individual thinks is in his interests. Thinking that the life of a movie star is in one's interests may result in one pursuing that option in a way that leads to success, a result that might not be possible if the individual did not have this belief.

Two additional complications are worth noting briefly. First, individuals may have preferences that go beyond their own interests, as when one wants to sacrifice oneself for the good of others or the environment. Doing so may conflict with an individual's interests overall, even though it is the case that contributing to valuable and worthwhile projects is in our interests. Second, individuals have an interest in deciding for themselves what lives to pursue, and it is in our interests to wholeheartedly pursue projects and relationships over time. One implication of this fact is that continuing to pursue a particular project or relationship may be in an individual's interests, despite the fact that it was not in the individual's interests to begin the project or enter the relationship in the first place. It may be contrary to one's interests to marry a particular person or to pursue the path of a cloistered monk. One's life may be better overall if one stays single or if one instead becomes a teacher. However, assuming that one has lived as a cloistered monk for 40 years (or been married to the same person for 40 years) it may, depending on the options that remain, be in one's interests to continue with that course. It may be that full commitment to this path is the best option, even though it was not the best option at the time it was chosen. Ill-chosen paths, if followed long enough, can become important commitments to the extent that continuing to pursue them may promote our interests.

Although purely subjective accounts of human interests face a host of problems, they offer a relatively straightforward way to answer the challenge of what makes it the case that those things that are postulated by the account to be in our interests are in fact in our interests. For example, a preference or desire satisfaction account of interests can explain why certain things are in our interests by pointing to the fact that we prefer or desire them (leaving aside for the moment whether this is a compelling explanation). Similarly, one might endorse a hedonistic account, according to which those things that provide us with pleasure are in our interests and those things that tend to introduce pain into our lives are contrary to our interests. In the *Protagoras,* Socrates and the great teacher Protagoras debate whether "to live pleasurably is good, to live painfully is bad."[19] Although the dialog ends with no clear resolution, Jeremy Bentham makes clear his views on the matter 2,000 years later, arguing that "nature has placed mankind under the governance of two sovereign masters, *pain,* and *pleasure.* It is for them alone to point out what we ought to do, as well as to determine what we shall do."[20] Here, Bentham is claiming that pain and pleasure determine what is in our interests (as well as endorsing motivational hedonism: pain and pleasure are the only considerations that motivate us to act).

To answer the question of why some things give us pleasure and others give us pain, hedonistic accounts could be more fully naturalized and appeal to explanations in terms of evolutionary theory and the evolution of our species.[21] Accounts of human interests that include objective elements have a more difficult time explaining why it is that some things are in our interests while others are not. As we just considered, anyone who espouses an objective list theory might argue that the question of why the list of what is in our interests includes some things and not others is no more interesting nor pressing than the question of why the list of the laws of physics includes the laws that it does. Because the account I endorse here includes objective elements, it will be worth considering briefly how this account might address the present challenge.

We can deny that all value depends on contingent mental states, without being forced to some fully objective theory, by tracing the value of human achievements to the kinds of individuals we are and the nature of our lives. Many things are in our interests because of the way in which they fit into our lives, into lives that are human and good for us. At this level, their goodness is not wholly independent of our mental states since it depends on the kinds of beings that we are, and the kind of beings that we are depends in part on the kinds of mental states that we have.[22] It is not so simple as to say that X is good because we say that it is or because we want it. Rather, X is good for us because it fits into our lives in certain ways, given the kinds of beings we happen to be. To oversimplify things a bit, this view holds that at least some interests are objective with respect to specific individuals, but are subjective with respect to the kinds of beings that we happen to be. Individuals do not decide what kinds of beings they are, hence, do not fully decide what is and what is not in their interests.

This line of reasoning underscores the extent to which the present account of our interests is based on an account of the preferable life. The assumption is that there are ways of filling in our lives that are preferable *for us*. And analysis of the content of this account reveals that what life is preferable for a given individual depends, to a large extent, on empirical facts about the individual's history and mental states, what the individual cares about, what the individual hopes for, what the individual is afraid of. The extent of the dependence on individuals' mental states is specific to the account of preferable lives for us. Whether this same account applies to other types of individuals is an empirical question that would require an analysis of the ways of life which are preferable for them.

This analysis raises further questions. What type of individuals are we in this regard? And which individuals are included in the set of individuals that includes "us" in the sense of being relevant to determining one's interests? Does the account of interests that I endorse here apply to dolphins, to plants? Does it apply to infants who are born with profound cognitive deficits? How would we go about determining whether it applies to aliens we might encounter? Briefly, the kinds of individuals we are has been determined by a long process of evolutionary change through natural selection and genetic drift. The fact that we have been shaped by our evolutionary history suggests the possibility of regarding the present account of interests as an account of human interests, and then appealing to the concept of our species to determine whose interests are in question here.

For present purposes, one can assume that the account endorsed here is an account of human interests and, for sake of clarity, I will often refer to it in this way. Although I will not argue the point, it is important not to conflate the question of how it is that we became the kinds of individuals we are (via evolutionary change) with the distinct question of who is of this same kind. We should, in other words, leave open the possibility that other kinds of individuals are like us in this regard and the same account of interests applies to them, despite the fact that they are not of the same species. The question of whether the present account of interests applies to dolphins is not settled in the negative by citing the fact that they are of a different species; the question of whether the present account applies to humans whose brains are profoundly and permanently different from ours is not answered in the affirmative by pointing out that they are of the same species.[23]

It will be worth considering briefly the view of well-being endorsed by Joseph Raz. Raz argues that "well-being consists in a whole-hearted and successful pursuit of valuable relationships and goals."[24] Because this account regards the whole-hearted and active pursuit of valuable goals as central to well-being, it will serve as an important contrast later. At that point, we will consider whether contributions made by very young children to valuable projects, including clinical research trials, can have positive implications for the children's lives, and whether such contributions can ever be in the children's interests, despite the fact that the children are too young to contribute to valuable goals whole-heartedly and sometimes are too young even to make active contributions. A conclusion that the whole-hearted and active pursuit of valuable goals exhausts the possibilities for increasing one's well-being (together with the assumption that one's interests refer to only those things that promote one's well-being) would preclude this possibility.

Here, Raz's account provides a nice example of an analysis of well-being that depends crucially on the mental states of particular individuals, but does not reduce to those mental states. Well-being on this account is determined by an individual endorsing certain pursuits or goals and actively pursuing and achieving them. Which goals an individual should pursue depends in great measure on what she cares about, what she finds interesting and worthwhile. To this extent, the well-being of an individual depends on her own mental states. Yet, well-being cannot be realized by pursuing and achieving whatever goals an individual happens to endorse. Some goals are pointless and others are evil, and the mental states of particular individuals cannot make it otherwise. For Raz, this more objective element is signaled by the fact that it is the achievement of only "valuable" goals that contributes to one's well-being.

Finally, we come to the question of what things or states of affairs are in fact in an individual's interests. Put in terms of the second-person perspective, what is it that we want for those for whom we care, say, our children, for their own sakes? James Griffin, the philosopher who has written perhaps more than any other on the question of human well-being over the past 20 years, argues that "There are prudential values that are valuable in any life."[25] He goes on to point out that not enough of these values exist to define one valuable life for everyone. It is not the case that every life would go best if it included the very same states of affairs as every other life. It is possible that I am better off drinking Beaujolais, while you are better off drinking Bordeaux. In addition, some of the things that are of value for all of us are necessarily vague and need "filling in" by the individual, and these "blanks" can be filled in different ways. It is valuable for humans to have projects or endeavors that they pursue over time. Yet, there exists a range of endeavors that might serve this purpose, and the specific one or ones that are best for a given individual may depend on her preferences and tastes, and on other facts about her life and situation. We all need projects and endeavors, but it is not the case that we all should be gardeners.

It is important to note that individuals' interests concern both the realization of particular states of affairs and the way in which these states of affairs are realized. Human are better off, all things being equal, in virtue of certain states of affairs being realized, including states of relative warmth and relative safety. Individuals' interests often are furthered or hindered by the way in which these valuable states of affairs are realized. Having a sufficient income may be in everyone's interests, but it furthers one's interests much more to earn one's income. Consuming a good meal may be in your interests, but typically only if you decide to consume it, not if someone else forces it down your throat (although that may be in your interests if you are starving and refuse to eat). Raz's analysis of well-being in terms of the whole-hearted pursuit of valuable goals highlights the importance of how desirable or valuable states of affairs are realized. To live a better life, we need to accomplish things, as opposed to having them fall in our laps.

We will return to the centrality of active pursuit when we consider potential objections to the present analysis of nonbeneficial pediatric research. I shall argue that it is in individuals' interests to contribute to valuable projects, including valuable clinical trials. Although this account provides a justification for some nonbeneficial pediatric research studies, it raises the obvious objection that it appears to justify our forcing competent adults to participate in clinical research against their will. The counterintuitive aspect of that proposal is accounted for by the fact that it would be contrary to the independent interest competent adults have in deciding for themselves the projects to which they contribute; it is precisely the same consideration that explains why the present account does not have this implication.

The claim that some states of affairs, as well as activities and contributions, can be valuable for us, independent of what we happen to value, will be central to the following arguments. Given the centrality of the claim, it will be worth considering reasons to think it plausible. In particular, I will argue that participation in a valuable nonbeneficial pediatric research study can be in the interests of very young children, even though they do not decide to participate and do not even understand or realize that they are participating in research. This claim may seem implausible because it divorces so clearly what can be in the interests of individual children from what they think, what they understand, and what they care about.

Philosophers imagine various experience machines and makers to support the plausibility of the claim that what we think is in our interests does not determine what in fact is in our interests. They argue, in effect, that we are better off living in the real world, with all its slings and arrows, than spending our existence in a virtual reality, fed pleasant and false experiences all the days of our lives. What we experience and what we want to experience does not necessarily determine what is in our interests. The most famous example comes from Robert Nozick, who imagines the possibility of living one's life on an experience machine. Nozick argues that this life would not be a valuable one for us because our goal is not merely to think that we have accomplished certain things with our lives, but that we want to actually accomplish certain things.[26] More mundane examples point to the same conclusion in a more limited scope. Engaging in difficult projects, running marathons, writing a book, can be more valuable for the individual than spending one's life lying on the sofa, watching TV, even if we assume that the latter, as experienced by the individual, would be more pleasant.

In a number of crucial ways, we are committed to the claim that certain things are of value for individuals independent of what they happen to want or care about. One instance involves the therapeutic context. To decide which aspects or features of a given life are candidates for therapy, we need to know more than the individual's personal goals. We need some account of what is a good life overall, what are the features of a good life for her, independent of her specific values and goals.[27] The appeal to elements that are not purely subjective makes sense of the possibility of asking whether what the individual desires is good for her. This is true not just for the professional therapeutic context, but also when one comes to reflect on the course of one's own life.

When one comes to ask whether the things one cares about are the kind of things one ought to care about, whether the causes, contributions, and projects one embraces are those one ought to embrace, one implicitly appeals to the fact that there are achievements and relationships which are valuable, all things considered, for oneself, independent of the things that one happens to care about (now). Perhaps the most famous perspective for asking these questions is the death bed perspective.[28] Lying in bed, at what one recognizes to be the end, powerfully highlights the extent to which it can make sense to ask whether it was a good thing for oneself that one got, during the course of one's life, the things that one wanted. The fact that one got what one wanted is not an answer to the question of whether one wanted what one should have wanted.

Moving closer to the present topic, the existence of valuable human achievements is vital to parenting. Parents do not simply take the view that they will keep their children healthy, see what values and goals the children happen to develop, and then help the children achieve those goals. Nor do parents take the view that children will be fine as long as they achieve whatever it is they ultimately hope to achieve. In one sense, the existence of independent values, of goals that are valuable for us, makes parenting more tractable. It is difficult enough to determine how best to raise a 1-year-old. It would be even more difficult if it were the case that 1-year-olds should be raised simply to prefer and achieve whatever it is that they end up valuing as adults. How would parents in that world decide what experiences to provide their child today?

One reason why the approach of merely catering to whatever preferences an individual child happens to develop would be inadequate is that the manner in which children are raised influences the goals and projects they come to endorse. In some cases, parents may decide to shape their children's goals based on their own interests, or societal interests, encouraging them to pursue a law degree because they value having a lawyer for a daughter, or they think the world needs another lawyer. But parents also shape their children's goals to further the child's own interests. The parent tries to direct the child toward certain lives and away from others on the assumption that some lives are better overall *for the individual*. It is better to have lived life A as opposed to life B, even if the personal values, preferences, and goals that one has in each case are equally satisfied or realized. This view of parenting makes sense only to the extent that it makes sense to talk about some things being, as a matter of fact, more valuable for us (or at least for certain subgroups of us), independent of what we think of the matter, and independent of what we happen to value and even experience.

Put differently, a general theory of value informs and partly shapes—although it does not fully determine—a theory of prudential value that influences parents' child-rearing decisions. This last point is crucial to avoid misunderstanding. Some commentators take the view that what is in our interests is independent, in all cases, from the preferences and values we happen to have. Our preferences and values may, if we are lucky, connect up in the right way with the valuable, but this is in all cases a contingent matter. It is important to note that the present claim that our interests are not necessarily tied to our preferences in all cases does not preclude the possibility that, in many instances, determining what is in an individual's interests will require some knowledge of his mental states, his preferences, values, hopes, or dreams.

For example, the following two claims regarding the previous point of pursuing projects over time may both be true. First, it may be in individuals' interests to pursue some projects, independent of their preferences and values, including their views regarding the value of pursuing projects over time. They may think that pursuing projects over time is a waste of time and, to that extent, what is of value for them does not depend on their own preferences. Second, it may be the case that the most valuable projects for an individual to pursue are those to which the individual herself is most committed. This too may be the case even though the individual denies it. But, this claim itself implies that the individual's preferences are relevant in one sense to determining what is in her interests. Her preferences help to determine which projects are (most) in her interests to pursue among the range of available options.

We can compare the present account of human interests to the account of human welfare developed by Sumner.[29] Sumner rejects all prevailing objective accounts of welfare and argues that we are left with only subjective accounts as offering plausible analyses of what is in our interests. When he labels an account of interests or welfare subjective, he means this "in the strict and proper sense of subjectivity, it only means one thing: that like colors, values of this kind are mind-dependent."[30] On this understanding of subjective accounts of interests, the present account also qualifies as subjective.[31] What is in our interests depends crucially on the kinds of beings that we are, and the kinds of beings that we are is determined to a large degree by the nature of our minds. Moreover, once we consider which ways of filling in or realizing the aspects of a valuable life will promote the interests of particular individuals, we need to appeal to their mental states. It is in our interests to have loving relationships. To determine with whom and how many of them will promote an individual's interests we need to know a great deal about that individual.

Sumner argues that welfare involves faring or doing well, and that welfare "more or less is the same as well-being or interest."[32] He also argues that welfare is a prudential value that concerns how well a life is going for the individual whose life it is.[33] To this extent, his account largely agrees with the present account. However, Sumner then argues that welfare is a matter of "authentic" happiness, which he defines in terms of the happiness of an informed and autonomous subject.[34] Here, he endorses a much stronger subjective account of interests. And it is here that his account diverges from the present account. I am assuming specific individuals, even autonomous and informed ones, can make mistakes, including profound mistakes, concerning what is and is not in their interests.

To be clear, it is important to distinguish what is in an individual's interests from the question of whether we should respect the life choices that individuals make for themselves. There are important reasons to respect the life choices that informed and autonomous individuals make, not least of which is the fact that, as we have seen, an important interest we have is being able to shape the course of our lives. Thus, once an informed and autonomous individual makes a life choice, we largely should respect that choice, although the extent to which we should accept the choices an individual makes for himself, and the extent to which we should try to influence his choices is a further question, and depends significantly on the relationship we have with him.

I have no business challenging the career choice of a stranger by asking a clerk at the store what she thinks she is doing with her life; in some cases, at least, that may be precisely what is called for in a close friendship. Once individuals make a particular choice, it may well be the case that continuing to pursue the chosen path will be in their interests. We considered this example previously with regard to the possibility that it might now be in an individual's interests to continue living as a cloistered monk given the fact that he has been doing so for 40 years. However, on Sumner's account, it appears that he is committed to the stronger claim that, assuming the individual was informed and autonomous at the time he decided to become a monk, it was in fact in his interests to become one: individuals' self assessments are, he writes: "determinative of their well-being unless they can be shown to be inauthentic, i.e., not truly theirs."[35] Unless one builds a great deal into the conditions on what qualifies as autonomous and informed, this does not seem to follow, not least because informed and autonomous individuals make mistakes regarding their own interests all the time.

With that said, the important point here is not to resolve these disputes but to recognize that the present account is objective in the sense that some of the things in an individual's interests can be independent of what he cares about. This account also can be regarded as subjective in the sense of basing what is in our interests (in answer to the second question on interests discussed earlier) on the kinds of beings we are, beings who happen to have particular kinds of minds. Many of the aspects of a better life, such as pursuing worthwhile projects and having enjoyable experiences, are open in the sense of being consistent with a range of different ways of realizing them. For this reason, the answer to the third question of what in fact is in an individual's interests depends a great deal on what that individual cares about, what he enjoys and dislikes, hopes for and fears.

We have been and will continue to evaluate what is in individuals' interests in part by asking how we ought to treat them. It is important to remember though that this is merely one way to try to determine what is better for the individual whose life it is. There are other ways to make this determination as well. Moreover, the proper way to treat an individual, although sensitive to what is in his interest, depends on a number of additional considerations. There are, as we shall see, conditions on what it is acceptable for us to do to others, independent of what might be in their interests. The question of how we ought to treat a given individual can further be influenced by social or policy considerations. Some individuals believe that committing suicide is unethical because of the implications for the specific individual. Others believe that we should take the view that committing suicide is unethical, even though it might be acceptable in limited cases, given the social or policy implications of allowing it. Put simply, it is important to be aware of the extent to which our intuitions and views on what are presented as isolated and individual cases can be influenced by our views on what constitutes an appropriate social policy.

Five Categories of Interests

We have myriad interests, and they relate to one another is complex ways. Contributing to a valuable project might be in an individual's interests, but also might pose risks of harm that possibly conflict with the individual's interests in maintaining physical health and avoiding doctor's bills. To keep things clear, it will be useful to develop a general typology of our interests in which different claims regarding one's interests can be located. This typology also will provide the basis for considering in what ways and to what extent participating in nonbeneficial pediatric research might be in the interests of individual children. Because our interests can be grouped and divided in different ways, one might develop a number of different typologies. The specific differences here will not be of concern for present purposes as long as those things we include in the typology are in fact in our interests.

In a somewhat rough and ready way, admitting of unclear cases and clear exceptions, individuals' interests (aspects of a better life for them) can be divided into five general categories. First, *biological needs*: in almost all cases, satisfaction of one's biological needs, such as for food and water, appropriate ambient temperature, and sufficient sleep, is in one's interests.[36] Labeling these interests "biological needs" is intended to mark the fact that they are more influenced by our biology and often are necessary conditions for a better overall life. This label is not intended to imply anything regarding the extent to which these interests are "genetic" or "innate."

Second, *experiential preferences*: a better or more valuable life involves having certain experiences or states of mind, and avoiding others. It is in everyone's interest to be content with oneself and the world, although this is not to claim that being content is valuable no matter what one's state, or state of the world. Sometimes a false conscience is worse than a bad one. Other experiential preferences vary across individuals and are not always clearly distinct from biological needs. The preference to avoid physical pain, for example, seems less important to some and seems at the boundary between a biological need and an experiential preference. In some cases, chronic pain can undermine biological as well as psychological well-being.[37]

Third, we have an interest in *meaningful relationships*. A life that includes meaningful relationships almost always is preferable to the same life without any meaningful relationships. We can have meaningful relationships with other persons, with animals, with the environment, or with specific projects, such as a project to build housing for the homeless or perform a great symphony. Part of the value and meaning that comes from participating in an orchestra that performs a great symphony is the contribution one makes to the performance. To this extent, one's contribution represents a valuable human achievement. But, the value for one's life is not exhausted by the contribution one makes to the outcome. Beyond one's contribution, the mere fact of being part of a worthwhile effort itself is valuable, connecting one with others and with a project of significance and meaning.

The possibility that one can derive value from the relationships, activities, and projects in which one is involved, independent of the contribution one makes to them, raises the question of what is required for it to be the case that one is involved in a relationship or project in the first place. In Chapter 7, we will consider the example of children participating in a political rally that leads to the overthrow of a despised dictator. Which individuals are part of such events, in the sense that is relevant to whether their participation has implications for their lives overall? What about the dictator's personal guards? Is the event in their interests, even if they simply are doing their jobs, or only if they assist the rally in some way? Or, consider bystanders who happen by, but do not know what is going on. Would we say that the bystander is part of the event and that being there at that time was in her interests?

Some of these cases are unclear, to me at least, and I do not have an account of the necessary conditions for it to be the case that one is part of a given relationship or project. Fortunately, sufficient conditions are easier to come by. In particular, whatever one's views on the bystander, it seems clear that one who is present and makes a contribution to a project is involved in that project to the extent that their contribution helps to sustain the project or helps to realize its ends or goals. The adult who helps to organize the rally is clearly involved, as is the adult who lends his support by being present and helping to make it a (greater) success.

The fourth category of interests in the present typology involves *personal goals*: a better human life involves achievement of (more of) one's worthwhile goals, understood broadly to include preferences, desires, hopes, dreams, projects, and goals. The qualification to worthwhile goals is important. Achieving goals that are not worthwhile does not further one's interests and often sets them back, although achieving nonworthwhile goals may have instrumental value in some cases, perhaps giving one the self-confidence needed to go on to achieve worthwhile things. A great deal of how well a life goes is a function of how well one pursues one's personal goals, and the extent to which one achieves them. A life that includes fully satisfied biological needs and experiential preferences is unlikely to be a horrible life, and may even be a decent one, but it will not constitute a truly flourishing human life. That requires sincere efforts to achieve one's worthwhile goals and, at least, a modicum of success. In Raz's terms, it requires the whole-hearted and successful pursuit of valuable relationships and goals.

Our personal goals have complex relationships to one another. Some goals are largely independent of our other goals, some overlap other goals, many are nested one within another, and sometimes our goals are contradictory. People may have the goal to exercise more because they enjoy the exercise itself; this goal may be consistent with an individual's other goals, or it may conflict with the desire to spend more time doing meditation. Others exercise because it puts them in the position to complete a marathon, which they may value in itself, or because prize money is on offer.

Sometimes the important thing is that a preference or goal is satisfied, essentially no matter how it comes about. One's goal of seeing the president can be like this. What matters most is that one sees the president. Here, the way in which the goal is realized is relevant largely as a negative constraint on acceptable ways to realize the goal (e.g., one should not harm others to realize it). More often, it is important that we do our best in trying to further our goals. It is often said that life is the journey, that it is the attempt or the struggle that matters, not the destination nor the outcome. This seems right to the extent that involvement in activities has great value for human beings. But, one might make too much of this advice, concluding that activity and striving are all that matter for us, that the extent to which our ends and goals are satisfied is irrelevant to our interests.

The ends for which we strive matter for how well our lives go (for us) in at least two ways. First, struggling for ends that are of no value is not the route to a better or more valuable life. We should not hope for and would not wish on those for whom we care, a life of pushing boulders up hills to no end, no matter how challenging the task might be. The ends matter, in the sense of it being (more) valuable to pursue valuable ends. Struggling for a valuable end connects us to things of value; struggling for valueless ends may have some value on its own, exercise perhaps, but connects us to things lacking in value. Second, although we want to make a good effort, whether we succeed, whether the state of affairs for which we are struggling is realized, is relevant to our interests. Working for a good cause is valuable not only because it is valuable to have a good end in sight while one struggles, and because striving for worthwhile causes puts one in contact with things of fundamental value, but because there is value in achieving or realizing valuable ends. The value of completing a poem or a marathon is not limited to the effort required, but includes the accomplishment. The person who struggles for 26 miles, but stops just short of the finish line may achieve a good many things, but finishing a marathon is not one of them.

Satisfaction of biological needs and experiential interests tends to feel good, and we feel better when we have these interests satisfied. To this extent, we can agree with Sumner's claim that "Nothing can make our lives go better or worse unless it somehow affects the quality of our experience."[38] However, when we consider personal goals it becomes clear that how our lives go can and does include things beyond our own experience. The reason for this is that the accomplishment of our goals is in our interests, and whether our goals are accomplished may, depending on the goal in question, not be something that we experience personally. The extent to which a first-grade teacher experiences satisfaction as the result of achieving her goal of helping students accomplish great things with their lives depends in large part on the extent to which she is touched, in one way or another, by their future accomplishments. The extent to which this goal is in fact realized does not depend on whether she is so touched; it depends on whether the students accomplish good or great things and whether those accomplishments are due, at least in part, to the efforts of their first-grade teacher.

Fifth, as suggested previously, there are *human achievements*, accomplishments and contributions that are valuable for us given the kinds of being we are. The fact that some individuals contributed to a project that saves the lives of millions of people is important and has value, largely independent (we will come to the qualification in a moment) of their personal goals and preferences.[39] This is a valuable human achievement and its being such does not depend on its being sufficiently rich to qualify as a meaningful relationship. All things being equal, a life that includes valuable human achievements is better than a life that includes fewer or no human achievements. Stephen Darwall asks us to consider:

> What kind of life you would want for someone you care about, for that person's own sake. Will it be a matter of indifference to you whether what the person herself takes to ground her activities' merit really has worth or not? If you are convinced that what she is devoting herself to is worthless, would you want this for her for her sake as much as you would if the thing she were devoted to were something you thought had worth?[40]

The point here is that what is of value or what is preferable *for an individual* is not necessarily exhausted by what the individual values, what she prefers, and what she wants to accomplish in or with her life. Our hopes for those for whom we care are not limited to their realizing their personal goals, whatever those goals happen to be. We also want them to have valuable goals and to achieve them (at least to some extent). We can explain this preference in terms of there being certain things that qualify as valuable human achievements. Valuable human achievements make for a better life, all things considered. But, as Darwall nicely points out, the preference here is not for some abstract better life compared to a worse life. Rather, the preference for a better life is a preference for the individual herself. This is so because having a life that includes more valuable achievements makes for a better life overall, and one of the things that is in our interests is to have a better life overall in this sense.

The possibility of arguing that participation in nonbeneficial pediatric research can be in the interests of even very young children begins to get some traction from the fact that clinical research studies often qualify as valuable human achievements. Briefly, health and well-being are fundamental to the pursuit of just about any plausible life plan and represent important interests. Because ensuring at least some level of health and well-being is in our interests, a project with the potential to help promote these interests is valuable, and contributions to the realization of that project can represent valuable human achievements.[41]

James Griffin asks us to reflect on the implications of the fact that Bertrand Russell devoted a good deal of his later years to the cause of nuclear disarmament. He writes:

> It would not have been at all absurd for Bertrand Russell to have thought that if his work for nuclear disarmament had, after his death, actually reduced the risk of nuclear war, his last years would have been more worthwhile and his life altogether more valuable, than if it all proved futile. True, if Russell had indeed succeeded, his life clearly would have been more valuable to others. But Russell could also have considered it more valuable from the point of view of his own self-interest.[42]

This seems right and provides a nice example of an important human achievement (in Russells's case it also would involve realization of an important personal goal). Part of what is in our interests is making important contributions; doing so leads to a better life for the individual and is in the individual's interests.

Commenting on this example, Sumner argues that Griffin conflates different modes of value. Sumner points out that a crucial difference exists between what is in Russell's own self-interest and what makes for a more valuable life. He writes that Russell "can think that a more successful life is a better life without thinking that he is made better off for it."[43] The distinction between what is in an individual's interests and what is involved in an individual having a more successful life is a crucial one for developing a complete and accurate account of individuals' interests. The fundamental point is that how well a life goes overall is distinct conceptually from how well the life goes for the individual whose life it is. To see this, imagine that an individual struggles against terrible and debilitating pain her entire life. Despite her courageous struggles, she suffers a great deal and, as she experiences it, her life is terrible. However, because of her courageous struggles, she inspires others to accomplish more with their lives. This individual's life may end up being an extremely valuable one overall, assuming she inspires enough people to do enough great things that otherwise would not have been achieved. This possibility is not inconsistent with the same life overall being largely terrible for the individual whose life it was.

Granting this distinction between the value of a life overall and the value of the life for the individual whose life it is, Sumner seems to neglect the point of Griffin's example. One of the things that is in our interests is to realize our personal goals. And some of our goals, including some of the more worthwhile ones, cannot be realized in the span of a single lifetime. Imagine that a public health advocate undertakes to ensure that all children receive the rotavirus vaccine. Because the vaccine is too expensive for most families and children in lower-income countries who need it most, this effort is likely to take a great deal of effort and may take more in years than the advocate has left to her. The advocate works effectively and diligently and, by the end of her life, establishes a consortium of governments, nonprofit organizations, and pharmaceutical companies devoted to providing the vaccine to all children who need it.

Imagine, after the advocate dies, all children who need the vaccine receive it as a direct result of her efforts. It would be a commonplace to say that those who see her efforts to fruition are doing it for *her*. This commonplace points to the deeper point that helping to realize the important goals for which she worked so hard is in her interests and in that sense truly is good for her. These examples, like the prior example of the interests of first-grade teachers being advanced by the future accomplishments of their students, provide an exception to Sumner's view that the obtaining of certain states of affairs, or the realization of specific projects or goals, can be in our interests only if their realization enters into our experience.[44]

We have been exploring the relationship between individuals' interests and their experiences. In particular, the fact that we have an interest in realizing our personal goals represents one way in which what is in our interests can extend beyond our experiences. With this conclusion in hand, we can now consider more fully the extent to which contributing to valuable human achievements is in our interests. In particular, to what extent can it be in our interests to contribute to significant human achievements when we do not experience the realization of the achievements personally?

One possibility is that we may adopt as a personal goal the realization of one or more significant human achievements. In that case, the realization of the achievements would be in our interests to the extent that it involves our accomplishing a worthwhile personal goal. This possibility raises the further question of whether this a necessary condition on it being the case that contributing to a particular significant human achievement is in our interests. Can it be in one's interests to contribute to a significant human achievement even if one never experiences the realization of the achievement and, moreover, one does not have the realization of the achievement as a personal goal? This possibility recalls the aforementioned distinction between how well a given life goes versus how well it goes for the individual whose life it is.

It seems relatively clear that making contributions to significant human achievements makes for a better life overall. A life that includes curing cancer is a better life than the exact same life absent that achievement. The more difficult question concerns what interest we have in having better lives overall. To what extent, if any, is it better for the individual whose life it is to have lived a better life overall? We shall consider in what follows the possibility that making contributions to significant human achievements can be in our interests, even when we do not experience the realization of the achievement and even when, more controversially, the achievement per se does not satisfy or realize a personal goal. I will argue that, all things being equal, it is in our interests to lead a better life, that our interest in contributing to significant human achievements implies this, and that this interest is independent of (in the sense of not relying on) our interests in having positive experiences and achieving personal goals. Put differently, the claim here is that, in standard cases, the fact that a life overall is better is itself in the interests of or is good *for the individual* whose life it is.

The postulation of this 5th category of human interests extends the present account beyond an account of human welfare strictly understood. One can understand our welfare as being a function of the first four categories of interests (biological needs, experiential interests, meaningful relationships, and personal goals). The extent to which these categories are filled and fulfilled by an individual's life determines that individual's welfare, how well that life goes to the extent that the individual experiences it and cares about it. The claim is that these categories, while vital for determining our interests, do not exhaust what is in our interests. Our interests, what is preferable or good for us, goes beyond our welfare to include the nature of our lives. Living a life that is preferable for us, given the kinds of beings we happen to be, also is in individuals' interests. It makes for a better life *for them*.

This claim is subjective in the sense that it is true in virtue of facts about us, about the kinds of beings that we happen to be, and the kinds of things that happen to be in our interests. I do not see any reason to think that having a better life overall is in the interests of fish or mice. This suggests that if we had been different, if our evolutionary history had gone differently, it might have turned out that a better life overall would not have been in the interests of the individual whose life it is, just as it might have turned out that having significant relationships would not have been in our interests if we had been very different.

The claim that having a better life is in our interests is also objective in the sense that it does not depend on, although it can be influenced by, the actual mental states—goals, hopes, dreams, values, preferences—of the individual in question. Given that the present claim is objective in this sense, it requires a response to the subjectivist challenge, voiced previously by Sumner. Briefly, the challenge is this: I hope to show that one of the things that is in our interests is for our lives to go better overall, and that the truth of this claim does not depend on the mental states of the individuals in question. The subjectivist challenge asks why specific individuals should care about how well their lives go overall, if how well their lives go is divorced from their experiences, preferences, values, and goals.

Consider average Joe who wants to feel good about himself, avoid pain to himself, avoid harming others, and provide for his children so that they can lead an even more fully pleasant life. Imagine that Joe does not think about and does not personally care about his overall life beyond these considerations. He does not care whether he ever contributes to any significant human achievements unrelated to his life or the lives of his children. The claim that I want to consider in what follows is that it would nonetheless be *good for Joe* if he in fact contributes to a significant human achievement (assume for the moment that this contribution does not otherwise affect Joe or his family). The subjectivist challenge asks how this could be the case. What import could this achievement have for Joe, given that it is not relevant to his personal experiences or goals? Put differently, what reason could Joe have to care about whether his life goes better overall as the result of contributing to a significant human achievement that is otherwise unrelated to him or his family?

Many commentators attempt to answer this question by developing an account of human interests that depends on the subjective mental states of the individuals whose interests are in question. Sumner, as we have seen, argues that something can be in an individual's interests only if it impinges on the individual in the sense of affecting his experiences. The virtue of this response is that it makes clear why individuals should care about those things postulated by the theory to be in their interests. It is plausible for individuals to care about what is in their interests because it is plausible to assume that individuals care about the nature of their experiences. Appeal to our experiences (or preferences or values or goals) makes clear the connection between individuals and what is in their interests. Put very roughly, the general intuition behind these views is that individuals care about things that affect them. While this is right, it does not exhaust the things that are important to us. In particular, and in addition to how things affect us, we care about how we affect others and the world. Our influence on others provides a different way in which things can have an important connection to us and a different reason why we care about them and why they are relevant to our interests.

A tempting response here is to point out that not everyone cares about making valuable human achievements. Not everyone cares about making the world a better place. Average Joe is just one example. This is true, of course, but it only begs the question of whether there is a sense in which such people are mistaken. The question roughly is whether we should adapt our theory to the existence of such people or try to adapt such people to our theory of what is in their interests. The latter possibility is highlighted by the subjectivist response to the existence of people who do not care about achieving their own goals or even do not care about their own experiences. The fact that some people do not care about their own experiences does not lead us to conclude that our experiences are not relevant to our interests after all. It leads us to conclude that these people are depressed and need help. Although this line of reasoning does not support the more expansive account of our interests that I am endorsing here, it does establish that we should not reject the theory merely because some people do not care about those things the theory postulates to be in their interests. Given the diversity of individuals, that approach would leave us with no theory at all.

What we care about for ourselves and for others is not simply that they have good or pleasant experiences. We care about both the impacts on them and the impacts they have on others and the world. Making the world a better place represents an important impact that individuals can have on others. Harming others is another kind of influence that we can have on others, and one that is relevant to us, independent of the extent to which the influence otherwise affects us. (To make average Joe plausible one needs to stipulate at a minimum that he cares about not harming others. To this extent he already cares about what happens beyond his own experiences.) In most cases, our influencing others also affects our experiences. But, this is not always the case. And, more importantly, the extent to which our influence on others and world is relevant to us is not exhausted by the extent to which making the contribution affects our experiences. It can be all too easy to harm another person and do so in ways that have negligible impact on one's own experiences. Of course, what it takes to have a successful life may conflict more or less with having pleasant experiences, or with satisfying our biological needs, or accomplishing one's personal goals. For this reason, as we shall see in the next section, these possibilities, like essentially all claims regarding our interests, come with "all things considered" qualifiers.

We have an important personal connection to the influence we have on others and the world. This is one way in which our contributions to significant human achievements have salience for us, one reason why how our lives go overall is in the interests of the individual whose life it is, independent of the extent to which these contributions are relevant to the individual's personal goals and experiences. A second reason for this is that the life in question is the individual's own life. In addition to the extent to which the overall quality of the life affects the individual's experiences, it affects quite simply the quality of the life that is the individual's life. Here is a different, but equally important personal connection. The overall quality of our lives is relevant to our interests because it is our life that is in question. This suggests that contributing to significant human achievements (the fifth category of human interests) is in our interests because making these contributions leads to a better overall life, and we have an interest in our lives going better overall. To have a valuable overall life is itself a significant human achievement and is realized by achieving specific human achievements that contribute to a better life overall.

The present section makes the point that whether a given occurrence, experience, or state of affairs is in our interests depends on whether it makes for a better life for the individual whose life it is. Many of the states of affairs that make for a better life for an individual are those that influence the individual's experiences. This is clear with respect to our experiential interests. Having positive experiences—some pleasure, happiness, and contentment with oneself and one's world—makes for a better life for the individual. Other states of affairs contribute to a better life for us by helping to realize a personal goal. The fact that realization of some of our personal goals does not impinge on our sensory organs implies that some states of affairs can advance our interests, can make for a better life for us, without it being the case that we experience them.

It seems plausible to assume, and many philosophers have argued, that our experiences and our personal (worthwhile) goals are essentially the only two routes through which it is possible to advance our interests. If a state of affairs does not influence your experiences and it is not relevant to one or more of your personal goal, it cannot promote (or thwart) your interests. The mistake this common view makes is to ignore the category of our interests that I have labeled human achievements. Contributing to or realizing a valuable human achievement leads to a better life overall. And it is better *for us* to lead better lives overall. The primary point of this section, then, is that a third way exists in which our interests can be promoted or thwarted. Our interests can be influenced by affecting our experiences, they can be influenced by realizing our personal goals, and they can be influenced by making our lives better overall.

All-Things-Considered Interests

The relationships among the five categories of interests are complex. For the most part, satisfaction of biological needs, experiential preferences, and the realization of human achievements are valuable and do not depend upon one's personal goals. But even with biological needs exceptions exist. Mountain climbers and endurance race contestants sometimes ignore their biological needs to satisfy personal goals. Indeed, ignoring one's biological needs seems to be part of what makes these activities valuable for some individuals. The goal, at least in part, seems to be overcoming, at least temporarily, one's biological needs.

The complexity of human interests and the complex relationships among them implies that essentially all claims regarding what is and what is not in an individual's interests come with implicit "all things considered" qualifiers. This is no less true in the present case. The claim that some projects are valuable and contributing to them is valuable for the contributors does not imply that it is necessarily in a given individual's interests, all things considered, to contribute to a specific project. At any given time, an individual may be presented with mutually exclusive options, such that the best course of action, all things considered, is for them to decline to contribute to some valuable project in order to pursue something else of greater importance or value for them.

Unlike biological needs and experiential preferences, the mere fact that one's personal goals are satisfied is not necessarily, even in standard cases, good for the individual (although the state of the world overall may be better as a result). There are several reasons for this. We saw previously that it often depends on how the goal is realized. In addition, (some of) our goals typically reach further into the world, they are broader in scope, than our interests (this aspect of the relationship between our interests and what we take an interest in was mentioned previously as one of the challenges facing subjective, especially preference satisfaction, accounts of human interests). I hope that children in the developing world receive the rotavirus vaccine. Yet, *my life* would not be better, any more valuable, simply as a result of their receiving the vaccine. It depends, as we shall see, on the process by which they receive it.

As we shall see, the converse is true as well; individuals' personal goals are not always rich enough to encompass all of their interests. We may take little or no interest in some things which, in fact, are in our interests. These qualifications raise the question of when it is the case that the satisfaction of those things in which one takes an interest is *in* one's interest. Put differently, which accomplishments or successes are in one's interests and, ultimately, when might contributing to a nonbeneficial research study be in one's interests?

Interested-in versus in One's Interests

Derek Parfit argues that our goals reach beyond our interests because one's interests are limited to those states of affairs that are "about one's own life," whereas one's hopes (one hopes) extend well beyond one's own life.[45]

Although this seems right, it leaves the challenge of determining which states of affairs are *about* an individual's life. James Griffin provides the beginnings of an answer when he argues that, in addition to what one experiences directly, one's interests include those states of affairs that one takes into one's "life as an aim or goal."[46]

Griffin's crucial insight is that mere desiring is not sufficient to ground an interest because it is too passive. Yet, taking on the state of affairs as a personal goal, as Griffin recommends, does not yet seem enough to yield an interest. Consider my previously discussed goal of worldwide provision of a rotavirus vaccine. We noted that realization of this goal does not make my life better even though I hope for such provision. And this conclusion seems unaffected by my adopting worldwide provision of the rotavirus vaccine as a personal goal. *My* life is not necessarily any better if the vaccine is provided to children worldwide.

The fact that I take on a particular goal makes the state of affairs referred to a part of my life in the sense that this is now one of my goals. However, it does not follow that the occurrence of the state of affairs in question necessarily has implications *for* my life. We would not say that I lived a better or worse life simply because this goal of mine is or is not realized; it depends on how the goal is realized. We assume, in standard cases, that once an individual takes on a particular goal, she will actively work toward realizing it. Yet, such activity is not required by the mere fact of having the goal—one can have goals that one does little or nothing to bring about (although the fact that one does absolutely nothing, especially in situations where doing something involves little or no cost, may provide evidence that one does not really have the goal in question; maybe I do not really want to learn Spanish).

Compare two different versions of my life. In both, I recognize that we now have effective rotavirus vaccines and adopt as a goal that children in lower-income countries receive the vaccine. Imagine that one version of me then undertakes to help bring about this end, perhaps I lobby politicians or pursue fundraising efforts, while the other version of me does nothing. Realization of this goal would not have the same implications for my life in both cases, even though the goal of realizing this state of affairs is constant across them. The reason for this seems clear: one version of me worked toward this goal, the other did nothing to bring it about. The effort itself, as we have seen, can be valuable for the individual. However, for the realization of this goal to also be valuable for the individual it must be the case that the individual's efforts made a difference. The individual had to make a contribution.

Put generally, working toward a particular goal and helping to realize it entails that its realization says something about one's life because it is now, in an important sense that it was not before, one's own project. One is now connected to the project and its value in a way that one would not have been if one merely hoped for its realization. One helped, assuming one was successful, to bring about the end in question. In this way, we can have interests in states of affairs that do not affect us personally, by working toward their realization. This line of reasoning can be pursued one step further by recognizing that the fact an individual works toward an important goal says something valuable about his life in what we might think of as an indirect way. It gives him a valuable project to pursue. This is valuable, and the fact that he pursued it says something about him, about the kind of person he is. But there is a more direct way in which the realization of some valuable state of affairs can be of value for one's life.

We can see this by asking, to the extent that we are concerned with an individual's interests, whether all we want to know is whether the state of affairs is valuable and whether the individual worked to realize the state of affairs. It seems that, in addition, we want to know whether the individual's efforts made a difference, whether he in fact contributed to the realization of the state of affairs. If he did, this fact says something about his life. He made a contribution to an important cause, and his life is better as a result. Put differently, he now has a personal connection not just to the fundamental value of the project, but to the value realized in the project's being attained or achieved.

How much a given contribution says about one's life, or how much it contributes to one having a better life overall, depends on the nature of the project in question and the nature of one's contribution to it. This includes the value of the project, the importance of one's contribution to the success of the project, and one's relationship to the contribution itself: how much one engages in the contribution, how much one embraces the contribution, and how important this goal is relative to one's other personal goals.

Consider again the two versions of me and their respective efforts to provide the rotavirus vaccine to children in lower-income countries. One version takes on this cause as a central project, spending a good deal of time planning his efforts and undertaking them. In addition, he considers the cause to be of vital importance and one of his most important personal goals. The other version takes on the goal but thinks very little about it otherwise and only once in an offhand way happens to mention the cause to someone at a cocktail party who, unbeknownst to that version of me, is a billionaire looking for an important cause to adopt.

Imagine that both versions of me had the same goal and their efforts in fact equally contributed to the realization of the goal. Nonetheless, it seems that the contributions of the first version of me say more about that life than the contributions of the second version, even though evaluated in objective terms the two versions had the same impact on the realization of the state of affairs. For simplicity, I will refer to this difference in terms of the extent to which the contribution "goes through" the individual's agency. All things being equal, the more a contribution goes through an individual' agency—the more they will it, intend it, understand, work for, and embrace the cause—the more it contributes to a better life overall for them.

Developing a complete account of the necessary and sufficient conditions for it being the case that a given contribution goes through an individual's agency would take us far beyond our present concerns, assuming it is possible at all. Fortunately, we have rough intuitions, sufficient for present purposes, concerning when a contribution goes through an individual's agency and to what extent. It is clear, for example, that the agency of the first version of me, the one that worked assiduously to raise funds, was more involved in the provision of the rotavirus vaccine than the second version. Of course, difficult epistemological issues will often arise here given that these comparisons depend on our making assumptions about the mental states and lives of the actors involved. Were they really interested in the goal? Did they intend the result, or were they focused on some other goal, perhaps fame or fortune? Were they working hard all that time, or mostly taking naps?

This line of reasoning raises the question of the extent to which a contribution must go through an individual's agency to have implications for his life overall. Is some minimal level of agency required for a contribution to have implications for one's life? Looked at from the other end, to what extent do passive contributions say anything about an individual's life? Nonbeneficial pediatric research is of theoretical interest because it provides a practical, not to mention extremely important, example with which to consider this question. Considering nonbeneficial pediatric research with younger and younger participants has the effect of progressively reducing and then eliminating the factors, including understanding and identification that connect a given contribution to the contributor's agency. The practical extreme is nonbeneficial research with infants, which involves what we might think of as purely passive contributions to a valuable cause. Infants in no way embrace, understand, appreciate, endorse, or strive toward the goals of the nonbeneficial pediatric research studies in which they participate. These contributions in no way go through the infants' agency.

The extent to which a given contribution goes through the contributor's agency should not be conflated with the distinct question of whether the contributor is part of the causal process that leads to the outcome in question.

By taking infants' blood and analyzing it for research purposes, say, investigators do not engage the infants' wills, but they do engage the infants' bodies. One possibility is that a merely causal contribution of this sort can have implications for an individual's life and that increasing the extent to which the contribution engages the individual and the individual's agency increases the extent to which it says something about her life, or the extent to which her life is influenced for having made the contribution. Alternatively, causal contributions alone may say nothing about the individual's life. It might be that the contribution has to go through the individual's agency to some extent. Perhaps the individual must realize she is making the contribution, or she must realize and intend to make it, or even realize, intend, and value the contribution for it to contribute to a better life for her.

One might assume that having a purely passive, purely causal impact on some state of affairs is not sufficient to qualify as a contribution. Infants may be a vital part of the causal process of nonbeneficial pediatric research studies to the extent that the research engages with the infants' bodies. However, unless and until they realize and actively embrace to some extent this role, or at least are physically active contributors, they cannot be said to make a contribution to the study and its findings. To assess these options, it will be necessary to consider the different ways in which we can make contributions to a project, goal, or state of affairs; what is required to make a contribution; and when is making a given contribution relevant to how we assess the contributor's life overall.

The Causal Nexus of Our Lives

Viewed in purely physical terms, the world consists of matter in motion, atoms, molecules, and objects moving in space, interacting with others and influencing and altering their courses. One object, the cause, interacts with another and has the effect of altering the object in some way—its speed, its trajectory, its shape. The cause (the object embedded in the causal process) itself had antecedent causes that influenced its characteristics. In the end, whether we describe an object or event (for present purposes the difference is unimportant) as a cause or effect will depend upon the frame through which we regard it in a given instance. The child is both the cause of the ruckus in the other room and the effect of his parent's decision to have and rear children.

Human beings, as physical objects, are very much a part of this causal nexus. We physically influence other objects in the universe, including other human beings, and are influenced by them. Once an individual influences another object as the cause of some effect, this fact becomes part of the individual's life story or narrative. It becomes a part of one's biography, and the individual's complete biography is told, in important part, by describing the causal relationships into which he enters over the course of his life. To push the point further, in the end, our causal narrative is one of the few truly unique aspects of our lives. No one else ever did or ever will have the same causal narrative, the same causal interactions over the course of his life. This narrative is mine; that (evolving) one is yours and uniquely yours. Furthermore, each of us has one unique narrative that encompasses all the relationships into which we enter over the course of our lives. We may privilege some over others, caring more about the influence we have on our families than the influence we have on the environment, what we do as adults compared to what we do as children, but all the interactions together are part of the single life that each one of us gets.

Because making a contribution is fundamentally a causal notion, we must consider briefly the concept of causality and causal factors to be in a position to determine when children's participation in a nonbeneficial research study qualifies as their making a contribution to the study in question. An enormous philosophical literature exists on causality, on what constitutes a cause, with many philosophers attempting to provide necessary and sufficient conditions on it being the case that a given process or event causes (is part of the cause of) another, and others familiarly arguing that causality is a figment of our perceptions or our expectations.[47]

The common notion of a causal interaction or relationship is of one factor influencing or affecting another, the child striking the white marble and sending it into the red marble. Wesley Salmon, who has worked over the past 30 years to provide a philosophical account of this understanding of causality and thereby save it from skeptical challenges, writes: "When there is an interaction between two processes in which both are modified, and the modifications persist beyond the place of intersection, this intersection qualifies as a causal interaction."[48] Beyond the details and various qualifications, this analysis highlights the extent to which causality involves interactions between two or more objects or processes. In many cases of causal interaction, we focus on one object, process, or event as the presumed cause and another object, process, or event as the effect. When the white marble and the red marble collide and move off at an angle from each other, we regard the white marble's moving into the red marble as *the* cause, and the red marble rolling away as *the* effect. Although this sketch can be useful for various purposes, it is important to note that it involves a simplification of the causal story.

Any causal interaction involves numerous contributing factors and a variety of consequent effects. The nature of the sidewalk and the air around it also serve as contributing causes to the effect in question. The small bumps in the sidewalk surface influence the speed and angle of the collision, as does the amount of humidity in the air. Although we may focus on a particular causal factor in a given case, depending largely upon our interests, these other causal factors also play a contributing role.

Often we focus on the active causal factor or agent as the cause of the effect in question. We regard the moving white marble as the cause of the effect of the red marble moving off rather than the slope and texture of the sidewalk. But the absence of activity or motion does not preclude these other factors from having a causal role. Consider again the case of the child stuck in the well and climbing out over the body of the thin man who was dangled down into the well. The thin man (or thin child) provides a vital contributing factor to the effect of the child escaping the well, despite the fact that the thin man is not an active or moving causal factor. Similarly, the surface of the earth is an important contributing causal factor to the injuries that result from Humpty Dumpty's fall, even though the surface of the earth is stationary (relative to Humpty Dumpty's movement).

To avoid confusion, it is important to be clear on the ways in which children are part of the overall causal process involved in clinical research. Imagine that a physician obtains some blood from a child as part of an experiment and gives it to another, sick child who, imagine further, is cured as a result. At the level of physical objects and physical processes, the donor child is clearly part of the causal process that leads to the cure of the sick child. A complete physical description of (this instance of) the experiment would include the child as a physical being, the child's arm, the child's skin, and the child's blood. Whether the child is part of the causal process as an agent depends on the further details of the case. Did, for example, the child understand and agree to take part in the study?

Whether children qualify as contributors to a study involving the evaluation of their medical charts seems less clear. Imagine that the information in the child's medical chart is the result of a physician observing the child and writing notes into a computer, which are then stored in the child's medical record. The study involves an investigator reading this part of the child's medical chart and comparing the information contained therein to the information contained in the medical charts of other children. Other physicians then read the published findings and amend their clinical practice accordingly. In this case, the child does seem to be part of a complete account of the causal antecedents to this change in medical practice. However, the causal connection here is sufficiently tenuous that it is less clear whether we would include contributions of this sort in the narrative of the child's life. The fact that the contribution on the part of children is clear in the paradigm cases will allow us to bracket the challenge of providing a complete account of when one is involved as a causal antecedent and when contributing causally is sufficient to constitute a personal contribution. The question here is whether and to what extent contributions in the paradigmatic cases of clinical research have implications for children's lives.

Salmon's analysis provides insight into the question of why the causal relationships into which we enter and the causal contributions we make can influence how we evaluate our lives overall. Why is it that our interests are so intimately connected to the causal contributions we make over the course of our lives? The answer lies largely in the fact that it is through our causal interactions that we have an influence on and are also influenced by the world and others. And, as the quotation by Salmon highlights, through these interactions we change the world and in the process are ourselves changed. Salmon's view highlights the crucial point that, in a causal interaction, change is not limited to the effect. The cause is also affected.

We typically think of causal factors as influencing or changing their effects. The white marble changes the position of the red marble. However, causal factors themselves are altered during causal interactions. The increase in the speed of the red marble (the effect) is mirrored by a decrease in speed of the white marble. Our lives similarly are altered by the effects we bring about in the world. The thin man is altered in a number of ways as a result of his causal interaction with the rescued child. His skin is pressed and the arrangement of some of his skin cells is changed temporarily. His life narrative is also changed by the addition of his serving in the role of a human ladder and being part of the process that saved a child's life.

The implications for inanimate objects of the causal interactions into which they enter are exhausted by the physical description of the events. The impact on the white marble of its collision with the red marble can be told in purely physical terms. The white marble's trajectory is altered by so many degrees and its speed by so many feet per minute. Humans, in contrast, can have causal influence on and be influenced as the result of causal interactions at different levels, based on the relationship that obtains between the individual and the causal effect in question. As Louis walks down the street, he has a causal influence on the environments through which he passes and on the people he passes. His body blocks the sun, casting a shadow on a moving patch of ground in the environments through which he passes. Many of these causal effects on his part occur at the level of purely physical objects. It is a matter of his shape and size and the angle of the sun that he casts the shadow that he does. And it is possible to be completely unaware of this effect, as we typically are of the fact that our movement introduces more kinetic energy into the environments through which we move.

In these cases, the effect we have is of little importance to us, but it might be of great importance to the objects we thereby influence. When the sun is low on the horizon, Louis walking past at just the right moment could shield a plant and imperceptibly alter its rate of photosynthesis. Depending on the health of the plant this impact could have no lasting impact or a catastrophic one. In the latter case, his movement was not the sole cause of the plant's demise, but it is one part of the complete description of the causes of that effect. We can make vital contributions to various effects without ever knowing about them, intending them, or caring about the result.

Louis also might be aware of this effect, but not care or attempt to alter it all. Or, he might be interested in this fact, know that it is occurring, but still not intend to do so. Further, he might intend to move his shadow about on the sidewalk without any real purpose in mind. Or, he might intentionally move his shadow about with the goal of achieving some relatively unimportant result, such as keeping his glass of wine out of the bright sun. Finally, he might intentionally bring about a result that is very important to him, has great value, and is part of a central project of his life. He might intentionally place his shadow so as to hide something of great value, thereby protecting it from harm. These different scenarios illustrate the possibility mentioned previously of the effects we have on the world going through our agency to differing degrees.

The spectrum of pediatric research spans essentially all of these possible levels of input to a given research study. Most older teenagers are able to understand most research studies and decide for themselves whether to participate and contribute to their goals. In these cases, investigators can obtain the voluntary informed consent of the participant. That fact is part of what makes it acceptable to then enroll the individual in research. Their informed consent also entails that the contribution they make to the project potentially has greater significance for them and their lives. It can be part of their overall life plan, and the fact that they decided to face risks for the benefit of other says something about them as persons. Here, the level of the causal input is defined by the extent to which making that contribution says something about the individuals' lives. The more of us that is implicated in making the contribution, the more relevance that making it has for an overall evaluation of our lives.

At some point in the process of considering the normative status of research with progressively younger children we fall below the threshold at which most of them are able to give fully informed consent. At that point, most research regulations specify that the investigators must obtain the permission of the parents and the agreement (often called the assent) of children who are capable of providing it. Of course, the fact that younger children cannot understand enough to give their own informed consent does not imply that they cannot understand anything about the research. Understanding and the ability to make one's own decisions comes in degrees. Younger teenagers often can understand the immediate requirements of research participation, including immediate pain and burdens. Although these children cannot give their own informed consent, their making a decision to participate, to face the pain and burdens that they do understand, implies that their participation says something about them and their lives.

This is important. Often, critics of nonbeneficial pediatric research will argue that enrolling children who are unable to give fully informed consent is necessarily unethical. Informed consent is important because it allows individuals to decide for themselves whether they participate in and contribute to a given project. Assuming that individuals make these enrollment decisions in light of the consequences for them, informed consent further allows individuals to protect their own interests. The fact that children are not able to provide informed consent implies that they are not able to make their own autonomous decision whether to participate and are not able to protect their own interests adequately. The ability to understand and to give voluntary informed consent is a threshold concept. An individual who does not meet the threshold, even one who is very close to sufficient understanding, is not able to give valid informed consent. In contrast, the extent to which one's decision to make a contribution to a valuable project goes through one's agency comes in degrees. One can understand more or less about the project and embrace it more or less wholeheartedly. Such contributions say more or less about the contributor's life overall.

To take a specific example, a child who does not understand the confidentiality risks the research poses will not be able to protect her own interests adequately. However, the same child may nonetheless understand a good deal else regarding the research, including its purpose and potential benefits and alternatives, and agree to participate (assent) on that basis. In this case, the decision to participate may represent an important contribution on the part of the child, despite the fact that she cannot give valid informed consent.

The mistake some critics make is to assume that the threshold for giving informed consent is coextensive with the point at which individuals are able to make a contribution to a given research project. Understanding why this is not so raises the possibility that younger children who cannot consent may still be able to make a decision to enroll that is in their interests, in the sense of going through their agency sufficiently to qualify as an active contribution to a valuable project. Imagine that a 6-year-old child sees an infant drowning in a backyard wading pool. The 6-year-old understands the benefits that she could provide to the infant by saving him and fully understands the option of doing nothing or running home and trying to summon adult assistance in time. Imagine, given the absence of any adults and the uncertainty as to how soon they might arrive, the 6-year-old decides to wade in, even though she does not fully understand how heavy the infant is and the risks of trying to rescue him. In this case, the 6-year-old should be lauded for the attempt and, if she succeeds, she has performed an enormously valuable service: She has actively saved a life, despite the fact that, in effect, she was not able to give valid consent to doing so.

The fact that one can make an important and active contribution before one can give informed consent reveals that agreeing to enroll in nonbeneficial pediatric research may qualify as a valuable contribution and, thereby, be in the interests of even relatively young children who cannot give informed consent. Ultimately, we come to toddlers who cannot understand anything beyond the basic aspects of the study, such as the requirement to sit in a particular chair, and then to infants who may not understand anything at all. The fact that infants cannot understand implies that they are no longer part of the causal nexus that is the research study in the role of a moral agent. They cannot understand and decide for themselves whether to participate. And the fact that they participate and contribute to a given outcome does not have any implications for our evaluation of them as decision makers, as agents.

The fact that infants are not involved as agents and decision makers does not, of course, remove them from the causal nexus. The infant who is involved in a research intervention or study is still very much a part of the causal process that leads to the outcome in question (again, focusing on paradigm instances of nonbeneficial pediatric research, such as investigators taking some of the infant's blood). And their contribution can have important consequences for the success of the project. The question for present purposes is what implications, if any, does having that type of purely causal impact on the project have for the individual's own life? When do such contributions become a part of the individual's life narrative, influencing to a greater or lesser extent whether the narrative is a good one or not?

Before trying to answer these questions, it will be important to say something about the relationship between causal responsibility and moral responsibility. One virtue of focusing on Salmon's account of causality is that it allows us to locate humans in the physical world and to understand the causal interactions we have with the world in a naturalized way, consistent with the analysis of causality as it pertains to inanimate objects and nonhuman animals. In many cases, we think of the causal impact we have on the world as being the same as the causal impact nonhuman animals have on the world. When the farmer kicks the lamp over and ignites a pile of straw, the causal relationship he has to the resulting fire is identical to the causal relationship the cow has when it does the same thing.

At the level of physical processes, we interact with the world and are causal agents in the same way as cows.[49] There also is a fundamental difference. Depending on the details of the case, the farmer may be morally (and possibly legally) responsible for the resulting fire, whereas the cow, we assume, is blameless. The farmer may have intentionally caused the fire, with full knowledge of and complete endorsement of its consequences. Or, he may have been guilty of negligence, which put him in the position to inadvertently start it. These differences raise the question of determining precisely the relationship between being causally responsible for a given outcome and being morally responsible.[50]

It is clear that agents can be morally responsible as the result of failing to act. Idle spectators sometimes are morally responsible even though they played no causal role in a given outcome. We sometimes hold individuals morally responsible when they could have and should have played a causal role, for instance, could have intervened, but chose not to. If it is true that Nero played music and did little else during the Great Fire in Rome, we may blame him and hold him partly responsible for the ensuing devastation (assuming he could have done something to prevent or minimize it). Analysis of his actions at a purely causal level would suggest that he had nothing to do with the fire. But, for the purpose of moral analysis, that may be precisely the problem. Notice that, in this way, negative causal judgments, especially when they lead to moral blame, also become an important part of one's biography. Similarly, one can be causally responsible for a given outcome, but not morally responsible. A person who is hypnotized against their will and then induced to commit a crime (assuming this is possible) would be causally responsible, but not morally responsible for the crime.

Some philosophers hold a very different theory of omissions. They point out that, in many cases, we ordinarily speak of someone who fails to act when they should have acted as *causing* the unwanted outcome. Imagine that Beth promises to feed your parrot while you are away on vacation, but intentionally and maliciously fails to do so, and your parrot dies. In this case, it would be quite natural to say that Beth was the cause of your parrot's dying. If she had fed your parrot it would not be dead, it would not now be an ex-parrot. While this way of describing the events seems natural enough, it leads to a problem. If the truth of the claim "if Beth had fed your parrot, your parrot would now be alive" is sufficient to identify her as the cause of your parrot's death, then just about everyone caused your parrot's death because it is true of them, as much as it is true of Beth, that if they had fed your parrot (the right food, in the right way), your parrot would now be alive.[51]

Some philosophers attempt to capture the idea that we can cause things by failing to act while avoiding the implication that essentially everyone causes everything. Judith Thomson attempts to distinguish Beth's causal responsibility for the death of your parrot from everyone else's by arguing that Beth caused the death of your parrot because she is at fault for its death (whereas everyone else is not at fault, hence, did not cause the parrot's death). This account of causality is relevant for present purposes because it effectively reverses the order of dependence between causality and responsibility. On the view I endorse, causality is the foundational concept that explains why individuals can be responsible for certain outcomes (they contributed to the causal process or failed to stop it) and, on the present account, why it is that participation in nonbeneficial research can have positive implications for the lives of the children who participate in it. It can have implications for their lives because they were involved causally, even if they were not involved morally. On Thomson's view, the normative concept is foundational and it accounts for the causal relationship. Beth should have fed your parrot, didn't and, therefore, caused its death. If this account of causality is correct, and if it provides a complete account of our causal relationships with the world, then the argument being considered here cannot get off the ground.

Compelling reasons exist to believe that these accounts of causality either are mistaken, or that they do not offer an exhaustive account of our causal relationships with the world. Although I will not argue the point here, I think these views of causation are mistaken precisely because they inappropriately reverse the explanatory relationship between causality and responsibility. The problem with these accounts is that causality as it applies to moral agents is seen as different from the relationship that inanimate objects and nonhuman animals have with the world. That, I think, is good reason to reject such accounts.[52] However, even if one endorses a normative-based analysis, it is clear that such an analysis cannot account for all of our causal relationships. We can have causal relationships in the way nonmoral agents do.

When Richard takes a walk through Sherwood Forest, he leaves a faint impression in the ground where his foot lands. He is the cause of the impression. If someone later comes along and asks for an explanation of why an impression exists at this particular spot, the answer will be that Richard walked there (and no forces impinged on the spot between his walking and the present to erase it). In this case, we determine the causal facts independent of normative considerations. To determine whether Richard was the cause of the impression one does not need to ask whether he should have walked precisely where he did, or whether he has any (legitimate) business walking in the forest at all. It is the physical facts that identify him as the cause of the impression. Similarly, infants enter into causal relationships before they are moral agents subject to normative evaluation. Imagine an infant, struck by the sudden iridescence of a wine glass, reaches for the glass and knocks it over, shattering it to pieces. It may be that the adult who was watching the infant, or the adult who placed the glass within the infant's reach, is responsible. Nonetheless, the infant is the cause of the glass being broken, despite the fact that he is not responsible in any moral sense for breaking it.

The fact that we can make physical contributions independent of our agency presses the question of precisely when an individual can be said to make a contribution. What, in effect, are cardinal signs of making a contribution to a given end or project? The use of action verbs to describe an individual's behavior often is a sign of the individual's having made a causal contribution, but not always. When we say that someone stirred the pot, it indicates that the person had a particular kind of causal interaction with the dish on the stove (or the activity in question). However, one also can play a causal role in cases in which one's contribution is not described using action verbs. In some cases, when you trip over my feet, I tripped you. In other cases, when I am standing where I have every right to be, with no intention of tripping you and no reason to think you might trip, you tripped over my feet, I didn't trip you.

But these cases are complex. In the case of Louis's shadow, he blocks the sun whether he does so unknowingly, having been standing in the same spot before the sun came out, or he intentionally moves to block the sun from some patch of ground. These cases reveal the complex relationship between whether we play a causal role in the sense of being part of the causal chain that brings about a particular outcome, and whether action verbs or moral judgments apply to our role. Cardinal signs, such as the use of action verbs, can help to identify possible cases of one's making a contribution. However, in the end, the only certain approach is to analyze what causal relationship, if any, obtains between the individual and the event or project of interest.

The implications that making a contribution or having a particular effect has for our evaluation of an individual and her life depends a great deal on the individual's preferences and goals, as well as the extent to which the contribution goes through her agency. To be in a position to consider the ways in which an individual's mental states influence the significance of a given contribution she makes, it is important to recognize the ways in which her mental states are irrelevant to her contributions. The fact that an individual does not embrace or even positively rejects something she did does not change the fact that the event in question happened. The Depressed Contributor (Chapter 1, Section "Outline of the Argument") rejects the contributions he made. However, that rejection does not change the fact that the contribution was made. It also does not change the fact that he made it. His taking the view that the contribution does not matter for him or his life does not imply that someone else made it. It is still part of his life, and we can ask whether it was a contribution to a valuable cause independent of what he thinks about it now or thought about it then.

We can also ask, independent of his attitude toward the contribution, whether the fact that he made it is part of a better overall life. His mental states, as we shall see, come in at the point, not of determining whether a contribution was made, not of determining whether he made the contribution, and not at the point of determining whether he made a positive contribution to a valuable project that is now part of his biography. His attitudes and relationship to the contribution influence instead the extent to which it went through his agency and, in turn, what significance it has for his life overall.

The Personal Significance of Making a Contribution: Five Factors

To determine the extent to which participation in nonbeneficial pediatric research might be in the interests of participating children, we need to consider which contributions have implications for contributors' lives (more precisely: which causal connections qualify as personal contributions), including which contributions qualify as human achievements for them. The ultimate goal here is to determine the conditions under which participation in nonbeneficial pediatric research represents a valuable contribution that has implications for our evaluation of the participants' overall lives. Does making a contribution as very young children have implications for the participants' lives? Or, do only contributions made after the participants can understand and agree to make them have such implications?

There are two aspects to evaluating an individual's contribution: the nature of the project to which the individual contributes and the extent to which a given contribution is in effect his contribution. We briefly considered the fact that, holding the project in question fixed, a contribution that involves doing more and working harder typically has more significance for one's overall life than a contribution that involves only a moment of thought and modicum of effort. This can be true even when the two contributions have the same impact on the project itself. The present section builds on these remarks to determine which factors or characteristics of a given contribution determine the extent to which the contribution has implications for the life of the individual who made it.

It seems plausible to hold that successfully accomplishing or realizing one's worthwhile goals contributes to one's overall well-being, flourishing, or quality of life, independent of the extent to which the realization of the goal itself contributes to the quality of one's life. We can think of contributions to realizing one's own goals as attainments, which involve contributing to one's own valuable ends. *Attainments* can be contrasted with *feats,* the paradigm example being feats of strength, which involve realizing one's own ends that do not have value independent of the process of realizing them. *Achievements*, as I use the term here, refer to outcomes that are of value independent of whether the individual values them or has them as a goal. The Depressed Contributor contributed to helping war refugees. The fact that he does not embrace or value his contribution implies that it does not constitute an attainment for him. But the fact that he does not embrace his contribution does not imply that the contribution was not valuable, and valuable for his life. It represents an important achievement—it made his life better, even though he does not see it that way.

Griffin regards accomplishments (what I call attainments) as central to prudential value.[53] Imagine that you accomplish your goal of painting a portrait for your friend's birthday. Presumably, the existence of the painting itself is a good thing, assuming that the portrait is good and the extent to which you experience it contributes to the quality of your life. This value you would have realized no matter who had painted it. Being the painter contributes further to the overall quality of your life, value that you would not have realized if you had not been the painter. Being the painter contributes in at least two ways. First, let us assume that you enjoy the process of painting and it is hard work, so you derive both satisfaction and the ability to exercise your talents. You would have realized these two values whether you ever finished the painting and whether it turns out to be of high quality. The fact that you did paint it and it does turn out to be of very high quality implies an additional source of value for your life. It implies that you achieved a very good or even great thing, and this adds to the value or quality of your life.

Portmore labels those who endorse this view "achievementists."[54] Although these writers differ in many ways, they tend to take the view that a successful achievement requires at least: 1) the end in question is something that the individual desired or valued (at the time the achievement is realized) and 2) the end in question is realized or accomplished. The view I defend here is similar to or related to achievementist views. It holds that contributing to valuable projects is, all things considered, in our interests. On this view, the first condition, the individual valuing the project in question, is not a necessary condition on it being valuable for the individual to contribute to the project. It depends on whether making the contribution in fact is valuable for his life. And this depends on the way in which making the contribution fits into his overall life, which, in turn, is influenced but not determined by his goals and preferences. This difference determines whether the individual's contributing to the project qualifies as attaining a personal goal (the fourth category of human interests) or realizing a human achievement (the fifth category). The rejection of the first condition has the virtue of allowing the present account to avoid the implication that it is in an individual's overall interests to contribute to whatever projects the individual happens to value, whether they happen to be valuable or not.

Scanlon avoids this implication by endorsing what Portmore calls a restricted Achievement View, according to which achievements contribute to one's welfare when they involve success in one's *rational* aims.[55] Raz, as we have seen, makes a similar move by talking about successfully achieving *worthwhile* goals. The present account endorses the second condition, according to which contributions to valuable projects contribute to one's overall life qua contribution only when the project is realized. The qualification here is intended to allow for the possibility that the process of attempting to make a contribution to a project that never is realized can have value for the individual in many ways (giving meaning to one's life, providing exercise or distraction, etc.). Achievement views often assume, implicitly or explicitly, that the individual's effort represents at least a significant component of the contribution that led to the realization of the achievement in question. I will talk about contributions rather than achievements largely to avoid making this assumption. For the most part, the extent of one's contribution influences how significant it is for the individual's life, not whether it qualifies as an achievement or accomplishment at all.

Whether one values or desires the realization of the project or goal in question also comes in, on this view, at the level of determining how significant the contribution is for the individual's life, and whether it says anything about the individual as a person, not at the level of determining whether the contribution has implications for the individual's life. That is determined by whether the individual in fact made a contribution and whether the project in question was valuable (and was not inconsistent with other things of value for him). This view holds that, all things considered, making contributions to valuable projects in itself has positive implications for the life of the contributor, it makes for a better life overall.[56] And, all things being equal, this is better for the individual, it is in the individual's interests because one of the interests we have is an interest in leading a better life overall.

With the central claim thus clarified, we need to consider next how significant a given contribution is for the contributor's life. What determines whether a given contribution says little or a great deal about one's life? We do not regard all causal contributions to a given project as equally important, even when the contributions all are necessary for the success of the project. Put differently, the importance of a given causal contribution is not merely a function of whether its presence is necessary to realize the outcome of interest. Some necessary contributions represent inputs of greater magnitude or importance for the purpose of realizing the success of the project in question compared to other causally necessary inputs. The driver of the race car makes necessary contributions to the ultimate victory, and we tend to focus on her efforts as more significant. Yet, the contributions of many others are also necessary. The individual who puts air in the tires at the pit stop also makes a necessary contribution to the ultimate victory. The victory would not have occurred, let us assume, if she had failed to put air in the tires.

From a purely causal perspective, there is little to distinguish the two contributions. Both are necessary, and the absence of either one would have prevented the victory. Despite this similarity, we make distinctions concerning the relative importance among even necessary causal contributions. Focusing only on the outcome, this practice may appear puzzling given that the contributions accorded less importance are nonetheless equally necessary to the outcome. This practice makes more sense understood as an estimate of the importance the contribution has for the individual, or the extent to which the contribution has implications for our evaluation of the lives of the individuals who make them. In this regard, a number of factors seem relevant to evaluating the significance of a given causal contribution for the individual who made it. A number of factors seem to account for the fact that we regard contributions like the race driver's to be more significant, compared to contributions like the pit stop crew member's, even though both contributions were necessary for victory.

MAGNITUDE

What I will refer to as the "magnitude" of one's contribution to a given outcome depends on a number of considerations, including the proximity in time of one's input to the outcome in question. In one sense, a given outcome is the result of all the causal inputs to it, including those stretching back in time. Yet, more proximate inputs typically are more salient or important for the outcome. The question of chronologic proximity distinguishes causal antecedents from causal contributions. A causal antecedent is any causal input that influenced the state of affairs or outcome in question. Causal antecedents, in principle, stretch indefinitely back into time. Actions by the race car driver's grandparents, especially their having children and perhaps how they reared their children, influence whether the driver exists and the career she chose. In this way, the actions of the grandparents represent a causal antecedent to the driver's victory. The driver's own actions are more important, in part because they are more proximate.

Whether a given causal input is necessary for a particular outcome depends on the specific or token outcome in question. Would this outcome have been realized even if the causal input in question had been absent? Evaluation of the relative importance of the necessary causal inputs to a particular outcome often is performed by considering its role with respect to the kind or type of outcome. First, with what frequency is this type of causal input associated with the type of outcome in question? In the racing example, filling the tires with an appropriate amount of air is rarely associated with victory. Thus, we consider this input to be of less importance to the particular victory even though its presence was necessary for that outcome in a particular case. Second, with what frequency is this type of causal input associated with different types or kinds of outcomes (i.e., how specific is the input to this type of outcome)? Although the grandparents having children was necessary to the victory, this type of input is often associated with very different outcomes.

One way to think about the account we are after here is in terms of the narrative of an individual's life and the question of which events are included in that narrative. Providing a causal input to a given outcome represents one way in which that outcome may become part of an individual's narrative (failing to do something that one should have done represents another way). The greater the magnitude of an individual's contribution, the greater its potential significance for the narrative of the individual's life. As we shall see later, the way in which and extent to which a contribution goes through an individual's agency can greatly influence how much, and what, it says about the individual's life overall.

In addition, there must be sufficient proximity for a given contribution to have implications for an individual's life overall. The proximity of a contribution is attenuated by the passage of time between the making of the contribution and the realization of the outcome. Although the success of the race car driver may have some implications for the lives of the grandparents, it has very minor implications at most. Although the passage of time tends to have the effect of diluting the magnitude of one's contribution, time per se does not have this effect. Rather, the passage of time is a proxy for the extent to which the outcome in question depends on the influence of other causal factors. In particular, the passage of time tends to be correlated with the intervening efforts of others. And these efforts can, in effect, screen off the ultimate outcome from having implications for the lives of those who made much earlier contributions.

This suggests a deep point about how we determine the narrative of an individual's life, what we include within that narrative. It suggests that this determination has a fundamentally comparative element. The determination that one made a contribution to a particular outcome, and that it says something about one's overall life, implies that this contribution says something about one's life rather than the life of others. Imagine that an individual places a message in a bottle intending to influence the lives of others in a positive way and, a hundred years later, following countless causal inputs that are necessary for the outcome to be realized, the message has its intended effect. The extent to which this contribution says something about the life of the individual who placed the message in the bottle depends, in part, on whether the other causal inputs are human ones or not. If the other inputs are merely effects of nature, tides, winds, then more of the input, in effect, traces to the sender's life. In contrast, if the bottle is moved around not by tides and winds, but rather by individuals picking it up and intentionally moving it around, then their contributions can diminish the extent to which the contribution says something about the sender's life. Whether and to what extent this process diminishes the individuals contribution depends crucially on the project in question. Some projects require the input of many individuals. Here, the input of others does not diminish the sender's contribution. Rather, their contributions make it possible for the sender to contribute to this successful project.

The interaction of other individuals does not reduce the significance of the message for the original sender, at least not to the same extent, when the content is especially unique and based on great insight or skill, factors we will consider later. Imagine that the message in the bottle contains the cure for cancer based on a vital insight the individual had during her dying moments on a deserted island. That contribution will have great implications for the individual's life, even if it takes the input of hundreds of others over the course of decades to see the cure realized. And the significance for the individual will depend on many factors realized after she dies, underscoring again the extent to which chance plays a role in the character of our overall lives, including the significance of the contributions we make with our lives. We considered the fact that the passage of time and the intervention of other agents tends to diminish the extent to which a contribution to an outcome has implications for the individual's life. But there are exceptions and variations here as well. In some cases, the passage of time may serve to magnify the significance of the contribution by underscoring the foresight or skill with which the contribution was made.

The magnitude of a given causal input determines the importance or the relevance of the input for realizing the outcome in question. However, the significance *for the individual's life* of making a causal contribution, the extent to which making the contribution has implications for the individual's life, is not determined solely by its magnitude vis-à-vis the outcome. Two causal contributions, one made with little effort, the other as the result of working diligently for years, may have the same level of importance for the outcome in question, but very different implications for one's life overall. The casual causal contribution may say little about your life; the concerted one says more. We saw this previously with respect to two individuals who contributed to the provision of the rotavirus vaccines, one by working assiduously, the other in a short-term and offhand way. At least several other factors are relevant to distinguishing the implications that these two contributions, similar in terms of magnitude, have for the evaluation of the individuals' lives.

AGENCY

The more a given causal contribution involves the individual's agency, the more it says about her overall life. As mentioned previously, we need to distinguish the extent to which making a contribution says something about the individual as a person from the extent to which it has implications for her life. To simplify a voluminous literature and complex topic, a given action says something about an individual as a moral agent to the extent that the individual is the author of the action, which depends, roughly, on whether she voluntarily, intentionally, and wholeheartedly performs it. If you coerce me to intentionally do X, in an important sense you are the author of X, even though I performed the action.

The question of agency as a factor in the extent to which a given contribution has implications for an individual's overall life is broader than agency as it pertains to moral agency. Imagine that Susan voluntarily and intentionally makes a contribution to a given project. Those factors are sufficient for the contribution to have implications for her life overall. How much it says about her life (the extent to which it has implications for her life) also depends on her attitude toward the contribution, the extent to which she embraces or identifies with the contribution, and her level of knowledge about and engagement in the project. These different factors taken together determine to what extent she is engaged in making the contribution in question. As I will use the term, a more "active" contribution is one in which Susan is engaged to a greater extent or degree, whereas more "passive" contributions involve her being engaged in them to a comparatively lesser degree.

In typical cases, the different factors influence the overall contribution in an additive way, the more of each factor that a given contribution realizes, the greater that contribution says something about the individual's overall life. However, in some cases, the contribution or not of a given factor can influence whether the satisfaction of the other factors has any significance for the individual or the individual's life. A contribution to a valuable project that satisfies all the other factors may nonetheless have no, or may even have negative implications, for an individual's life if that individual made the contribution for the wrong reasons. If one ends up inadvertently aiding someone in need in the process of trying to take advantage of them, that contribution may not say anything positive about one's overall life. Instead, we may view what was done as illustrating and reinforcing a problem with the individual and her life. The fact that she intentionally tried to cause harm has negative implications, and the fact that she focused on causing harm precisely in a situation where someone was in need seems particularly offensive.

Evaluation of cases like these can easily lead one to conclude that whether a given contribution to a particular cause has implications for one's overall life depends entirely on whether and the ways in which the contribution issues from their agency. One might conclude that positive contributions have positive implications for one's overall life only when one knowingly or intentionally undertook them. If this were correct, it would follow that positive contributions to valuable projects can have no implications for the lives of very young children who are not in a position to understand. I want to consider here the alternative possibility that conclusions drawn from examples that involve contributions made by autonomous agents do not reveal the necessary conditions on contributions having implications for one's life in all cases. Instead, these examples reveal the conditions on which contributions have implications for autonomous agents. Our intuitions are greatly influenced by the alternative possibilities in a given case. When the example involves a competent adult, we evaluate the significance for them and their lives of what they did—inadvertently helped someone in need in the process of attempting to take advantage of them—in light of what they could have done otherwise—intentionally assisted someone in need.

SKILL LEVEL

A causal contribution that takes great skill says more about one's life than a contribution that involves less skill. Imagine two individuals who save priceless paintings. The first does so simply by placing his body between the painting and would-be thieves. The second does so by devising and carrying out a complex plot by which the thieves are induced to unwittingly return the painting to its rightful owners. In the two cases, the value of the contribution for the world in general may be the same, and the two individuals may have provided the same level of input toward saving the paintings. Nonetheless, the more skillful contribution has more significance for the overall evaluation of the contributor's overall life, compared to the less skillful one (ignoring for the present example the possibility that the less skillful contribution was better in some other way, more courageous perhaps). All things considered, we would prefer to have made the second contribution as part of our lives than the first. From the second-person perspective, we would prefer the more skillful contribution to be part of the life of someone for whom we cared for their own sake, including our children.

Part of this preference involves the extent to which making a more skillful contribution reveals the skill level of the contributor. But, this epistemological significance is not the only way in which the level of skill that goes into the contribution is relevant to the individual's life. Even when two individuals are known to have the same skill level in some regard, making the more skillful contribution says more about their lives, in addition to the extent to which it says something about them as skilled individuals. Someone who has all the skill in the world but rarely, if ever, puts it to use has a less valuable life than someone who has slightly less skill but exercises it for the good.

LEVEL OF EFFORT

Making a given contribution may require more or less exertion, and more or less time. Some contributions require an individual to simply be present, as in the case of a security guard. Other contributions require a great deal of effort at a given time, and others require effort over a span of time. The overall level of effort is a function of the degree of exertion required at a given time and the duration of one's exertion. All else being equal, contributions one makes over several years say more about one's life than momentary contributions. They say more about one's life because, in effect, they comprise more of one's life. The description "contributing to helping war refugees" covers both those who write a single check and those who spend a lifetime promoting the cause. It is the very different exertions and time that determine the significance of the contribution for one's life, not the similar description.[57]

Portmore denies that level of effort per se influences the extent to which a given achievement contributes to one's welfare. He argues that this intuitively plausible claim implausibly implies that, other things being equal, we should adopt goals that require more productive effort to achieve, and we should expend more productive effort to achieve our goals. If this were right, one could add to one's overall welfare simply by taking the long way round. The painting you completed for your friends begins to look like a more significant accomplishment for you if you painted it while standing on one leg rather than two. This argument effectively refutes, I take it, any view that claims expending more effort always implies that one has made a more significant achievement. The lesson for present purposes is that we should not assume that we can determine how much each of the factors considered here influences the significance of an individual's contribution independent of the context or the presence of the other factors. Sometimes making a contribution that requires more effort is more significant. In other cases, it is silly or wrongheaded. With that caveat in mind, the level of effort required often does influence the significance of one's contributions to a valuable project or goal.[58]

UNIQUENESS

A contribution may be more or less unique to the individual who makes it. Some contributions require only the performance of a task for which just about anyone is equipped. Others require skills, talents, characteristics, or properties possessed by a smaller number of individuals. This in part explains the difference in our evaluation of the contribution of the race car driver compared to the contribution of the pit stop mechanic who fills the car's tires. Although both contributions are necessary for the ultimate victory, filling the tires with air could have been performed by just about anyone. Driving the car, in contrast, represents an achievement that could be accomplished by very few individuals.

This example highlights the often close connection between uniqueness and skill level. A very skilled action typically is one that few individuals could perform and, therefore, is necessarily somewhat unique. But, the converse is not also the case. A contribution can be unique even though it requires little, if any, skill. This possibility is exemplified in the clinical research context, in which individuals can make unique, but not skilled contributions. An investigator may need a few samples of human blood, or the investigator may need a few samples of blood of a type that can be provided by only a few individuals. One instance of this involves the great interest in so-called "long-term non-progressors" of HIV. These individuals have been infected with the HIV virus for years, even decades, but do not display any of the characteristic symptoms of AIDS, despite receiving no treatment. It is assumed that these individuals have some fairly unique immune system characteristics which, if identified, might provide a way to treat the disease. All else being equal, the more unique a contribution, the more it says about the individual's overall life. The relevance of uniqueness as an independent factor reaffirms the point made earlier of the extent to which the narrative of an individual's life involves a contrastive element. Whether this person did it depends, in part, on the fact that others did not and, perhaps, could not.

These five factors concern the nature of the contribution that an individual makes to a given outcome, and the extent to which that contribution has implications for the individual's life, meaning the extent to which the contribution becomes part of the narrative of the individual's life and makes that narrative a better or less good one. When we turn to nonbeneficial research, these factors help us to evaluate the extent to which participation is in a child's interests. This evaluation, developing at least some estimate for the extent to which participation is in a child's interests, will be vital to determining the level of risks to which it can be acceptable to expose a child in the context of nonbeneficial pediatric research.

It bears repeating that the value or importance of the project itself also is relevant to determining how significant the contribution is for the individual's life. No matter how skillful and effortful a contribution is, and no matter how engaged one is with making it, contributions to projects with little value are in the contributor's interests to only a slight degree. An important implication of this fact is that making a contribution to a project with little value will be in an individual's interests, all things considered, only when the alternative courses of action available to the individual are even less promising. A second implication, vital in the next two chapters, is that making a contribution that satisfies only one or two of the five factors, and those only slightly, can nonetheless be in an individual's overall interests when the project has great value. This is especially true when the alternative courses of action available to the individual, when the options of what other things the individual might do with her time, are very limited, as often is the case with young children.

SIX | Our Connection to Our Contributions

The Present Chapter

In the previous chapter, we considered what is in our interests, what is involved in making a contribution to a given project or state of affairs, and factors which influence the extent to which making a contribution has implications for an individual's overall life, in the sense of being relevant to an evaluation of that life, to how good or preferable the life is overall. It was argued that we have an interest in leading a better or preferable life overall, and that realizing valuable human achievements is part of a better life overall. It follows that realizing valuable human achievement is in our interests (this is the sense in which the present account of our interests is broader than an account of human welfare). This background puts us in position to consider the specific question of the extent to which participating in nonbeneficial pediatric research might be in the interests of individual children.

Earlier chapters introduced the possibility of developing an account of when nonbeneficial pediatric research might be acceptable based on the relevance for the participating children's interests of the value of the study. The present chapter pursues this suggestion by considering whether participation in nonbeneficial research can be in children's interests, to the extent that such participation involves their making a contribution to an important project which, at least in some cases, constitutes a valuable human achievement that advances the individual's own interests by yielding a better life overall for him. To clear the ground for this analysis, consider first a skeptical challenge to the effect that contributions made as children, no matter how valuable for the individuals as children, have no implications for how we evaluate the value of their lives overall.

Our (Tenuous?) Connection to Childhood

In what follows, I will often talk as though what happens to us at different stages of our lives is on equal footing with respect to its implications for our overall lives. That, in effect, we have one life and the significance for our lives of the contributions we make is independent of the phase of life in which the contributions happen to be made. Characterized in this way, one might object to even the possibility of showing that the contributions we make as children have implications for an evaluation of our lives overall. The contributions we make as children have no implications for how we evaluate overall lives for the simple reason that they occurred while the contributors we were children and, to that extent, are childish.

Michael Slote argues that the value of what happens in one's youth, in effect, stays in one's youth.[1] His view is based on the claim that some goods are time relative. Whether something is good for you or not depends on when it occurs in your life. To understand Slote's claim, it is important to distinguish it from an unobjectionable and, for present purposes, irrelevant sense in which personal goods are time relative. The unobjectionable sense involves the fact that whether certain occurrences qualify as good for a person can be a function of when they occur. Marriage is one example. Getting married can be good for one, but only if it occurs at certain times and not others. Getting married at age 8 is not good for one and may even represent a minor evil for the individual (reminder: all claims regarding what promotes one's interests carry an implicit "all things considered" clause; it may well be in one's interests to marry at age 8 if the alternative is to live a life of constant deprivation). In contrast, as long as one marries (well) at an appropriate time in one's life, then it is true that the marriage is good for that person.

The unobjectionable sense, then, is that whether certain states of affairs are in one's interests depends on when they occur; some things are good if they occur at certain ages or stages of life, and not good, perhaps even bad, if they occur at other ages or stages of life of the person in question. The goodness for an individual of certain states of affairs also can be relative to the timing and ordering of other states of affairs in the same life. This is true because the value for the individual of some experiences derives from their being aptly situated within an overall project or series of experiences. Sadness typically is not a more valuable experience than pleasure, but it can be when it serves as an important part of one's appropriate response to viewing certain films.[2] Experiencing some sadness while viewing *The Bicycle Thief* can add to one's overall experience of the film; finding it all humorous can detract from the overall experience.

Granting that personal goods are time-relative in these two senses (relative to the age in life in which they occur, and relative to the timing of other events in that life), it seems that if one experiences a good at the appropriate time it follows that this experience is good for the individual's overall life; it makes for a better overall life for the individual. Put differently, although (some) personal goods are time-relative, their goodness, assuming they are good for the individual whose life it is, has transtemporal significance for the individual's life. Marrying well at the appropriate time is good for one at that time. Furthermore, it is good for the person's life overall that he got married (at an appropriate time). This conclusion seems to follow from a plausible general principle: if an occurrence is good for a person at a given time in his life, then it is true that that occurrence is good for the person's life overall. This implication seems to follow from the mere fact that it is the same individual's life. Thus, it seems that at any given time in the individual's life, even 30 years later, he should be glad that the good in question occurred at the time it occurred and that it now forms a part of his life's narrative.

Slote calls into question the general move from the goodness of an achievement at one time in an individual's life to the conclusion that it is good for that individual's life overall. He considers the possibility that some goods are good for us at certain times of our lives, but not necessarily good for us all things considered, or good for our lives overall. This possibility is relevant to our purposes because Slote focuses a good deal on what he considers the time-relative goods of childhood. He argues that certain accomplishments may be good for us when we are children, but that, as adults, they are not necessarily good for us, our lives are not necessarily better overall, as a result of the fact that we achieved these things when we were children. Some, perhaps many, of the accomplishments of childhood do not count toward the betterment of our lives overall once we become adults.

Reflecting on a child who works hard to become captain of the basketball team, Slote writes: "We may say, in other words, that such things have value for, or in, childhood, but not value *überhaupt,* i.e. not value from the perspective of human life as a whole."[3] The intuition Slote is appealing to here is one which holds that being captain of the basketball team was good for the individual at the time she was a child, but is not good for the individual's life overall, once she becomes an adult. The reason for this, Slote argues, is that "the facts of childhood simply don't enter with any great weight into our estimation of the (relative) goodness of total lives."[4] And further: "What happens in childhood principally affects our view of total lives through the effects that childhood success or failure are supposed to have on mature individuals."[5]

Before proceeding, it is worth noting the extent to which Slote apparently qualifies these claims. He says that what happens in childhood "principally" affects our view of total lives through the effects on mature individuals and that the facts of childhood do not enter with "any great" weight on our estimation of the goodness of total lives. This seems another example of claims that focus on our autonomous actions, and autonomous stage of life, as being the most important in our lives. These claims seem largely correct as far as they go, until they are conflated with the distinct view that these contributions are all that matter, and other things matter not at all.

If the individual's being captain of the basketball team makes her comfortable in the limelight and that sense of comfort leads her to great things as an adult politician or actor, then becoming captain as a teenager indirectly contributes to the value of her overall life. But, the achievement itself does not have implications for her overall life. A related example involves the possibility, considered previously, that children who participate in nonbeneficial research will realize an educational benefit, and this benefit will help them in their later lives. One who endorses Slote's view could grant the possibility that research participation as a child may indirectly improve the child's life overall in this way. However, on Slote's view, in the absence of such influences on the individual as an adult, the accomplishments of childhood are not relevant to a proper evaluation of one's life overall. The fact that these events occurred in the individual's life do not imply that her life is better. They do not have transtemporal significance for the evaluation of one's life overall.[6] If this claim is correct in general with regard to the accomplishments of youth, it would undermine the possibility that participation in nonbeneficial pediatric research might be in children's interests in the sense of contributing to a better life for them overall. It would undermine the possibility that such contributions can be in individuals' overall interests (as adults).

The plausibility of this challenge rests on the fact that accomplishments attained during childhood tend to be childish, yet we judge the value of one's life largely from the perspective of mature adult goods. Certainly the fact that, at 8 years of age, one is a very good finger painter may well be a good thing for one's life as an 8-year-old. However, the fact that one made impressive finger paintings at 8 years of age will not say much about the individual's life overall.

Imagine someone who, for the rest of his life, regards the finger paintings he made at the age of 8 to be his crowning achievement and perhaps keeps them displayed about his home as an adult. We tend to believe that there should be more to an adult life than this and, it seems plausible to argue, with Slote, that these accomplishments do not say anything at all about one's life once one becomes an adult (recognizing again and bracketing the possibility of indirect influences: the accolades the 8-year-old received influence him in positive ways that resonate throughout his adult life). To put the point negatively, the individual's life would not be in any way less impressive or flourishing if we later discovered that he had not made the finger paintings at all. Perhaps the paintings were done by an older sibling, found their way into his baby book, and were remembered as his own.

Although the present example supports Slote's view, it suggests an instance in which childhood accomplishments might have positive implications for the individual's life overall; in essence, when the accomplishments made during childhood are not childish. Imagine that the finger paintings were not just impressive accomplishments for an 8-year-old, but were themselves impressive as pieces of art. In that case, the paintings do seem to have positive implications for the individual's life overall, even though they were completed when the individual was 8 years old. A life that includes creating artistic masterpieces is, all things considered, a better life than the same life without those accomplishments, no matter the stage of the life at which they occur.[7]

Claims to the effect that this or that accomplishment or contribution is in an individual's interests in the sense of making for a more valuable life overall for him will be central to the remainder of the text. Thus, it will be worth reminding ourselves of the three different perspectives from which we might evaluate the accuracy of such claims. These perspectives, first-, second-, and third-person, were mentioned in Chapter 1. Briefly, to evaluate the plausibility of a claim that making a given contribution is in an individual's interests, we can ask whether, all things considered, we would prefer to have that contribution be part of our lives; whether, all things considered, we would prefer to have that as part of the life of someone for whom we cared for their own sake; and whether we consider a life in general to be better, to have gone better, if it includes the contribution in question.

The claim that making artistic masterpieces is in the artist's overall interests, even when they are made when the individual was 8 years old, seems plausible by these three tests. Most people would prefer to have their lives include having made artistic masterpieces, rather than not. Granting that point, it does seem that making such a contribution as an adult would say more about an individual's overall life compared to making the same contribution as a child. Presumably, to consider the five factors evaluated earlier on the personal significance of a given contribution, the adult who makes the contribution likely will better understand the significance of what he is doing, he will be more thoroughly engaged in making the contribution (compared to a child making the same contribution). In this way, the factor of "agency" on the personal significance of our contributions implies that making the contribution as an adult would have greater implications for the individual's interests.

Here, too, it is worth mentioning some possible counterexamples to remind ourselves that claims regarding one's interests always depend on the case and the circumstances. One can imagine preferring that one not have done great things as a youth, to the extent that those accomplishments haunt one in adulthood. To take a somewhat more complicated case, impressive accomplishments in one's youth may influence how we evaluate one's lack of accomplishments later in life. Compare two individuals who do little with their lives as adults: one who similarly did little as a child, whereas the other accomplished great things in youth. The latter life might seem worse in some cases, despite its including some impressive feats not present in the former life, because it effectively declines or goes down hill over time. We might think, for example, that the latter individual's life is worse overall, despite including more impressive accomplishments, because it involved wasting more ability or potential than the former individual who might have done as well as he could do with the skills and opportunities he was afforded in life.

These examples, which establish that accomplishments in youth do not always yield a better overall life, are useful to keep in mind, but do not undermine the present thesis. The claim we need to establish at this point in the argument is only that accomplishments in youth sometimes can contribute to the value of one's life overall. And this seems clear. To consider a different example, imagine two lives that go well in adulthood, one of which included nothing but pointless and immature activities in youth. The other included a fair share of immature and youthful activities, but also included instances in which the individual, as a youth and as a teenager, helped others in important ways, perhaps volunteering for Habitat for Humanity or teaching younger children to read. The life that also includes some valuable achievements in youth seems, to a slight extent, better overall. Presumably, it is the life we would prefer to have lived and seems clearly to be the life that we would prefer for our children, for their own sakes.

The conclusion that youthful accomplishments sometimes are relevant to our evaluation of lives overall is likely to be of little practical significance to artists and the art world. Rarely do individuals have the choice of whether to create a masterpiece as a youth or as an adult. And, if one does have that kind of talent and control, the choices are unlikely to be mutually exclusive. One can simply do both. In contrast, as we shall see, the present analysis has important practical significance for nonbeneficial research. At least in some cases, investigators need to enroll only a limited number of individuals, and they have a choice whether to enroll adults or children. In these cases, the consideration of the individuals' own interests provides one reason to prefer enrolling adults over children, to the extent that the adult contributions can go through their agency and thereby have greater implications for evaluation of their overall lives.

The possibility of making what we might think of as nonchildish accomplishments as a child may seem far fetched when it comes to great art. However, clinical research affords children, even infants, the opportunity of being involved in projects with significant value, as judged from the perspective of an adult. Most regulations require that pediatric studies be judged valuable by adults before children may be enrolled in them. We do not decide whether a given clinical trial is valuable by asking a panel of 8-year-olds to assess it from the perspective of what an 8-year-old values (although we might do well to ask a panel of 8-years-olds to assess the psychological risks and stress of participating in the study[8]). Pediatric research is ethical only to the extent that it has value as judged by informed and mature adults, not necessarily because it will benefit mature adults. But the benefit has to be something that adults consider valuable. It has to be the case that the study has the potential to improve health and well-being for some individuals, possibly children.

Put differently, clinical research does not aim at the childish values that children often endorse and toward which their actions often aim. These Slote wants us to cast off as we reach maturity. Instead, clinical research focuses on values with transtemporal significance, such as contributing to projects that help other children to avoid disease and death, and to live healthier and longer lives. The point here is not that the children realize these benefits as a result of their participation in nonbeneficial research. Rather, by participating in nonbeneficial research, children contribute to the realizing of increased health and well-being for others. And making such contributions is not simply of value to children. This is underscored by the fact that many adults dedicate their lives to contributing to these goals, and they are widely esteemed for doing so. The development of the rotavirus vaccines required the efforts of children and will (hopefully) be used to benefit children, but that is not at all a childish accomplishment. Indeed, it may turn out to be one of the more valuable developments in clinical research over the past several decades.

A different skeptical challenge concerns not the nature of the contributions we make, but the nature of ourselves when we make the contributions. Ordinarily, we think of an individual as having one life and it being the case that the different stages of one's life are equally stages of the same life for the same individual. The infant is the same individual as the man he grows up to be and the old man he becomes. This standard view of personal identity implies that it is better for me to make a substantial contribution many years ago compared to a relatively minor contribution very recently. Precisely how long ago the contribution was made is irrelevant for the purposes of evaluating the contributions I have made, since both contributions are made by me (at different times). The extent of changes that occur over the course of a lifetime makes this standard and seemingly indubitable view somewhat puzzling. In particular, what makes it the case that the different stages of a life are different stages of life of the *same individual?*

Derek Parfit famously challenges the standard view of our lives. He points out that we value two types of relationships that obtain between the different times slices of our personal history.[9] *Psychological continuity* involves the extent to which an individual's past psychological make-up flows into his present psychological make-up, which then flows into his future psychological make-up. Barring a dramatic and sudden break in psychological make-up, one's psychological states (e.g., thoughts, beliefs, hopes, intentions) at a given time largely are continuous with one's psychological states at immediately prior and subsequent times. The fact that our psychological states change over time implies that, despite the fact of psychological continuity, the content of our psychological states at one time point may be very different from the content of our psychological states at a distant earlier or distant later time. Parfit refers to this relationship as "psychological connectedness."

Parfit points out that we care about both psychological continuity and connectedness. He writes: "I want my life to have certain kinds of overall unity. I do not want it to be very episodic, with continual fluctuations in my desires and concerns. Such fluctuations are compatible with full psychological continuity, but they would reduce psychological connectedness."[10] Parfit argues that the importance of psychological connectedness undermines the extent to which one has prudential reasons to care about what happens to time slices that are psychologically continuous with, but which have little psychological connectedness to oneself now. The fact that the individual has your numerically same body in 30 years, or your numerically same brain does not provide reason for you to care much about that individual's welfare if no psychological connectedness exists between the two.[11]

An important implication of Parfit's view is that personal identity is not an all or nothing matter as we tend to assume. Rather, we are more or less closely related, more or less the same person, as different times slices of ourselves depending on the degree of psychological continuity and connectedness between us (now) and those instances of ourselves. This view seems to undermine the extent to which contributions made by earlier versions of oneself redound to one's present credit. These same worries also might seem to undermine the view that one single perspective exists from which we can view one's overall life, one single narrative into which all the exploits of one's life fit. Instead, an increasing discount rate applies to the relevance of past contributions to our present lives and, at some point, as the degree of psychological connectedness gets sufficiently low, the contributions of the past individual have essentially no implications for the life of the present individual.

We tend to assume that writing an individual's life narrative in real time is accomplished by adding new chapters as the individual ages. Parfit's view of personal identify implies that this feat also requires the deletion of earlier chapters as the individual loses psychological connectedness with those time slices. Given that there is essentially no psychological connectedness between the adult and the 1-year-old infant, it seems to follow that the contributions made by an infant in the rotavirus vaccine studies say nothing about the overall life of the individual as an adult. The infant in the study is not the same person as the adult. By the time the individual who participated in the rotavirus studies as an infant becomes an adult, those earliest chapters are no longer part of his personal narrative.

An enormous literature exists on personal identity theory in general and Parfit's view in particular. For present purposes, the important point is to notice that regarding the contributions of the child as having no implications for the overall life of the adult would undermine the present justification for some nonbeneficial pediatric research. It is also important to notice that acceptance of this view would enormously expand the challenge that we have limited to nonbeneficial pediatric research. Consider a study that poses risks to a 3-year-old child, with the potential to allow the child to avoid some devastating disease in adulthood. We assumed, at the beginning, that this study does not raise significant ethical concern in the way that nonbeneficial research does, provided the risks are justified or outweighed by the potential for future clinical benefit. The reason is simply that we assume the risks and potential benefits apply to the same person.

On Parfit's account, this type of research poses essentially the same ethical concern as nonbeneficial research since little, if any, psychological connectedness will exist between the individual who faces the risks and the one who enjoys the benefits. Treating a child in a research study with an experimental medication that might reduce the chances of a disease in later life is seen as another instance of nonbeneficial research, one in which an individual is exposed to risks for the benefit of another individual. The challenges that acceptance of Parfit's view would pose go even further. Pediatric research raises concerns because it exposes children to some risks for the benefit of others. This concern is standardly contrasted with pediatric clinical care, which exposes children to risks for their own sake. Yet, many of the interventions in the lives of children are not for their immediate benefit, but for the benefit of the adult we assume they will become. The adult who is psychologically and physically continuous with the child is importantly not the same person assuming a loss of psychological connectedness. Much of pediatric clinical care on this view raises the same ethical concerns raised by nonbeneficial pediatric research. Medical interventions that will benefit children as adults are seen as ones that expose one individual to risks for the benefit of another individual.

Or, consider treatments for pediatric cancer, such as chemotherapy and radiation therapy. Although these treatments are often very effective, they typically pose future risks, such as an increased risk of developing other cancers as an adult. On standard views of personal identity, we need ask only if the benefit from the treatment justifies the future risks to the same person. On Parfit's view, we get the puzzle of whether it is acceptable to provide benefits to this person in exchange for risks to a future individual, a kind of reverse of the dilemma posed by nonbeneficial pediatric research, in which present individuals face risks for the benefit of future individuals. Many nonmedical interventions in children also are intended for their future benefit. We force children to get an education and take piano lessons not for their immediate benefit. Instead, we assume that the present burdens of the activities will be justified by the appreciation of the adult for music and the greater opportunities from the education.

These examples reveal that acceptance of Parfit's account of personal identity would require us to completely rethink the way we live our lives and the ways in which we treat others. The fact that we may ultimately regard these changes as very negative ones raises the question of whether the metaphysical facts about our lives that Parfit cites, even if we accept them, necessarily have implications for how we should view our lives and what we should care about morally and prudentially. The radical implications this view would have, and the extent to which they run counter to how we think we ought to live our lives, provides at least some reason to reject them, at least as an account of what is important to us, what counts in our lives.[12] Consideration of this point would take us far beyond the scope of the present analysis. The important point is that, if one rejects the present argument concerning the justification of nonbeneficial pediatric research based on Parfit's account of personal identity, one will dramatically expand the number of practices for which some justification is required. On that view, nonbeneficial pediatric research does not stand in need of special justification, any more than many widely accepted ways in which we treat our children.

This analysis regarding the transtemporal significance of one's contributions leaves us with an important qualifier. If a child's contribution to a clinical research study represents a valuable one that makes for a better life overall at the time the contribution is made, then the contribution can continue to have positive implications for the child's life as an adult, assuming the study has important social value and, adding in the caveat from Parfit's analysis, that we regard the adult to be the same individual as the child with whom he is physically and psychologically continuous (I will bracket cases in which psychological continuity and connectedness are lost between the child and the adult). This conclusion leaves the question expressed by the antecedent clause of whether the contributions that children make to clinical research studies as children have implications for their lives overall. Put differently, is it in individuals' overall interests to contribute to nonbeneficial research as children?

The Value of Youthful Contributions

The possibility that children may gain valuable lessons (e.g. learn to be altruistic) reveals one way in which participation in nonbeneficial clinical research may be in children's overall interests. The previous skeptical argument regarding this claim granted that such educational benefit might be in a child's interests, but pointed out that the potential for this type of educational benefit is present for only some children, at some times in their lives, and likely only for some types of studies. This argument clearly does not justify nonbeneficial pediatric research with infants and may well not justify such research with children younger than age 10 or so. Although it is an empirical question, it may turn out that children learn lessons of altruism only at certain ages and only in certain contexts, involving certain types of experiences and interactions. Thus, if the educational argument is the only justification for nonbeneficial pediatric research, future empirical research on the development of altruism may reveal that a good deal, perhaps most nonbeneficial pediatric research, including a good deal of research currently being approved and conducted, is unethical.

The intuition that it can be acceptable to enroll children in nonbeneficial research, provided the research is important and the risks sufficiently low, provides reason to think that the educational argument is not the only justification for nonbeneficial pediatric research. For example, this argument does not capture the intuition that it can be acceptable to pose extremely low risks to infants, taking say a minute amount more blood during a clinically indicated blood draw, as part of important projects that cannot be conducted in any other way. The educational impact argument provides a very limited justification for nonbeneficial pediatric research because the educational benefit must be realized at the time the children participate in the research. They learn the value of helping others in the process of participating in the study. The problem, as we have seen, is that some children are not in a position, at the time they participate, to learn this lesson—they may not possess the necessary concepts, for example—and other types of research are unlikely to provide this type of lesson to children. This suggests that an alternative approach to consider is the impact that participation in clinical research has, not on the children themselves, but on the children's lives.

At a minimum, it seems clear that making a contribution can be in an individual's interests even when it does not have a positive impact on him; for instance, even when he does not enjoy making the contribution and does not learn from it. Making a contribution can be in an individual's interests when it represents an important accomplishment for him. Put in terms of the five categories of human interests, making a contribution to a valuable project can be in an individual's interests when it represents a valuable human achievement or involves a meaningful relationship, even when making the contribution does not satisfy the individual's experiential preferences or realize her personal goals (as described previously, one way to understand this claim is in terms of the fact that it is possible to promote an individual's interests without advancing her welfare. To evaluate the extent to which such contributions might have positive implications for the children's overall lives, consider a controversial example of children being enrolled in a pharmacokinetic study, which involves their taking a single dose of a new experimental medication and undergoing a series of research blood draws.[13]

These children are certainly making an important contribution to the study. Put in terms of Salmon's analysis of causal interactions, the children are very much a part of the causal process of testing the medication and giving blood in order to collect the information needed to answer the scientific question posed by the study. Does the importance of the contribution for the study imply that the contribution has significance for the children's overall life, hence, is in their interests? Put differently, do these contributions qualify as important accomplishments for the children?

Recall Sumner's claim (in response to Griffin's example of Bertrand Russell's work for nuclear disarmament) that an individual may regard an accomplishment as leading to a more valuable life overall without thinking that it leads to a better or more valuable life for the individual whose life it is. It will be crucial as we proceed to keep this distinction in mind. At least in some cases, it is in an individual's interests, it is better for the individual whose life it is, that his life is better or more significant. We saw this with respect to the fact that it is in an individual's own interests for his life to include some valuable human achievements. It also can be contrary to an individual's interests for his life to include certain valuable human achievements. For example, some morally impressive achievements may nonetheless be counter to an individual's interests overall when the value to the individual of the achievement does not compensate for the losses incurred (jumping on a grenade to save the lives of many others may be one instance of this, at least for many individuals).

For Sumner, impressive accomplishments are in the individual's interests only when they influence or have an impact on the individual's own experiences. We considered earlier reasons to think this account too limited. One example involved the teacher whose own success depends in part on the future success of the children she taught, even though she may never personally experience their success. But rejection of this account will not be sufficient to establish that human achievements when young may be in an individual's own interests. It may be, not that individuals must experience their triumphs, but that they must be of a certain age or maturity, they must be able to contribute to the achievement in a particular way.

In Chapter 5, we considered five factors relevant to determining the significance of an individual's contribution to a given project or state of affairs. They are: the magnitude of the contribution, whether and to what extent it "goes through" the individual's agency, the uniqueness of the contribution, the level of skill involved in making the contribution, and the level of effort required. Coming back, then, to the example of the children's participation in the pharmacokinetic study, this study does not involve much effort on their part, nor does it require any skill. The investigator gives them the medicine and takes their blood. To make the case a difficult one for the present analysis, imagine further that the study enrolls healthy children, so that there is little uniqueness to the children's contribution; the contribution they are making is one that could have been made by hundreds of millions of children.

One caveat is worth noting in this regard. Children who are unable to give consent typically should not be enrolled in nonbeneficial research that could be conducted just as well with adults or older teenagers who are able to make a competent decision regarding the research in question. For this reason, nonbeneficial pediatric research that must enroll children provides a rare opportunity for children to make a contribution to an important project, one that typically cannot be made by adults. This aspect of nonbeneficial pediatric research provides a kind of comparative uniqueness to children's participation. Even when the study could enroll any of several million young children, the study needs to enroll children as opposed to teenagers or adults. When this condition is not met, investigators typically should not enroll children.

Nonbeneficial pediatric research interventions and studies typically involve only a few children, sometimes as few as four or five, implying that the magnitude of participating children's contribution to the study in question will be substantial. However, as we have seen, most nonbeneficial pediatric research studies are preliminary ones, removed by years and a series of future studies from the realization of any useful treatments. Pharmacokinetic studies, like the present example, are necessary preludes to future efficacy studies, hence, necessary in many cases to developing improved treatments. But, many steps are needed from these initial studies to the realization of the value of a new and improved treatment. Thus, relative to the ultimate value to be gained from the study, the contribution made by individual children tends to be necessary, but relatively minor with respect to magnitude.

Finally, the extent to which the children's contribution to the study goes through their agency depends, most importantly, on how mature the children are at the time of their participation, which is roughly, although inexactly, a function of the children's ages. Existing empirical data suggest that most children over age 14 are able to make decisions regarding enrollment in clinical research roughly on a par with adults.[14] Taking a standard account of informed consent, teenagers are able to understand sufficiently the essential elements of the research (e.g., risks, potential benefits, alternatives), they are able to appreciate how this information applies to them, and they are able to make a voluntary decision whether to enroll. If we assume that the children are asked to provide their agreement (assent) to enroll in the study, and they do so, it follows that their contribution to the research represents a competent decision on their part. Competent decisions come in degrees, and the extent to which the contribution goes through individuals' agency will depend on how much they understood and the extent to which the decision was voluntary.

The contributions children make to nonbeneficial research studies once they are competent have positive implications for their lives; they qualify as valuable contributions. In this case, the children's lives are somewhat better overall with this contribution than the same exact lives absent this contribution. First, the fact that they autonomously made such a contribution represents a valuable achievement for them. It says something valuable about them, and about their lives. They chose, despite the risks and burdens, to contribute to the significant project of helping to improve the lives of others by helping to identify improved medical treatments. Second, making this valuable contribution engages the children with significant values. By participating in the research study, they engage with the values of health and well-being, and with the critical significance of recognizing and engaging the value and importance of others.[15]

One way to understand this aspect of the example is in terms of individuals' interests in having significant relationships, not all of which necessarily are with other individuals. In the present case, participation in research provides children the opportunity to enter into an important relationship with things of real value. It follows, in this case, that making the contribution is directly or intrinsically, rather than instrumentally, in the children's interests. The value does not depend on the impact that making the contribution has on the children at some future point in their lives. It does not depend, for instance, on what they learn from making the contribution, from any educational benefit they realize. Instead, when the contribution goes through the children's agency, the fact of making the contribution itself is good for their overall lives and, all things considered, good for them.

Saying Something Positive

The fact that a contribution has implications for the evaluation of an individual's life is not sufficient for it to be the case that contributing to the project is in an individual's interests. For the contribution to be in the individual's interests (as opposed to possibly being contrary to his interests), it must have *positive* implications for the individual's life. It is not enough that the individual engages in making the contribution; the project or state of affairs to which the individual contributes must in fact be valuable or worthwhile.

If the project is horrific or even somewhat harmful, the more the individual contributes to the project, the worse her overall life is for it. The fact of having made an active contribution rather than more passive ones, or no contribution at all, is not overall better in all cases. Better to sit on the sofa and watch bad TV than to go out and struggle mightily to make the world safe for scoundrels and despots. When the project or goal is not especially horrific, there seems a sense in which making the contribution itself may be valuable. An assiduous effort to a project that turns out, despite the individual's intentions to do good, to degrade the environment to a slight extent may in itself be valuable even though the ultimate consequences of the contribution are negative in the sense that they outweigh the value of the effort itself. With contributions to horrific projects, in contrast, we are less willing to distinguish the effort from the effect. We are disinclined to credit someone with making a good effort when that effort leads to significant harm or loss (although this depends, to some extent at least, on whether the person is responsible for the loss).

In some cases at least, whether a contribution says something positive about the individual's life depends on whether the individual values making the contribution (often I will not take the time to distinguish valuing making the contribution from valuing the project to which one contributes). My efforts to promote and sustain a close relationship are valuable in large part because *I value* the relationship. This suggests, then, a preliminary analysis for it being the case that making a contribution is in an individual's interests in the sense of saying something positive about the individual's overall life in a way that is valuable for the individual: the individual engages in making the contribution (as determined by the five factors considered previously), the individual values making the contribution (values the project), and the project, cause, goal, or end is itself valuable.

In standard cases, we assume a specific temporal relationship between the first two conditions. The individual actively contributes to the realization of the state of affairs because she antecedently values making the contribution or believes that the state of affairs obtaining would be a good thing. If this sequence represents an independent necessary condition on a contribution saying something about an individual's life overall then, for young children at least, making contributions to clinical research studies will not have positive implications for their lives overall because, at the time they make the contributions, they are not able to understand and value them.

Consider someone who, in the course of going about her job, ends up contributing, willy-nilly, to several valuable projects, all the while regarding the projects with indifference. Imagine that later on in life she comes to value these projects, and views her earlier contributions in a positive light. She comes to have a positive attitude regarding the contributions she made, and she incorporates them in her personal life narrative. In this case at least, it seems that the fact of having made the earlier contributions may be valuable for her life overall, even though she did not value making the contributions at the time she made them.[16] One way in which this may be the case is through the process of what I will call "embracing" the contributions.

To appreciate this possibility, it will be important again to distinguish our evaluation of the individual from our evaluation of the individual's life as a whole. The fact that she made these earlier contributions at a time when she regarded them with indifference suggests that the fact of having made them says nothing about her as a moral agent (and may have negative implications to the extent that she failed to recognize their value at that time). And this fact has important implications for which attitudes are appropriate toward the individual and her contribution. It may not be appropriate, for example, to praise her or thank her for having made these contributions. Nonetheless, it seems that making contributions at a time when one does not value them can be in one's interests in at least two ways. First, the fact of having made the contributions may have future effects on the individual as a moral agent. The individual may become a better person in part because she made these earlier contributions. She may, in effect, decide to become the kind of person who is consistent with having made these contributions.

Part of the effect here might be described as a kind of delayed educational effect. The individual may, when thinking back on the contribution, come to see it as an important and valuable contribution and decide to be more of that type of person in the future. This delayed educational effect may be significant in individual cases. However, to the extent that the benefit is purely educational, the contribution need not have been made by the individual. All that is required is that *someone* was enrolled in a valuable study, and she later learns about the contribution of that individual and is inspired by it. We can learn lessons from the example of others just as much as learning from our own.

In another sense, it is crucial that the contribution was made by oneself. This is the possibility of the contribution influencing the person's future behavior through a kind of psychological consistency. For the most part, psychologically healthy individuals strive to see their lives, or at least distinct segments of their lives, as more or less of unified wholes, so that the things they did in the past are consistent with those they do in the future. Here it is important that the previous contributions are mine, rather than being made by someone else. I am inclined, to some extent, to live consistently with past contributions that I made, but not past contribution made by others (although, again, the contributions others make may inspire me).

One's own contributions also may become a part, even an important part of the individual's own view of herself and her life, in addition to the extent to which it influences her future behavior. The individual may come to embrace these contributions as a valuable feature in the narrative of her life. The Report of the International Bioethics Committee of UNESCO points out that a child who participates in clinical research may later be "grateful to learn that the use of his data, or his participation in a trial, facilitated the discovery of a new treatment or increased understanding of a dreadful disease."[17] Although it is an empirical question, it may be that adults later come to value (some of) the contributions they actively made as young children, even though the contributions were made at a time when the child did not fully understand what they were doing.[18] Presumably, the more active the contribution was at the time, in the sense of the individual being more fully engaged in pursuing it, the more likely it is that the individual will embrace it later as her own.

Uncertainty over whether an adult will come to embrace a contribution made as a child implies that parents cannot be confident that making decisions for their children on these grounds will promote the children's interests. The level of uncertainty is increased by the fact that individuals can embrace previous contributions only to the extent that they are aware of having made them. Thus, the individual needs to make the contribution at an age when he is old enough to understand and remember it. Or, someone, most likely the child's parents, will need to explain to the child the contribution he made previously. These considerations reveal that enrolling a child in nonbeneficial pediatric research on the grounds that it may influence him later in life and he may come to embrace the contribution represents something of a gamble on the part of parents.

Granting this point, we should not equate parental gambles with parental mistakes. Parents must take chances all the time when deciding how to raise their children. Will the piano lessons be worth it? Or, will they lead to rebellion and rejection of all (good) music? The fact that these are real possibilities does not imply that putting one's child in piano lessons is a mistake, provided a sufficient chance exists, given the burdens and options foregone, that the child will ultimately embrace the piano as a result of the lessons. Similarly, the possibility that an individual may embrace a contribution made as a child provides some justification for enrolling children in nonbeneficial research. This possibility alone reveals that nonbeneficial pediatric research is not necessarily unethical.

We have, then, one response to Ramsey's challenge. This justification, unlike the potential for educational benefit, does not rely on the conceptual abilities of the children at the time they are enrolled in the research. Thus, in principle, this justification applies to the enrollment of all children. At the same time, this potential is uncertain at best and it may turn out that, in fact, few children embrace these contributions in the sense required here. Recognizing its limitations, the present justification of embracing one's contributions does provide one justification and also points to the possibility for a more general justification for nonbeneficial pediatric research, namely: making a valuable contribution can be in an individual's overall interests, even when the individual does not embrace or perhaps even recognize having made the contribution. This conclusion is suggested by an analysis of the conditions that must be met for it to be the case that one can embrace a contribution that one made previously.

Roughly, the argument to be made is that one can embrace a contribution made earlier in life, perhaps even at a time when one did not know one was making it, because the making of a valuable contribution does not depend on one's recognizing that one is making it. In effect, embracing a given contribution does not make it mine in a physical sense, and embracing the contribution does not give it value. Rather, the fact that the contribution was mine and has value explains the possibility of my embracing it, thereby giving it more value for my life. This provides support for the primary argument to come, namely, that the fact of contributing to valuable projects, including valuable nonbeneficial pediatric research studies, can itself be in individuals' interests, independent of whether they learn from the experience, are changed by the experience, or later come to embrace it. Even when none of these benefits are realized, the fact remains that the individual contributed to a valuable study as a child.

We have now three distinct ways in which contributing to a nonbeneficial pediatric research study might be in a child's interests. First, if the pediatric participants are old enough they may be able to make an active contribution to the study, they may be able to understand the study and voluntarily decide to contribute to it. In this way, participation would represent a valuable achievement for them, and assuming that participation in the study does not conflict with any important interests, participation would be directly or intrinsically in their interests overall. Second, the experience of participating in the research itself may have a beneficial impact on the child. The example most frequently noted here is the possibility that they may derive some educational benefit. This is typically understood in terms of benefits of learning altruism, from the child learning to help others. Other possibilities include learning about medicine and science while involved in the study. Third, the individual may later come to embrace contributions made as a child, seeing them as one element of what makes his life valuable overall and possibly leading him to further valuable accomplishments in the future.

Finally, the importance of the value of the project or end to which an individual contributes highlights an additional factor on the extent to which a contribution is in an individual's interests in the sense of making for a better life overall for the individual. All things considered, it is better to contribute to more-valuable projects compared to less-valuable ones. There are at least two reasons for this. First, contributing to more-valuable projects connects the contributor to greater or more significant fundamental values. Second, a contribution to a more-valuable project represents a more significant accomplishment. Again, one primarily wants to do one's best. But, all things considered, we prefer to make a difference as the result of our striving, and making a greater difference is preferable to making less of a difference.

Are Contributions Necessarily Active?

The analysis thus far has assumed a number of necessary conditions on a contribution counting as an active one that is in the child's interests in the sense of directly making for a better life overall for him (as opposed to being in his interests by saying something valuable about him as an agent or person): the contribution engages the individual (a function of at least five factors: magnitude, agency, uniqueness, skill, and effort), the individual values the project (or his contribution to the project), and the project itself is valuable.

These may seem in every case to be necessary conditions on a project being directly or intrinsically in an individual's interests in the sense of representing a valuable achievement or contribution. We shall see in the next chapter that, in fact, a contribution can have positive implications for an individual's life even though the individual does not value it and does not actively make the contribution. To see this, it will be important again to distinguish the extent to which a given contribution has implications for the individual, or implications for his character, or him as a moral agent, versus the extent to which it has implications for his life overall in a way relevant to how well his life goes. Helping young children learn to read is a valuable human achievement. However, in most cases, whether we consider an instance of helping young children learn to read to redound to one's credit, it must be the case that they actively did so and valued the process. Someone who helps because she is forced to do so does not get credit; it does not represent a valuable achievement for her as an autonomous individual.

We do not say that the individual was better than she might have been otherwise on the grounds that she helped young children learn to read as the result of a threat to her bodily integrity. Depending upon the details, we might even think that this instance casts a shadow on the individual's character; she had to be forced to help. Similarly, for a contribution to have positive implications for one's character, it needs to be the case not only that one voluntary contributes, but that one regards the end as valuable. We are not impressed with those who voluntarily help young children learn to read based on the false belief that doing so will harm them.

A good deal of what constitutes a better overall life depends on actively pursuing and realizing, to some extent, one's (worthwhile) personal goals. For this reason, most analyses of the causal relationships into which we enter with other humans and the rest of the world focus on the subset of causal relationships that go through our actions and agency. And this focus can lead to the implicit assumption that only this subset of causal relationships matter or count for a given individual's life overall. This attitude helps to account, I suspect, for the intuition that the infants' participation in the rotavirus vaccine trials does not have any implications for their lives. The infants did not know they were making this contribution, did not understand the project to which they were contributing, and did not make the decision to participate. In this sense, their involvement represents a purely passive contribution, one which did not go through their agency and does not have any implications for them as agents or individuals. We do not praise the infants for their contributions to the rotavirus vaccine studies.

This line of reasoning seems to imply that it was not in the infants' interests to participate in the rotavirus trials. For present purposes, the important point is this: the claim that making a contribution is in an individual's overall interests only when the individual actively contributes to a project he endorses is plausible to the extent that one thinks of evaluating the individual as a person or moral agent. For the contribution to have positive implications for him *as a moral agent,* it must be the case that he actively contributes. But, once we see that there is a distinct way that making a contribution can be in an individual's interests, we will need to consider whether these conditions are necessary in that context as well. The fact that he made a particular causal contribution may have implications for his overall life—his life may be better or worse overall—independent of whether it has implications for his character, or for him as an autonomous agent, and those implications for his life may promote his interests. The argument to be considered here is that purely passive contributions, ones that do not go through the individual's agency at all, nonetheless can have implications for his life overall in a way that is relevant to the individual's interests. This can be the case because one of our interests is having a better life overall.

Consistent with the previous considerations, a good deal of our intuitions that oppose this possibility focus on autonomous individuals. For autonomous individuals, we typically do not regard contributions made against their will as redounding to their credit. But, notice that in these cases, much of our concern traces to the possibility of things going differently. Rather than being forced to help children learn to read, the individual could have embraced the opportunity and pursued it willingly. Given this possibility, we tend to be less than impressed by autonomous individuals who help unwillingly and may even consider such contributions as having no or perhaps even negative implications for them and their lives: they did not care, they had to be forced to help. What does that say about them as a person, given that they could have cared, they could have helped willingly?

The existence of alternative, more willing courses of action is relevant to our evaluation of autonomous adults, but not to contributions made by very young children. Again, to evaluate the implications that participation in nonbeneficial pediatric research might have on children's lives, we need to keep in mind the fact that they are not autonomous and refrain from judging them according to standards appropriate for adults. Central to the task of taking seriously the fact that children are not autonomous is recognizing the fact that they do not have available to them the option of making fully active contributions.

We can begin to get a sense for the possibility that participating in nonbeneficial research may be in younger children's interests by recognizing that the existence of different categories of individual interests implies that all value, even for specific individuals, does not trace to their autonomous action. Indeed, sometimes it may be valuable for an individual to be forced to do what is in his interests. Depending upon the details of the case, forcing someone to take his medication or a drink of water that will save his life may be in his interests overall. Roughly, it depends on how comprehensive the personal goals are that one thereby contradicts. If someone was refusing to drink for a narrow or limited goal that meant little to them, forcing them to drink might be in their interests. Here the biological needs, and the opportunity to remain alive and fulfill many other interests, may take precedence over the immediate personal goal of avoiding the forced outcome and avoiding being forced to realize it.

This example establishes that some things can be in an individual's interests in at least an instrumental sense, despite not going through—indeed, being opposed by—the individual's agency. Keeping the individual fed and alive puts him in a position to promote his interests further, in more intrinsic ways.

This example supports some of the accounts we considered previously in which participation in nonbeneficial research might promote children's interests by inspiring them to go on to accomplish great things autonomously. It does not yet establish that an individual's interests can be promoted intrinsically (independent of the downstream consequences on their other interests) in virtue of making contributions to valuable projects that do not go through the individual's agency. Nonetheless, this simple case makes the point that not everything in an individual's interests need go through his agency. We will pursue this possibility further in the next chapter.

SEVEN | The Value of Passive Contributions

Striving versus Contributing

To clear some conceptual space for the possibility that passively making a contribution to a valuable project may be in an individual's interests, it will be helpful to analyze more carefully examples in which individuals later come to embrace a prior contribution. For the most part, we judge individuals based on the effort they make, how hard they try, how conscientiously they strive. An individual who works hard and stays at a difficult and worthwhile project because she recognizes it to be valuable does something valuable and deserves our praise, independent of the outcome. All that we can control is our own efforts, and these say a lot about us. There is a tendency, especially when instructing children, to say that this is all that matters, our efforts and our attempts. For the purpose of evaluating the individual as an agent, to the extent that we evaluate her moral character, this makes sense. We evaluate her based on what she can control and what she tries to do. And because outcomes tend to figure too prominently in our own evaluations of our efforts, whether we win or lose, it makes sense, as a therapeutic move, to emphasize the value and importance of the effort itself.

This focus on agency makes sense to the extent that one's goal in characterizing our interests, in delineating what constitutes a better life for us, is to instruct, to provide guidance on how individuals ought to live. Instructions on how to live one's life make sense and have practical import only to the extent that they involve actions that one can control, and these largely are actions that go through one's agency. Thus, to the extent that one regards the philosophical project as that of providing instructions on how autonomous individuals ought to lead their lives, it makes sense to ignore the possibility that contributions independent of one's agency may have implications for one's life. Even if they do, so what?

Granting all this, it would be a mistake to think that the level of effort is all that matters in our attempts. Imagine individuals who cared only about their own efforts toward a given project. As far as they are concerned, evaluation of what they do stops with the effort itself. How they feel about their actions and their lives in general, their preferences, hopes, and dreams, is limited to whether they sufficiently tried to bring about worthwhile ends. Although we might understand the appeal of such an approach, it nevertheless seems odd. When we think of ourselves as agents, we simply want to try our best, perhaps. But, when we think about the narrative of our lives, it is not the case that all we care about is trying hard and doing our best, even though those things are important. We, at least sometimes, want to make a difference, we want our efforts to come to something, we want to have an impact on the world independent of ourselves and our efforts. We do not want merely to strive, we want to contribute.

These two views can be understood as taking in different aspects of our lives: the one focuses on us as agents and evaluations of our character, the other takes in our lives and evaluates the overall goodness of them, the extent to which they constitute flourishing lives. For this latter judgment, it matters what difference, if any, we make in the world, what the result is of our striving. When one strives assiduously for good causes for the right reasons one is a good person and one is related to significant values in making the attempt. When one's efforts actually help to realize a valuable outcome or state of affairs, one has an additional and valuable relationship to that value, a relationship that does not obtain for those who strive without ultimately making a difference.

Consider two individuals who donate bone marrow to patients with cancer. Both make the decision to donate to someone else, recognizing the burdens and risks (bone marrow biopsies can be painful and involve some risk of serious infection) but coming to the conclusion that it is important to make this contribution. If both individuals make the same sacrifice, they are both to be praised equally for doing something important and truly heroic. In addition, making the donation connects both of them to significant values of recognizing the importance and needs of others. But, imagine that one of the bone marrow recipients goes on to live a full life after the infusion of the donated bone marrow, whereas the other recipient ends up dying in the process of receiving the donated bone marrow, through no fault of the donor.

This fact influences the nature of the donors' contributions and thereby influences the extent to which making the contribution says something positive about the donor's overall life. To see this, one need ask only whether we would be indifferent between the two outcomes for ourselves *as donors*. Certainly, we want the recipients to survive for their own sakes. In addition, the recipient's survival has implications for the nature of the contribution the donor made; hence, it affects what implications the contribution has for the narrative of the donor's life. Both made important attempts to save the life of another, and their lives are better for it. The life of the one donor also includes having saved another's life.

The lesson of this example is that the value our contributions have for our lives and, ultimately for us, is not determined exclusively by factors within our control. Factors outside our agency also influence whether an active contribution says something positive about our overall lives. This is so because the value of our contributions, for us, can depend on their ultimate consequences. And the consequences of our action often are outside of our personal control. Coming back to Sumner's distinction, this is not just a matter of saying that the life is overall better in some way irrelevant to the donor whose life it is. It is better, in this case at least, for the donor that his overall life goes better in this way. It is better, all things considered, *for the donor* to have lived a life that included the saving of another life.

Once we divorce, to even this extent, the value of a given contribution for the agent from the extent to which the agent controls the contribution and its consequences, we begin to create conceptual space for the possibility that passive contributions may have implications for how we evaluate individuals' lives overall. This is not to say that the present analysis gets us to that conclusion. Here we have seen that the effects of contributions that go through our agency can have implications for our lives, even when the ultimate effects are not completely within our control. To show that participation in nonbeneficial pediatric research can be in the overall interests of even nonautonomous children, one must establish that our contributions can have implications for our lives, they count as our contributions or our accomplishments, and they can influence how well or not our lives go for us, even when we do not control, not just the consequences of the contribution, but the fact that we made the contribution in the first place.

The argument to be made is that passive contributions can have implications for how we evaluate overall lives, whether the life in question is more or less flourishing, and this can be relevant to the interests of the individual whose life it is. One reason why this possibility seems counterintuitive is that we tend to conflate the value or implications of a given contribution with what it says about the contributor as a person. When we consider examples of autonomous agents, it also is the case that making active contributions tends to be preferable. Thus, in comparison to that alternative, less-active contributions (e.g. an autonomous adult being forced to help children read) seem, at best, unimpressive. One way to avoid these confounding factors is to begin with an example that does not involve agents at all.

Imagine, for instance, that the rotavirus vaccine studies enrolled children who die at age 3, before they develop any sense of autonomy or agency. These children never have the opportunity to learn about these contributions, much less the opportunity to embrace or learn from them. The contributions did not derive from their agency and have no impact on the children's agency. In this case, it seems at least plausible to argue that the children's lives are better for having made this contribution than not. For present purposes, we need not determine whether, in fact, this is the case. A life that ends at age 3 but contributed to a study of incredible value may be better or preferable to a life that ends at age 3 without having any such impact on the world or others. Similarly, we can imagine that the parents, given the choice between having children who die at age 3 having made such a contribution, or children who die at age 3 not having made such a contribution, might take the view that, for the children's own sakes, the former option is better. This is not to argue that, in fact, it is in the interests of infants who die at age 3 to have contributed, however passively, to a valuable project, rather than not. The claim here is the more modest one of whether the logic of making a contribution, and the value of doing so for an individual, necessarily requires that the contribution be an active one. The possibility that contributions made by 3–year-olds have value for them supports the claim that a contribution need not be active to have value for the contributor.

Whether this in fact is the case depends on a number of additional considerations. Most prominently, it depends on whether infants who die young have the same interests as those who make it to adulthood. That is a further and difficult question that we need not address for present purposes.[1] The present argument will focus on children who become adults and, by implication, the proper treatment of children whose parents ex ante have reason to believe will make it to adulthood. This example provides some reason to think that purely passive contributions might have implications for an individual's life, independent of the extent to which the contributions go through the individual's agency.[2] The remainder of the chapter provides support and argument for this conclusion and addresses a number of objections to it.

The Causal Asymmetry Thesis

The present argument is based on the claim that, in principle, all the causal relationships in which we are involved can have implications for our lives overall. One can think of this thesis as part of a more general view that considers and takes seriously the implications of the fact that we are not merely autonomous and feeling individuals, we are embodied ones. As a result, much of the narrative of our lives involves our physical selves and the ways in which we interact, in physical space, with others and the world. This thesis gains prima facie plausibility from the fact that the causal relationships into which we enter are part of our overall lives. A comprehensive telling of one's life story would include the causal relationships into which one entered over the course of one's life. Thus, it makes sense that the causal relationships into which we enter can have implications for how well our lives go depending on their normative valence, on whether they are positive or negative.

In telling the story of a life, one may be more interested in certain aspects, hence, focus on one or more subsets of the causal relationships into which the subject entered. One might be especially interested in the individual as a moral agent and focus on those causal relationships over which one had control or responsibility. But, this particular interest and consequent focus does not imply that the causal relationships thereby omitted were not part of the narrative of the individual's life. Our agency is an embodied one, realized in physical space. We interact at a physical level with other embodied beings and change, sometimes for better, sometimes for worse, sometimes due to our agency, sometimes not, the course of their lives and ours.

This view raises the possibility that even purely passive contributions may have implications for our overall lives. The most obvious objection to this claim is perhaps the fact that passive contributions are not within one's control. Thus, it seems odd, even unfair, to regard such contributions as having implications for our lives. The infants involved in the rotavirus study were not in control of, or even aware of their contributions at the time they made them. This suggests at least two grounds on which one might defend the claim that such contributions have no implications for how we judge their lives overall. First, the causal relationships into which we enter may have implications for our lives only to the extent that we are to some extent in control of them. Or, it might be the case, more narrowly, that the *contributions* in particular that we make to relationships, ends, goals, projects, activities, can have implications for our lives only to the extent that we have some control over them, or they go through our agency. To properly qualify as one's contribution in the first place, it must be the case that one was in control of what one did.

To consider the first option, the claim that the causal relationships into which we enter can have implications for the goodness of our overall lives only to the extent that we control them or they go through our agency, implies that causal connections independent of our agency cannot influence the value of our lives. This thesis is contradicted by the fact that the causal *inputs* to an individual's life can have negative consequences for that life, making the individual's life less good overall and less good for the individual, even when the inputs do not go through the individual's agency or will. The way each of us is reared and the historical circumstances into which each of us is born can have a profound impact on our characters and our lives. Many are born in a time and at a place that does not allow for greatness.

This may seem unfair, but it is not for that any less true of our lives. Similarly, an accident that has the effect of eliminating my ability to have close friends would diminish to some extent the overall goodness of my life for me. I may come to accommodate myself to the consequences of the accident (a real possibility: our powers of accommodation often outstrip our powers of projection[3]) and disdain friendships for myself, if I ever valued them in the first place, and go on to accomplish many things not dependent on having them. Although this accident does not preclude the possibility of my ultimately having a good life overall, it does reduce to some extent how good my life can be unless, perhaps, I have the ability and the inclination to pursue a life plan—being a cloistered monk, perhaps—for which having friends is irrelevant or even inconsistent. But, even here, whether I have those abilities and inclinations itself depends on factors outside my control. Not everyone can be a (successful) monk.

The claim that this causal input would have negative implications for my overall life is independent of whether I was in any way responsible for losing my ability to have close friends. The mere fact of losing this ability, independent of how it occurred, is bad for my overall life and contrary to my interests. A finding that I was also responsible would add a second way in which it has negative implications for my life. Put generally, the implications that a given causal effect or impact has for an individual's overall life is not determined strictly by whether the individual had control over the causal input that led to that effect. The reason for this is straightforward. The effect itself has consequences for the individual's interests independent of the cause that brought it about. Having some close relationships typically improves one's life overall. Hence, an inability to make close friends diminishes the overall quality of most lives, independent of whether one is responsible for lacking this ability. To deny this, one would have to deny that some things are good for us given the types of beings that we are (e.g., one would have to deny the existence of valuable human achievements), or one would have to insist that we can always fully overcome the loss of any characteristic, object, or property of value.

A related debate asks whether it can be acceptable for deaf parents to intentionally have a child who is deaf. Some argue that being deaf is not a deficit, but simply a different way of being, and that being deaf allows one to be part of a culture that is closed to those who are hearing. Opponents argue that being deaf represents a deficit to which one can adjust, but for which one can never fully compensate. Recognizing this fundamental disagreement, both sides agree that whether deafness constitutes a deficit does not depend strictly on whether the individual in question had a hand in being deaf. Causal inputs that are independent of our agency and beyond our control can nonetheless have an impact on the quality of our lives. The fact of being deaf may be a deficit for the individual who was born deaf to the same extent that it is a deficit for the individual who becomes deaf as a result of irresponsible personal behavior.

Granting this conclusion, one might argue that causal *contributions* that are beyond our control do not have any implications for our overall lives. That is, one might argue that there is a causal asymmetry to the relevance for our lives of the connections into which we enter. It makes sense that causal inputs can have implications for our lives even when they are independent of our agency because the impact or the effect of the input may influence our lives in positive or negative ways (including, in Bernard Williams' words, the possibility of "constitutive" luck). It seems less clear that the causal contributions we make can affect or have an impact on our lives. If someone causes me to be deaf, they have affected my life in a dramatic way, even if the input and its effect were beyond my control; I am now deaf as a result of the causal input. It seems less clear that my life is altered if I cause someone else to be deaf in a way that is completely outside of my control. There seems, in this way an important causal asymmetry in our judgment of the personal implications of the causal relationships into which we enter over the course of our lives.

In the Valley of the Kings

The intuitive plausibility of a causal asymmetry depends, I suggest, not on the implications of causal interactions, but on the ways in which we tend to evaluate them. Recall the example of the white marble moving into the red marble and causing the red marble to change position. The white marble is the cause of the event in question (the changed position of the red marble). In this case, we tend to focus on what impact the cause had on the effect and, thereby, tend to ignore the impact that the interaction had on the cause. This often hidden aspect of causal interactions was highlighted by Salmon's definition according to which a causal interaction involves an interaction between two processes, in such a way that both are changed. The white marble does influence the position of the red marble. But, in so doing, the white marble, its position and velocity, is also affected. To make this point less abstract and begin to apply it to the normative status of nonbeneficial pediatric research, we need to move from marbles to people and consider some of the logic of contributions—the extent to which being a cause can affect us.

The Valley of the Kings is situated on the west bank of the Nile, opposite Luxor, in Egypt. It was here from approximately 1539 bc to 1075 bc, in what was then Thebes, that the kings and nobles of the New Kingdom of Ancient Egypt were buried in vast, ornamental, and often treasure-filled tombs. To visit the tombs today, one walks through thousands of years of human history. The experience, for some at least, is profound, and one gets the urge to see what a several-thousand-year old tomb feels like, to touch the walls, to literally be in touch with that history. Individuals have been coming here for centuries, and many of them have been giving in to this urge and touching the walls, an act harmless in itself, but devastating in the aggregate, over millions of visits and millions of touches.

When I was there, I visited a number of tombs and met people who had visited tombs on their own, with no guard and no cameras around. Some of them had a desire to touch the walls. They were confident that they would not get caught and that their individual touching, seen in isolation, would have no appreciable impact on the tombs. Despite these individuals' beliefs that their touching the walls would satisfy a personal desire and would have no negative impact on the walls, they declined to do so. On one level this behavior is puzzling. What was holding them back? The only way in which the action of touching the walls would influence them seems to be the fact that it would satisfy their desire to learn what an ancient tomb feels like. If our interests are exhausted by our experiences, it seems irrational for them to restrain themselves. Similarly, if our interests depend only on our preferences, it seems that the only relevant interest is to have an experience that depends on touching the walls. Yet, at least some refrain.

The individuals I met wanted to experience touching the walls, and they had a strong preference to know what the wall felt like. But, they also realized that, in doing so, they would thereby become part of the process by which these monuments to history are slowly being destroyed. It is not just that these individuals do not want the tombs to be harmed. They independently do not want to be part of the process that harms them. They do not want to be part of and connected to that effort. In this case, the individuals want to avoid the causal connection that involves them in the destructive process. Of course, if they choose to touch the walls, they become part of that process, both as agents and as physical beings. But, we can imagine, these individuals also did not want, for themselves, to innocently bump up against the walls, even when doing so would have satisfied their desire to feel the walls. They do not want to have even purely physical connections to a destructive process.

A defender of a preference satisfaction theory of interests can explain all of this. It is contrary to the individuals' interests to touch the walls because they do not want, all things considered, to touch them. They have a preference to know what the walls feel like, but this desire is less important to them than the competing preference to avoid being part of the process that harms the walls. Although this account is consistent with the facts of the example, it does not provide an accurate picture of the relationship between the facts. On this account, the existence of the preference explains what is in the individual's interests. It would be bad for the individuals to touch the walls because doing so contradicts the strong preference they have not to be part of the process by which the walls are being degraded.

In fact, these individuals had the preference not to touch the walls because they regarded it as contrary to their interests to do so. They took the view, rightly I think, that being part of the destructive process would be bad for them, not because of some prior preferences, but because it is bad, all things considered, to contribute to the destruction of priceless historical treasures. In their view, the belief that it would be bad to contribute in this way applied to everyone. It did not depend on the preferences the individual happened to have. This example highlights the extent to which the fact of making a contribution can have implications for our interests, independent of our experience and preferences. While this conclusion is important, we still are within the realm of autonomous individuals who are aware of what they are doing. To come closer to the example of nonbeneficial pediatric research, we must examine a case in which an individual who makes the contribution is not aware of the negative contribution he is making.

The Virtuous KKK Member

Consider an individual who is raised to believe that the cause of the Ku Klux Klan (KKK) is a worthwhile one, and all those with whom the individual has interactions endorse and praise the KKK and its members, and shun those who should be shunned, according to KKK lights. We would not be at all surprised to learn that these inputs to the individual's life resulted in the individual living what we would regard as a less good life overall. It may be that the individual ends up being narrow-minded and simply holds many false beliefs. That, in itself, would amount to a less good life overall and a less good life for the individual. The individual also may lead a narrow and shallow life as a result, missing out on the richness of experience that can be gained from interactions with and understanding of a broad range of groups, cultures, ways of life, and individuals. In this case, the individual leads a comparatively diminished life overall as a result of these causal inputs. The effects of these inputs change the way we evaluate the individual's life.

This conclusion is consistent with the previous analysis, which suggested that causal inputs beyond our control can have implications for our interests. Now consider the possible implications of the impact of causal *contributions* that this individual makes over the course of his life. We would not be surprised if the consequences of the way in which this individual was raised went beyond the immediate impact on his life to influence what he did with his life. He may end up harming others as a result of the beliefs with which he was raised, in minor or more significant ways. It seems clear that an individual who also did these things lived a worse life than an individual who was raised in the same way yet never had the opportunity to harm others. This conclusion seems to hold even if we are willing to grant that these individuals are not to blame for the beliefs they hold—perhaps they were never given an opportunity or never had the chance to evaluate the correctness of the KKK belief system.

How negatively we judge the individual's life will depend on how much he advanced the cause of the KKK, how active he was in this pursuit, and how much he is to blame for his efforts.[4] But, the question of moral blameworthiness is not a necessary condition on whether we judge the individual's overall life differently in light of what he did. And the disvalue of these contributions does not attach in some abstract way to the individual's life, independent of him as a person; it is worse for him that his life includes these contributions. It is bad enough for one's own sake that is one is a racist; it is even worse to make contributions to racist causes.

Once we turn to the question of evaluating overall lives, the engagement of one's agency is no longer necessary for it to be the case that actions which have negative consequences thereby can have negative implications for one's overall life. Like the white marble, the causal relationships into which we enter have implications for our lives, even when we are the cause rather than the effect. Specifically, the causal contributions that one makes become part of one's overall life, they influence and change the narrative of one's life in ways that can be bad for the individual. In the process of influencing and affecting others, our own lives are thereby influenced and changed in ways that can promote or thwart our interests.

The present analysis is consistent with the views we take of our children's interests. On the input side, we hope that those for whom we care are able to avoid causal inputs, accidents say, that curtail their lives in important ways. We have hopes for their lives on the output side as well. In addition to our concern for those who may be harmed, we hope that those for whom we care, for their own sakes, do not end up contributing to harmful causes. Of course, we do not want our children to embrace the cause of the KKK, we do not want to them to be responsible for furthering the projects of the KKK. We also do not want it to be the case that they contribute to the cause of the KKK through no fault of their own.

A second aspect of the virtuous KKK example is also worth noting. This example establishes that the causal contributions we make can have implications for our lives even when the circumstances are such that the individual is not morally responsible for making those contributions. Notice also that the implications these contributions have for the individual's overall life do not necessarily depend on the individual's attitude toward them. Presumably, the virtuous KKK member embraced and endorsed (through no fault of his own) the harms he was causing. It follows that a given contribution can be negative and have negative implications for one's life even though the individual does not regard the contribution as negative. There is an independent normative evaluation of our contributions and the impact they have on our overall lives that is independent of the contributor's own normative evaluation of them.

By hypothesis, the virtuous KKK member was not responsible for his views regarding the moral status of individuals from minority groups. Thus, in one sense, the negative contributions that he made did not go through his agency. However, in another sense, he was clearly in control of the contributions he made. According to the example, he made these contributions as a competent adult, fully aware and in control of what he was doing, despite the fact that he may not be responsible for the beliefs on which his actions are based. Younger children, in contrast, are not responsible for their actions even to this degree. We need to consider, then, whether this difference implies that the contributions children make do not similarly have implications for their overall lives.

Nazi-era Children

The Hitler Youth included children as young as 10 and later in the war still younger children as desperation and the state gained increasing control over individuals' lives: "While their fathers and Hitler Youth leaders went off to the Front, the [younger] boys were to supplement the depleted workforce and plug the gaps at home."[5] Although the Hitler Youth was limited to males, females also were recruited, dragooned, and coerced into helping the cause. By 1940, 100,000 girls were helping to keep the Nazi railway system functioning. Some of these trains were merely transporting ordinary citizens from place to place, but others were involved in transporting prisoners to concentration camps and soldiers to the front. The overall effort was enormous. By the latter stages of the war, "some 6 million young people were working in industry and agriculture, the majority in arms and munitions factories."[6] Importantly, and tragically, the efforts of these children, some as young as 8 years of age "contributed significantly to the prolonging of the war."[7] These children made the bullets that Nazi soldiers used to commit atrocities.

What implications these contributions to the Nazi war effort have for the lives of the individuals who made them depends a great deal on how old the children were, what they knew, and what they could possibly have known. Especially for the younger children, it seems clear that they were not morally responsible and what they did does not reflect negatively on them as moral agents. We do not blame an 8–year-old who could not possibly have done otherwise, who did not even know what she was doing in an important sense, for supporting the Nazi war effort. Nonetheless, as in the case of the virtuous KKK member, these causal contributions have negative implications for the children's lives even when we do not blame the children for the beliefs on which they acted. Even if the children fully supported the Nazi cause and contributed to it on those grounds, we do not blame them. In addition, unlike the virtuous KKK example, there is a deeper sense in which the children were not responsible for the contributions they made. They were too young to know better; they also were too young to know what they were doing.

At the same time, these efforts are part of the children's lives, they form some part of the children's biography, and it goes without saying perhaps that, all things being equal, one would prefer a life, would prefer for one's children a life, that did not include making the bullets that Nazis used in their atrocities. This very intuitive claim seems puzzling if one assumes that our interests are influenced only by the contributions we make as autonomous adults. One could regret that the war was prolonged, that more people were slaughtered, but there would be no reason, on this view, to independently regret the fact that one contributed, as a very young child, to the prolongation and the slaughter. On this view, there is no reason to prefer that someone else's child had made the same contribution. Another way to put this point is that the nature of the contributions we make is not defined solely based on what we know and what we intend at the time we made them. These examples underscore the possibility that what we do even as very young children can have these deeper and more direct implications for our overall lives, the possibility that the causal connections we make can have implications for our lives independent of the extent to which our moral agency is implicated in making them.

Children were enrolled in the Hitler Youth by their parents or even required by the state in the later years of the Third Reich to participate in the program and thereby contribute to the Nazi cause. These younger children had been reared and lived their whole lives within the embraces and teachings of the National Socialist party and its adoration of Adolf Hitler. Many of them at least had no meaningful choice; they knew no better, they could not have known any better, and they are not to blame for this being the case. Recognizing these factors, recognizing that the contributions they made to the Nazi war effort were made by unknowing and immature children, one history of the Hitler Youth ends with the following observation:

> As they grew older and looked back, they found it easier to face the memories of their place in this dictatorship, including the contributions that they themselves had made—a dictatorship which oppressed, maimed and killed millions, and, if they were honest enough to admit it, had damaged their own souls.[8]

These individuals recognized, as clearly as any in history, that contributions made to a horrific project can have negative implications for one's life, for one's soul, even when those contributions were made at an age at which one cannot be blamed for them, at an age at which the contributions go through the individual's agency only in the minimal sense that the individuals willingly contributed and knew what they were doing under some purely physical and morally innocuous descriptions—helping at the train station, working at a factory. They did not and could not have understood what they were doing under the description that has such devastating normative implications—supporting the Nazi cause, helping to eliminate innocent lives.

What we might think of as unknowing but active contributions to horrible projects can have negative implications for our overall lives and to that extent can be contrary to one's interests. This conclusion reveals that the age range for active contributions having implications for our interests is broader than one might otherwise have assumed. Previously, we saw that an active contribution can have implications for a child's life provided that the child understands the project and voluntarily agrees to participate because he wants to help. The individual need not understand the project in a robust sense for his contribution to nonetheless have implications for his life. In particular, a contribution can have negative implications for one's life and one's interests, even when one is not capable of understanding the project and one's contributions to it under the relevant normative descriptions.

The claim that this view is consistent with the first-person perspective on our interests is movingly exemplified in "The Mascot,"[9] the story of Alex Kurzem who, 50 years after the fact, vividly confronts the contributions he made to the Nazi cause while a young child. At the age of 5, Alex's family and most members of his village were slaughtered by the Nazis. The boy survives first by running into the woods and then as a result of his unofficial adoption by a group of Latvian police who subsequently become integrated into the Latvian SS. The unit dressed the boy in a uniform and took him along as they carried out a series of atrocities.

Alex was charming, and he came to the attention of high-ranking officers in the Latvian SS who gave him a starring role in a Nazi propaganda film. The book describes Kurzem watching the forgotten film 50 years later, in the basement of the Latvian archives, and struggling with his emotions and his response. His struggles echo the difficulty we considered briefly in the first chapter. It is not only moral philosophers who have difficulty explaining the significance that blameless but harmful contributions have for our lives. Initially, the now much older Kurzem feels guilty for what he did as a young child, but then concludes, partly convinced by his son, that he was too young to be responsible for what he did, for the contributions he made. Alex agrees but continues to be disturbed by his role. He deeply regrets the contributions themselves even though he recognizes that he is not to blame for having made them. Of note, Kurzem does not adopt the strategy that Sumner offers to Russell posthumously. Kurzem does not, that is, conclude that these contributions were worse for his life, but have no relevance for him or his own personal interests. He recognizes that these contributions touch him and his own interests; they are relevant to how well his life went for him. He wishes, for his own sake, that his life had not included contributing to the Nazi cause.

In the cases considered thus far, the contributors were active in the physical sense of doing something as part of the contributions they made. The virtuous KKK member did things to harm others; the Nazi-era children actively worked to help the trains run on time; Alex Kurzem went on patrol and acted in a Nazi film. To this point, then, the argument is potentially relevant to nonbeneficial pediatric research using children who actively participate. This argument may help to justify a good deal of nonbeneficial pediatric research. It may justify nonbeneficial pediatric that involves children who are active and understand to some extent what they are doing—children who run on a treadmill or answer an investigator's questions.

In contrast, the argument thus far does not apply to participation in nonbeneficial pediatric research that is physically passive on the part of the children. It does not apply to research with infants and research in which investigators take blood from physically passive children. To consider whether and to what extent the argument might extend to these types of research, we must consider whether being physically active is a necessary condition on a given contribution having implications for one's life and one's interests. We need, then, an example in which an individual makes a purely passive contribution—passive both with respect to the will and with respect to the body—to some cause.

The Reluctant Propagandist

In October of 1937, Irmgard Hunt was 3 years old and living in Berchtesgaden, Germany, already famous, if not yet infamous, as the site of Hitler's mountaintop headquarters at Obersalzberg. One day, while out walking with her family, a crowd approaches Irmgard and out of it appears Hitler. Startled and frightened, Irmgard tries to hide, but her mother, who reveres the dictator, pushes Irmgard out and on to Hitler's knee, allowing his oft-present official photographer to snap a picture of him with this "perfect picture of a little German girl with blond braids and blue eyes" wearing a blue dirndl dress.[10] Later in life, Irmgard worries that the picture and by implication herself might have been used by Nazi propagandists to increase Hitler's popularity, on which so much of the Nazi effort was based, and that she in this very, very minor way might have contributed to the horrors to come.

Irmgard's concern makes sense despite the fact that the possible contribution she made to the Nazi effort was completely passive on her part. Indeed, in some sense, she actively attempted to avoid making the (possible) contribution in question. The concern she has retrospectively regarding the possible contribution she made is not for those who might thereby have been injured. By the time she is an adult, considering what happened, the number and degree of atrocities has been fixed and is past. The answer to the question she faces, whether she in fact served as part of an influential piece of Nazi propaganda, will not influence the number of lives ruined (apart from her own) or lost. And she is not concerned for the value of her life in some abstract sense, how well her life went overall independent of her own, personal interests. She is concerned about whether *she made* this passive contribution. She recognizes that it would be worse *for her* if she had done so.

This example illustrates the extent to which even the most passive and even reluctant contributions can have implications for our overall lives in a way that can be relevant to our interests, to how our lives go for us. Passively contributing to a horrific cause is not as bad as doing so actively and energetically. The latter contribution says more about one's life, and says something about one as a person. Nonetheless, even purely passive contributions to horrific projects become part of one's life narrative and thus can influence how we evaluate that life overall and, by implication, how well the life went for the individual whose life it was.

This conclusion regarding the possible implications of purely passive contributions is consistent with the first-person judgments we make about our own lives. For Irmgard, she strongly hoped that her life did not include contributing to the Nazi effort (she never learns whether it did), even though her contribution would have been passive in the sense of lacking physical activity on her part and also lacking willing or even knowing agency, and including a level of uniqueness only as an instance of a general (mythic) type. It is not that she worries that she might somehow be to blame for taking that walk or not resisting her mother with enough force. Rather, she does not want it to be the case that she helped, that her life includes within it contributing to, the Nazi cause. She does not want it to be the case that she had that influence on the world. She is worried whether she contributed to those harms because she recognizes that the fact of having made such a contribution would be bad *for her*.[11]

This view makes sense from a second- and third-person perspective as well. We would hope for those for whom we care for their own sakes that they not in *any way* contribute to the Nazi cause, actively, passively, or otherwise. And, all things considered, we judge a life to a certain extent based on all the causal contributions that emanate from that life, and regard, all things considered, a life to have gone less well when it involves contributions to, what in Irmgard's case is a vastly euphemistic description, negative projects. The factors that determine how active a contribution is and how much it engages the individual do not, as one might otherwise surmise, determine whether a contribution says anything at all about one's life. This is determined by whether one makes a contribution and the value of the project in question. These factors (how active is the contribution, how much it engages the individual) determine *how much* a contribution says about our lives and whether the contribution has implications for us as moral agents, for our characters. It follows that even purely passive contributions can have consequences for the goodness of our lives and, by implication, can have consequences for our own interests.

The Normative Asymmetry Thesis

The examples considered thus far have involved contributions of varying degrees to negative relationships, projects, or causes. The fact that these contributions can have implications for our lives, independent of whether we were in control of making them, undermines the postulation of a causal asymmetry in the significance of our causal connections. Both the causal inputs and causal outputs (e.g., contributions) to our lives can have implications for our interests by influencing the goodness of our lives, even when they are beyond our agency, beyond our willing and knowing.

One might accept the argument to this point, but hold that *positive* contributions, unlike negative ones, can influence our interests only to the extent that they go through our agency. Negative contributions may cast a shadow over our lives, even when we are not responsible for them. However, positive contributions do not shed positive light on our overall lives if we are not responsible for them. Hence, they cannot influence our interests. To evaluate this view, we need to consider whether positive contributions can have implications for our lives—and for us—in the same way that negative contributions do.

We have seen that a contribution to a negative cause can have negative implications for our lives because it becomes part of our life narrative, even though our agency was not implicated at all, at least with respect to the outcome under the description for which it says something about one's life (e. g. "assisting the Nazis"). This finding allows us to make sense of our judgments of the lives of those children who contributed to the Nazi war effort at an age and time when they could not possibly have known better. Why should the fact that they made these contributions reflect negatively on their overall lives if we are assuming that they are not responsible in any moral sense, but responsible only in a causal sense for these contributions? The fact is that the negative causal contributions we make become part of our lives, they become part of our biography, and thus have implications for our overall lives. Positive contributions that we make also become part of our life's narrative, providing some minimal support for the claim that they too have implications for our overall lives, even when they do not go through our agency. Considering examples to this effect brings us close to nonbeneficial pediatric research.

Previously, we considered the case of Ted Lilly, pitcher for the Chicago Cubs, who fouled off a pitch that then fractured the skull of a 7–year-old fan. In the actual case, Lilly felt a connection to the accident that he wished were not part of his life. Given the choice between the boy's skull being fractured as the result of what Lilly did, versus it being fractured as the result of a freak accident, Lilly certainly would have preferred the latter option. We saw in the first chapter that this kind of reaction is a commonplace in our lives. Although this aspect of the example was not discussed at that point, the outcome of Lilly's actions was negative. Thus, a proponent of the normative asymmetry objection might grant everything I have said about that case, but deny its relevance for nonbeneficial pediatric research, which involves contributing to a valuable cause.

To begin to consider the objection, imagine that Lilly's foul ball had instead led to a positive outcome. Imagine that the boy had brought his glove to the game and caught the ball, which then served as an inspiration to his going on, many years later, to become a great philanthropist. I will modify the example in a moment, but this version of it is useful for illustrating how aspects of the examples we choose here influence our intuitive responses. In this modified version of the case, it seems unclear at best whether we would say that Lilly contributed to the good deeds that the boy goes on to do with his life. In this case, the contribution Lilly makes seems too unrelated to the later good works which, we assume, require an enormous amount of work and the input of countless other individuals. Previously, when considering whether a causal antecedent qualifies as a causal contribution we noted that the intervening efforts of many other people can screen off (in the contribution sense) one's life from the ultimate outcome.

The important lesson of this possibility is the extent to which determining the narrative of a person's life is comparative or, perhaps better, contrastive: the contribution was made by this person rather than that person. I suspect that this phenomenon may account for some of the intuition that supports the normative asymmetry objection. In standard cases, it is difficult to inadvertently bring about a very valuable result. Important philanthropy takes a great deal of work to accumulate the necessary funds and to distribute them wisely. Bad outcomes, hitting someone on the head with a baseball, running someone down in one's car, seem, by comparison all too easy—and all too easy to trace to the actions of one person.

Although this is a common feature of contributing to valuable projects, it is not a necessary one. Imagine that we revise the Lilly example. This time the ball hits a man on the head, knocking him to the ground, just as he is about to kidnap the boy. Imagine that the blow is just enough to stun the man into inactivity until security guards arrive and take him away. Here, the causal connection between Lilly's actions and the outcome are just as clear and just as direct as the case in which his foul ball fractures the boy's skull. What should we say about this case? If the foul ball that leads to the negative outcome is part of the narrative of the batter's life, it is difficult to see how we can avoid drawing the same conclusion regarding the positive case. With that said, it is important to note that many factors are at work here that modify in various ways our reactions to these cases.

In the modified case, there may be a good deal of teasing of Lilly and mock adulation for the great thing he has done. In part, this teasing plays a similar role to the many expressions of support that Lilly receives in the actual case, where the hit led to the fractured skull. In that case, it was important for Lilly not to make too much of his relationship to the outcome. It is especially important for him not to conclude that he is morally responsible for the outcome in any way. A similar need exists in the positive case to keep clear the significance of the outcome for the hypothetical Lilly. It is important that he not conclude that he deserves credit, for example, for having done something great. It was luck, and that fact significantly modifies how Lilly should feel about it and how we should feel about him.

Giving credit for accidental successes and blame for accidental mistakes also has the potential to undermine the subtle but powerful incentive mechanisms built into our social practices. Society offers countless ways to provide incentive for individuals to act properly and further mechanisms to provide recognition for appropriate behavior. Making too much of the accidents in our lives, both positive and negative, can undermine these mechanisms, especially when it comes to the actions of autonomous agents. We emphasize autonomous action because it is central to the moral life, to who we are, but also because it is the type of behavior that is susceptible to these mechanisms.

This is but a brief consideration of a complex topic. For present purposes, the challenge is not to determine all the different factors that result in downplaying our accidental contributions, whether negative or positive. The point instead is that these factors influence what we say about the significance of the contributions for the agent. These factors do not influence whether the contribution in fact comes from the individual. That is determined by the causal structure of the event. In fact, several of the mechanisms are based on recognition of the fact that these contributions are made by the individual. We downplay the importance of the lucky contribution because we recognize that the person in fact did make it, but we also want to emphasize its relative unimportance compared to those contributions that go through the individual's agency in richer ways.

This conclusion is reinforced by considering cases in which it is clear that the worrisome implications are not in place. In the actual case, it is absolutely clear that Lilly did not intend the negative result. No one could intentionally have brought about such a result. And the player clearly feels terrible for what occurred. In that case, one might ask why we simply do not conclude that he was not part of the causal nexus at all. Indeed, there are, as we have seen, good policy reasons to adopt this view. Focusing on the fact that the individual is causally responsible may deflect attention from the fact that, in this case, the appropriate response, if one is called for at all, is a societal one. We could forbid children from going to games, allow them in certain seats only, or require a glass partition between the fans and the game (this is not to argue in favor of these measures; the risk is sufficiently small that it seems worth accepting for the benefits that can be realized by taking children to baseball games, without intervening and interfering glass partitions). Despite these considerations, it is nonetheless the case that Lilly is, in part, causally responsible for the outcome. There is a limit in these cases on the extent to which we control what does and does not have implications for our lives. The response here is similar to the appropriate response to the stoic ideal. Leaving aside the question of whether it represents a better life, it simply is not an accurate account of what is important in our lives.

One might accept the revised Lilly case as a counterexample to the simple normative asymmetry objection, but then use the example to develop a refined objection. One might conclude from the Lilly example that even positive contributions that we do not intend and do not foresee (Lilly did not foresee the possibility of knocking out the kidnapper in the revised version of the case) can have some implications for our lives. Yet, one might argue that the contribution in this case is not relevant to nonbeneficial pediatric research, at least with infants. Although Lilly did not intend or foresee the consequences, he was nonetheless acting purposively in fouling the ball off, even in the revised example. The contribution then went through his agency to that extent, whereas nonbeneficial pediatric research does not involve very young children making contributions that go through their agency.

There is a strong intuition that passive contributions to valuable projects do not contribute at all to one's interests. Given that negative passive contributions can have implications for our interests, proponents of this view must, at least implicitly, endorse a normative asymmetry in the implications of our contributions. To this point, we have considered a number of theoretical reasons that tell against a normative asymmetry. The causal similarity between negative and positive contributions provides no reason to think such an asymmetry exists. Are there other reasons to endorse such an asymmetry in the implications that the effects of our lives have for our interests?

Contributing without Trying

Although I am unaware of any positive arguments for a normative asymmetry with respect to the relevance for our interests of the causal effects of our lives, some authors seem to endorse this view. The clearest and most explicit example of which I am aware comes from Joseph Raz, who asks us to consider two pairs of cases:[12]

> *Passive contributions*: 1.1 Mary is photographed without her knowledge and the photograph is used to become a vital element in a great work of art. 2.1 Rather drunk, Mary falls asleep with her body blocking shut the (fire) door, thus saving many people from the fire which erupted accidentally on the other side.
>
> *Active contributions*: 1.2 Mary takes a photographic self-portrait and incorporates it in a great work of art she was creating at the time. 2.2 Aware of the danger the fire poses, Mary stays by the fire door pressing it shut, thus saving many lives.

Raz points out that in all four cases "a good or valuable episode involving Mary occurs. However, he writes:

> She is active in the episodes of the second list, while passive in those of the first. That difference explains why neither episode in the first list can be good for her, whereas those in the second list can be. Episodes in which we are passive, as well as ones in which we do not feature at all, can be good for us only indirectly, through their contribution to another valuable aspect of our activities. Only active episodes can be directly good for us.

In a footnote, Raz points out that "Oddly, the same is not true of what is bad for us. Events in which we are totally passive can be directly bad for us. They can violate our integrity, dignity, etc." Here we seem to have a clear endorsement of the normative asymmetry thesis. Raz argues that we can benefit directly, our interests can be advanced, only when we are active, and this is so because episodes that are good for us directly "consist in an appropriate response to value."

The qualification to benefiting *directly* here may suggest that no real disagreement exists between Raz's view and the claim being considered here.

A direct impact on our interests involves a state of affairs being realized that is itself in our interests. Nothing else needs to follow for our interests to be promoted. Indirect promotion of our interests occurs when one state of affairs leads to another, and it is the second state of affairs that promotes our interests. This is the sense in which participation in nonbeneficial research can be in children's interests by providing them with an educational benefit. The participation itself does not promote an interest of the children. Instead, that participation leads to them learning important lessons. And these lessons may directly promote their interests; the children may be better off for having learned these things. As well, these educational benefits themselves may also be indirectly in the children's interests by putting them in a position to do further things (e.g., pursue a career in medicine) that promote their interests.

The claim to be considered here is that participation in nonbeneficial research can be in children's interests to the extent that such participation, contributing to the study in question, results in a better life overall, and all things considered, one of our interests is to have a better life overall. This is a slightly different way in which some events can be in our interests, via the impact they have on the goodness of our lives overall. Whether this impact qualifies as direct or indirect in the sense intended by Raz is less important, for present purposes, than the question of whether the examples he provides support a thesis regarding our interests which denies the possibility that passive and positive contributions can be in one's interest in any way, even "indirectly" through the interest we have in leading better lives overall.

Consider the examples Raz offers of passive and positive contributions: Mary being photographed without her knowledge; a drunken Mary accidentally blocking a fire door and saving many lives. Again, it is important to keep in mind the extent to which our evaluation of specific cases is influenced by the available alternatives. This is especially true of our evaluation of autonomous agents who are, or who should be aware of the available alternatives. Our evaluation of what implications Raz's examples have *for Mary* depends in part on the alternatives available to her. This is clearest in the second passive contribution in which Mary blocks the door as a result of being drunk, blithely unaware of the fact that she and many others are in grave danger. In this case, we can easily imagine a sober Mary in the same situation, a Mary who is able to respond to variations on the danger in question. In the actual case, if Mary had happened to fall asleep just short of the fire door, she would not have noticed and everyone would have died. Thus, two descriptions of this case are possible, which bring out very different aspects and possibly lead to very different normative evaluations.

The first description would be one in which Mary does a good thing, albeit out of sheer luck. She blocks the door and saves many lives. A second description would be one according to which Mary acts very badly. She gets drunk and thereby impairs her ability to respond to a dangerous situation in a way that could have imperiled the lives of many people. The fact that things just happened to turn out for the best does not mean that this alternative is irrelevant to how we judge the case with respect to Mary's interests. The problem, as this alternative highlights, is that our judgment of autonomous agents take into account more than simply the outcomes of their actions. We consider not only what they did, we consider what they should have done.

To eliminate this element from the examples and better focus on the passive contribution itself, we need to consider cases of what we might think of as innocent instances of making a passive contribution. As mentioned previously, there is passivity with respect to the will and passivity with respect to the body. It will be useful to include in the example both aspects of our actions. And, to evaluate the normative asymmetry thesis, we need to consider two versions, one involving a positive contribution and one involving a negative contribution. Cases of innocent shielding provide a source of such examples. Imagine, then, that while on a visit to Washington D.C., Mr. Magoo goes for a stroll and innocently finds himself in a group of unfamiliar and well-dressed men. What Magoo does not know (and let us assume could not have known) is that he has wandered into the President's entourage at just the moment a team is trying to kidnap him.

> *Negative version*: Magoo innocently shields the President from his security team for a moment, allowing the kidnappers to succeed.
>
> *Positive version*: Magoo innocently shields the President from the kidnappers for a moment, allowing his security team to rescue him.

In the negative version of the case, Magoo unwittingly contributes to a terrible project and, it seems clear, that contribution is a negative thing for Magoo overall. All things considered, a better life overall, and a better life *for Magoo,* would be one in which he does not, however innocently, contribute to the kidnapping of the President. It would be better for Magoo not to causally contribute to that effort. And we can well imagine Magoo preferring that the shielding contribution, if it has to be made at all, be made by someone else or by an inanimate object. He would strongly prefer it to have been the case that the shield be provided by a toppled tree as opposed to being provided by his body.

In the positive version, Magoo is, albeit inadvertently, an important part of the group that saves the President. A life that involves that contribution seems a better one, all things considered. And it seems better for Magoo to have been part of that group; it is better for him. We can imagine Magoo preferring that his life includes this contribution on the grounds that making this contribution, being part of the group that saves the President, is valuable for him. He would prefer that he, rather than someone else or an inanimate object, make this contribution. Finally, to make these cases analogous to nonbeneficial pediatric research, imagine that, in the negative version, the kidnappers grab Magoo and place him in the shielding position; in the positive case, the security team, not having time to explain what is going on, grabs Magoo and places him in the shielding position. In these cases, like research with children, others are intentionally deciding for Magoo that he will make the respective contribution. They decide that Magoo is part of the effort in question, either positive or negative. The fact that the decision is made by someone else does not eliminate the fact that Magoo makes a physical contribution in the two cases. This is evident in the fact that, in both cases, someone is using Magoo. If they use him successfully, then he has made the contribution in question. That is what using him involves in this case. Put differently, the intentional efforts of others do not, in these cases, completely eliminate Magoo's contribution to the ultimate effect. The reason is that their efforts involve precisely that of using Magoo.

The innocent shielding cases support the claim that purely passive contributions can have implications for our lives. They do not say a great deal, and they do not say anything about the individual as a moral agent. They do not show that Magoo is a good or a bad person. And, taking Magoo's life in consideration as a whole, they say very little about that as well. They are, we might say, interesting and potentially amusing footnotes to the narrative of Magoo's life. They are a very minor part of the story and for that reason have only very minimal relevance for Magoo's interests.

The innocent shielding cases deny that a normative asymmetry necessarily exists with regard to the implications for us of our passive contributions. These examples suggest that passive contributions to valuable causes can have implications for how well our lives go and, in that way, can promote our interests. Raz rejects this possibility when it comes to the passive (and positive) contributions made by Mary. The cases of innocent shielding suggest that our evaluation of that example may be influenced by the alternatives available to Mary. As we have seen, in the case of blocking the fire door while drunk, we can imagine a better scenario in which Mary retains her wits and is capable of responding to the extant circumstances as well as responding to slight changes in those circumstances (e.g. the door won't close so she has to wake everyone up and get them out). A second factor is that the examples are under-described, so that we have little sense for the extent to which the contributions Mary makes engage the five factors for determining how relevant the contribution is to how we evaluate the individual's life. We can remedy these shortcoming of the example by considering a real case, one that is strikingly similar to Raz's case of Mary being photographed without her knowledge.

More than two decades ago, Antonio Carlos (Tom) Jobim was sitting in a café in Rio as a woman walked by, inspiring him to write a great pop song: *The Girl from Ipanema.* This woman's actions were purely passive with respect to the contribution she ends up making. She did not know she was making this contribution, she did not intend to make it. Granted, she was walking at the time. But, with respect to the contribution in question, she was passive. She did not know she was being watched by a song writer, and his presence did not alter her behavior in any way. And it is not the case that Tom Jobim was admiring something that the woman intentionally cultivated over the years. He was not, for example, inspired by some aspect of the woman's walk that she developed over years of practice. She gets no credit for inspiring him. Thus, if our knowledge and intentions, the extent to which things go through our agency, defined the implications of our contributions for our interests we would conclude that she did not contribute to the writing of this song, at least in any way that promotes her interests.

Again, we do not praise the woman for making this contribution. But, a theory that implies that the contribution is irrelevant to her and her life forces us to miss a fundamental aspect of the story. She made this contribution and, although she made it unknowingly, it is part of her overall life's narrative. One of the consequences of her life was that this great song was written which, let us assume, would not have been written otherwise (readers who are unimpressed by the value of the project in question are invited to substitute Beethoven and his Ninth Symphony for Tom Jobim and *The Girl from Ipanema*).

The contribution in this case is not in any way comparable to the contributions considered earlier, helping the Nazis, harming individuals from minority groups. Still, her life did have this positive effect and it seems that a life with such effects is better than the same life absent those effects. Finally, it seems plausible to conclude that it was a good thing for her that she made this contribution. Making this contribution is in the interests of the woman who made it, it says something positive about her life, despite the fact that she did not intend or even know at the time that she was making it. This reading of the example is supported by the historical reactions of the woman herself. When the (by then) woman from Ipanema learned that she was the inspiration for the song, she regarded it as a contribution she made and one in her interests to have made. She clearly preferred her life with that contribution, to her life exactly the same but without the contribution. It was good *for her* that she made the contribution.

Imagine that the alternative story is one in which Tom Jobim is even slightly more impressed with her and that this extra degree of appreciation keeps him from writing the song. She bewitches rather than inspires him. It seems clear that the woman would prefer, for her own sake, the actual world to this alternative. Indeed, she came to embrace the contribution and came to regard it as a valuable part of her life. We may be more or less impressed by this contribution, and we may debate how much the contribution alone says about her life. But, she can embrace this contribution in a way that, for anyone else, would represent delusion or confusion. This contribution may serve as an important lesson for some other woman, but only the woman who was in fact the Girl from Ipanema made the contribution and can embrace it.

There are at least three crucial differences between this example and the Mary photography example considered by Raz. First, Raz provides us with an alternative in which Mary is the artist rather than the subject. This immediately provides a much more significant contribution against which being a mere and unknowing subject seems unimpressive. In that case, there does not seem much reason to spend time considering whether any residual benefit accrues to Mary in the passive case. Second, the meager description of the passive case tells us only that Mary's agency was not engaged in the case. It provides no way to evaluate whether Mary's contribution involves any of the other factors relevant to the importance of a contribution. As a result, assuming that these factors are necessary for a contribution having relevance for the individual, the sparse description yields the impression that the factors are not present at all.

In the Girl from Ipanema example, Tom Jobim is influenced by what he sees as the grace and beauty of the girl. We can thus see this instance as having some significance for her because it engages her as a somewhat unique individual. In Raz's example, by contrast, the meager description of the case begs the reaction that Mary's passive contribution to the final artwork does not involve her as an individual at all, hence, says nothing about her life. Instead, it says something about the photographer's life. He was able to use Mary as the subject in a way that yielded a great work of art.

This aspect of the example raises an important contrast that we will consider in a moment. But, first, note that this example involves an aspect of many passive contributions which influences our judgment of their value for the individual. When we are passive and someone else in effect uses us to good effect, we are inclined to give all the credit to the individual who was active. Yet, the Girl from Ipanema example highlights the fact that being active is not the only way to enter into the causal chain as an individual in a way that has implications for one's life overall. We can make a contribution by the fact that the good outcome depended, in part, on some aspect of us as individuals. Although this aspect of passive contributions to valuable goals may not be present in every case, it typically is present in the case of nonbeneficial pediatric research. Clinical research studies invariably have inclusion and exclusion criteria such that only some individuals can contribute to a given project. Thus, the investigators rely on the properties of those children who allow them to satisfy these requirements, whether it is an unusual protein in the blood; a specific age, weight, and drug history; or perhaps the fact that the child has the right combination of properties to serve as a normal control.

Finally, our intuitions can be influenced in these cases by the possibility that the subject is being exploited without their knowledge. Raz explicitly mentions that Mary is unaware of the fact that she is being photographed. Imagine, then, that Mary is sitting chatting with a friend when the picture is taken. Just before the photographer takes the picture, he asks her if she is willing to serve as his subject in this way, and she indicates that she is willing. This change in the example does not influence Mary's actions in any way with respect to the quality of the resulting art. She continues to be physically passive, although she is now active in the sense of willing her contribution to the project in question. She continues to act just as she would have if she had not been asked, and the picture turns out just the same. Imagine that the photographer asks Mary to "behave exactly as you were just before I approached you" and she succeeds. In this case, a stronger argument can be made that this contribution promotes Mary's interests. All things considered, a life that involves serving as the knowing and willing subject of a great work of art is better than the same life without that element.

The only difference between this case and the original Mary is that here she agrees to serve as the subject, thus taking away concerns of her image being inappropriately taken. But notice that the contribution she makes to the great work of art, the extent to which she is physically passive and in effect does nothing physically, is the same in both cases. This suggests that the original example may not tell against the personal significance of passive contributions so much as it points to possible concern, in cases of passive contribution, of being used without one's knowledge. When it comes to the passive contributions of autonomous individuals, often the better alternative is available of getting the individual's active agreement and participation. That possibility can influence our judgment of the actual case. In the Girl from Ipanema example, this seems less of a concern since the song writing is not taking her image literally and is, in any case, clearly celebrating her as an individual.

The finding that contributions made independent of one's agency and even knowing can have implications for one's life begins to make plausible the claim that purely passive contributions, ones that do not even satisfy the uniqueness and activity conditions, can have implications for an individual's life. To consider this possibility, we will have to evaluate examples that involve individuals making purely passive contributions to a valuable cause. If these contributions can have positive implications for the contributor's life, participation in nonbeneficial pediatric research by very young children, even infants, may be in their interests in the sense of saying something positive about their lives, in the sense of it being the case that a life that includes such contributions is better or more preferable overall to the same life absent those contributions.

To this point, we have seen that our intuitions regarding passive contribution cases are sensitive to the ways in which the examples are described, and the relevant alternatives to them. The cases in which autonomous agents make a passive contribution often are those in which they might instead have made an active one. It is not just that Mary could have made a more valuable contribution by agreeing to the photograph. The passive aspect of the contribution in effect magnifies the failure that results in its not being an active one. Mary passively contributes to the work of art because the photographer did not ask her permission, thus failing to respect her as an autonomous agent. She passively saves the lives of many people because she got drunk and thereby failed to keep her wits in a way that would have allowed her to respond appropriately to slight changes in the circumstances. The extent to which our intuitions regarding these examples are sensitive to the details and the alternatives available to the actors in them undermines the extent to which they can be used to argue for a normative asymmetry with respect to our passive contributions. This, of course, is not to say that no such asymmetry exists, only that these examples may be unable to establish it as a fact about the nature of our contributions. In the next section, we consider examples that undermine the postulation of a normative asymmetry by providing instances of passive contributions that seem to redound to the life of the agents who passively make them.

Consideration of children in these examples is relevant to the present task of evaluating the acceptability of nonbeneficial pediatric research and also allows us to remove a number of the aspects of the prior examples that influence our intuitions, especially the fact that the agents are autonomous and were in a position to make an active contribution if only they, or someone else had behaved better. To set the stage for these examples, it will be worth considering how one might begin to develop a positive argument for the normative asymmetry thesis. This consideration serves to highlight the commitments that might lead one to this view and thus underscores the commitments that one would be giving up by accepting the present analysis on which passive contributions can have implications for our lives overall.

A plausible view of our lives holds that a better, preferable life for an individual involves one in which he develops, pursues and, to some extent, achieves worthwhile goals. This analysis has the virtue of leaving it up to the individual to decide what things he values. This can be taken too far, however. Some things are bad for one's overall life, for how well one's life goes, no matter one's personal attitude toward them. It is a bad thing for one's life overall to violate the rights of others, to harm the innocent, to make the world a worse place. The account to which this plausible line of reasoning tends is one in which there are, in effect, side constraints on the pursuit of our own ends.

It is up to us to decide the positive account of what makes our life go better. But independent constraints exist that we should not violate. On this analysis, violation of the independent constraints is bad for us, no matter what our personal attitude toward them happens to be. Even passively violating these constraints can be bad for one and for one's life. But what is good for one depends on actively pursuing one's own worthwhile ends. This account supports a normative asymmetry with respect to passive contributions. The important thing for present purposes is to note the commitments that get one to this asymmetry. Specifically, one gets to this account by assuming that a more objective account exists of at least some of the things that are bad for us and for our lives. It is bad, independent of what we happen to think, to violate the rights of others. In contrast, there is no matter of fact about which goals it is good for us to actively pursue (other than those we endorse). That part of the good life is up to us to decide, to fill in as we please.

Considering this sketch of an argument is useful because it highlights an implicit assumption that might be behind some of the intuitive pull of the normative asymmetry thesis with respect to passive contributions. We allow individuals to decide the positive content of how they should live their lives within certain constraints. There is good reason to treat autonomous agents in this way. Allowing them to make what they want of their lives is an important way to show respect for them. But, it is also important not to confuse this account of how we should treat other autonomous agents with an account of what is and is not in their interests overall. If there are more objective facts about what is contrary to a life well lived, then the primary theoretical objection has been removed against there being more objective facts about what promotes a life well lived. At a theoretical level, it is no more puzzling to claim that there are some things that are good, all things considered, for all of us to accomplish than it is to say that there are some things that, all things considered, are bad for us to accomplish. It is bad if one's life includes killing the innocent, and it is good for one's life to save them. And this fact does not, as we shall see in the next section, depend on determining first whether the contributions leading to those outcomes are active or passive ones. Those considerations come not at the point of whether the contribution was made, and not even at the point of whether the contribution was a good thing or a bad thing for one's life, but at the point of deciding to what extent it was a good thing or a bad thing for one's life.

Our intuitions on the value for an individual of contributing to a positive cause and contributing to a negative cause also may be influenced to some extent by an intuition about the comparative implications of doing good versus doing ill. It seems, in some sense, to be worse to do something bad than it is good to do something beneficial. For present purposes, the point is not to consider this possibility in depth and determine whether it is right, but instead to note this possibility and the extent to which it may be informing our judgments of the plausibility of the normative asymmetry thesis.

Compare two cases, one in which Susan intentionally reduces Richard's well-being by 10 utils and a second case in which Susan intentionally increases Richard's well-being by 10 utils.

Imagine that the cases are the same in all other relevant respects. Or, compare one action of electronic theft of X dollars from Richard's bank account versus the electronic gifting of X dollars into his bank account. It seems that the negative actions are more significant for how we judge Susan and her life than the positive actions. This difference is reflected in the typical social responses in the two cases. Stealing money often leads to a few years in jail; contributing the same amount of money to a worthwhile cause often leads to a pat on the back. This difference is worth nothing here to the extent that it lends plausibility to the normative asymmetry thesis. It may be that doing bad has, or at least seems to have greater implications for one's life than doing good. Yet, even if this view is correct, it does not imply that doing good things, even passively, has no implications for one's life, only that negative contributions are more weighty with respect to our evaluations of contributions and the lives of the contributors.[13]

Children in Opera, Infants at Political Rallies

Our lives are defined, to a great extent, by the causal interactions we have with others and the world, the causal inputs that shape and influence us and our lives, and the causal influence we in turn have on others and the world. All of these causal connections taken together help to uniquely define our lives and define our lives as unique. As we have seen, how well things go for us, our welfare or well-being, is distinct from, but influenced by how well our lives go in general. Each of us has an interest in our lives going better, and one way in which we can promote an individual's interests is to increase the goodness of his life overall. In evaluating the ways in which we can promote an individual's interests by increasing the goodness of his life overall, it is important to remain cognizant of the ways in which the available options to a given course influence our evaluation of it.

This is a fundamental difference in how we can promote our own interests versus how others can promote our interests for us. In many cases, the extent to which the road taken promotes our interests is independent of the extent to which our pursuit of the road not taken would have promoted our interests. The extent to which becoming a librarian promotes your interests depends on the consequences of that life course. And this is largely independent of the consequences that would have been realized had you decided to become a farmer instead, although, even here, the alternative can influence our judgments—whether the choice of librarian was wise or foolish for instance depends on the available alternatives.

When we make decisions that influence the overall goodness of the lives of others, the alternatives available to us when we act can have a dramatic influence on how we evaluate the choices we make. In particular, as we have seen, an individual's interests are vitally influenced by his own pursuit and attainment of valuable goals. Therefore, when possible, we should promote the overall goodness of the lives of others by going through their agency. At first glance, one might think that going through the individual's agency will merely increase the value of the achievement. In fact, in many cases failing to go through his agency has the effect of robbing the achievement of any value for him, since it did not go through his agency. If you secretly paint the picture I have been planning for years, you may increase the value of my life by introducing into it a work of art that otherwise might not have been realized. However, you rob me of the opportunity of accomplishing this goal, of having painted this work of art.

Accomplishing things for others can do even more than merely rob those things of their value for the individual. Doing things for others can have positive disvalue when we could have gone through their agency, but failed to do so. Such cases can disrespect or dishonor the individual in ways that fully taint the accomplishment. We saw this possibility with respect to Raz's example of Mary's photograph, unknown to her, being taken and included in a great work of art. If Mary could have taken her own picture and made the work of art, the result would have had dramatically greater value for her. This possibility is exemplified by the alternative example Raz provides, possibly draining the original contribution of its value. The thought that the photographer could have asked Mary whether she was willing to serve as the subject of the painting, but failed to do so, raises concerns of disrespect or improperly taking advantage of her in the original case. With this option in mind, we might conclude that making the actual contribution has no value for Mary at all.

When we evaluate examples of individuals making contributions to valuable projects or goals we almost implicitly make these evaluations based on what we think of the contributions, what implications they have for the life of an autonomous agent. And, in that case, the alternative is typically present of the individual choosing for himself to make the contribution or, least, for him to be asked whether he is willing to contribute. When we evaluate the contributions that young children make, including the contributions they make to clinical research, we need to keep in mind the paucity of options typically available to them.

CHILDREN IN OPERA

Central to Bellini's opera *Norma* is a secret love affair between the Druid seeress Norma and the Roman official Pollione. Their relationship produces two children who are young at the time the story opens, at which point Pollione has decided to throw off Norma for a younger woman. The presence of the two young children is vital to at least some stagings of the story. The children are a physical manifestation of their love and the costs of Pollione's treachery.

Presumably, the child actors who play the parts of Norma's children take some risks: they may become petrified, they may trip or be accidentally hit by one of the soldiers, they may be disturbed by Norma's plan to kill them, and those risks should be minimized to the extent possible. Especially shy children should be excluded, as well as those who strongly resist or might be particularly disturbed by the planned, although not executed sacrifice. In addition, participation poses not insignificant burdens on the children. They must attend several practice sessions and be present for an opera performance that seems long, even to many adults.

Recognizing these risks and burdens, it seems possible, in certain cases at least, that the risks to the children will be sufficiently low that it can be acceptable for them to participate in the opera.[14] This seems acceptable even if the children at the time are too young to have any understanding of opera and do not value it, or even value the arts in general. The presence of the children has value for the opera to the extent that it makes real their existence and the costs of Pollione's treachery. To make this point, the children need not do anything in the opera. They do not have to show any special abilities or qualities. They do not have to be active at all.

Enrolling even very young children might be justified on the grounds that, as the children get older, they may come to embrace the fact that they were part of this artistic production, seeing it as an important and worthwhile part of their overall lives. This experience may also have an important educational impact on the children and influence their interests and pursuits. They may be more likely to pursue an interest in the performing arts. These potential future benefits might justify the risks and burdens to which the children will be exposed, to the extent that overall the ex ante probabilities are in the child's interests. In addition, enrolling the children may be self-reinforcing, increasing the chances that they will come to embrace their participation. Of course, there always exists the potential for rebellion; the fact that the parents enrolled the children may be precisely the spur that leads the children to reject this contribution and artistic endeavors in general. But the long-term effects of rebellion likely are minor compared to the chance that the child will come to be shaped by this and similar experiences, thereby increasing the chances that they embrace this contribution. Consistency has psychological as well as logical force.

Presumably, children may learn valuable lessons even if they make mistakes on stage to the extent that their performance detracts from, rather than enhances the opera. To this extent, the value of being in the opera for the children does not depend solely on the value of the opera and the nature of their contribution to it. In contrast, as mentioned previously, the possibility of the children appropriately embracing the contribution they make to the opera does depend on the prior fact of its being a valuable contribution to make. The children cannot embrace a contribution made by others, nor can they appropriately embrace as valuable a contribution that was not valuable.

Imagine that this performance comes to be regarded as one of the great opera performances of all time. The fact that the children contributed to this project and its value seems to have positive implications for their overall lives. All things considered, a life that involved contributing in a positive way to a valuable artistic project is better than the same life absent that contribution. And the fact that the contribution is positive and says something positive about the children's lives grounds the possibility of their later coming to embrace it, and seems to be positive or of some value for them as individuals. This conclusion suggests that making a positive contribution to a valuable project can be in children's interests, even when the contribution is made at a time when they are not autonomous.

To recall a point made by critics of nonbeneficial pediatric research, notice that this conclusion does not require that making a contribution to the opera involved the making of a gift on the part of the children. One cannot be said to offer a gift unless one understands what one is doing. Ramsey is right about that. However, as the present example reveals, making a gift is not the only way to contribute to valuable projects. One also can make a valuable, albeit passive contribution. And the making of a positive, although passive contribution to a valuable project can have positive implications, all things considered, for the contributors' lives and can, to that extent, be in the contributors' interests.

We saw in the example of Irmgard Hunt that purely passive contributions to negative causes can have negative implications for one's overall life, even when the contributions occur when one is a young child. Contrary to the causal asymmetry thesis, the present example suggests that purely passive contributions to valuable projects similarly can have implications for our lives, even when they occur when one is a young child, and even when they do not involve active contributions in any sense. Such contributions can nonetheless have implications for our lives by virtue of the fact that they become part of our lives and the value of a life is determined by the aspects that go into it, including the causal relationships into which one enters and the causal contributions that one makes. One final example will support this view and put us in a position to apply the present analysis to nonbeneficial pediatric research.

INFANTS AT POLITICAL RALLIES

An infant's parents decide to take their infant to a large public protest aimed at the overthrow of a dictator. The parents have good reason to believe that the number of protestors will be an important factor in determining the success of the rally, and that the presence of children may be especially influential in bringing about the dictator's downfall. In particular, there is reason to believe that the public is willing to tolerate the dictator's continued rule for the remainder of their own lives, but they are unwilling to accept the dictator's rule when reminded of the long life ahead for and the innocence of the infants.

Notice that the level of the infants' engagement in this contribution is very low, to the extent that it qualifies as a purely passive contribution. The infant who attends the political rally in her parent's arms literally has no idea what is going on and does not at that time value the cause in question. Although the child may be a proximate causal factor in the sense that her presence has some influence on a successful outcome, the other factors of causal contribution we have considered—agency, uniqueness, skill, effort—are largely, perhaps wholly, absent. The contribution is one that any child could make, thus uniqueness is very low; no skill is required, nor any effort on the part of the child; and the decision to contribute does not go through the child's agency in any way. Finally, assuming that a massive turnout is needed for success, even the magnitude of the child's individual contribution is very low.

Granting these considerations, the child's presence may have some impact on the outcome, in which case the child would qualify as a contributor to an important political cause. It seems reasonable for parents to take their children to the rally on these grounds, even when the parents could have left the children at home in safety and doing so would not have altered the nature of the contribution that the parents make. The possibility of contributing to such a valuable project seems in the infants' interests and can justify the parents' decision. In the present case, one might be tempted to make an even stronger argument. It is not simply that the parents have the authority to take their children. In some cases at least, it seems that the parents positively should do so.[15]

Imagine that the rally comes at a historic moment, one that is unlikely to return in the children's lifetime. Opportunities are time sensitive and, in these cases, there is no opportunity for the parents to simply play it safe and argue that nothing is lost if the child does not attend the rally. Something may be lost, namely, an opportunity to contribute to a vital cause to the extent that parents who decline to take their child may be positively making a mistake as far as their child's interests are concerned. They have failed to provide their child with what might have been an important and valuable opportunity. History has conspired in such a way that the child is not in a position to make this particular decision for himself. The child has the opportunity to contribute to possibly overthrowing a dictator. However, this opportunity comes at a time when the child is not able to decide for himself whether to make this contribution. The parents must decide for the child.

Imagine that the parents decide to take the child to the rally, knowing that there is a very small chance of harm to the child. Perhaps this is a march in Stockholm, not Seoul. Would we say along with Ramsey that the parents are abusing the child, making decisions for the child that the parents have no right to make, placing the child at risk for the benefit of an alien cause, and thus using the child as a mere means? These descriptions seem inapt. Indeed, this seems a reasonable decision for the parents to make, this rally can be attended, this cause contributed to only at a time when the individual is a child.

Ramsey claims that: "Only if one discovers some medical interest in treatment or research for a particular child, or some grounds in the moral nurture of the child or capacity in the child to give supplementary consent (which Bartholome believes exists at a quite early age) can consent be given to experimental research with the child without doing violence to the deputyship of parents and guardians."[16] This seems right, but the present account suggests that the interests of children need not be limited to their medical and educational interests. Children have interests in contributing to valuable projects, even when they are very young, because such contributions can have positive implications, all things considered, for their overall lives, and it is in our interests to live better overall lives.

In casual conversation we might describe the sense in which these contributions were valuable by claiming that the experiences were valuable for the children themselves. In some cases, this description is literally accurate. In the case of the opera, the children may enjoy the actual experience at the time they were involved. Alternatively, the experience might have been a good one in the way that persevering through adversity can be a good experience, one that teaches important lessons and highlights the value of the contribution and the project by contrast to the difficulty of its attainment. In the case of infants, these uses become metaphorical. We do not mean that the experience itself will be enjoyed or appreciated by the individuals either at the time it occurred or in retrospect. Here our citation of the experience provides a somewhat crude mechanism for referring to the contribution itself, not the way the child felt or experienced the contribution, but the fact that the child made a contribution to a valuable cause. The contribution was a good thing for the child because it was a good thing for the child's life overall. We appeal to these indirect ways of referring to the contribution itself because we rarely focus on the nature of our causal contributions independent of what they say about us as autonomous agents. We do not focus on them because we primarily are concerned, for good reason, with the way in which agents should lead their lives. And this focus influences the vocabulary we have available for describing the importance of our causal contributions.

The claim that participating in the political rally can be in the children's interests is independent of any chance that the child might personally learn from or later come to embrace the contribution. Of course, embracing the contributions that one makes as a child can enhance the value of making the contributions for one's life. But, as we have seen, doing so does not determine that the contribution has value for one's life. The fact of making valuable contributions is itself, all things considered, in our interests. We can confirm this conclusion by evaluating it from the three perspectives on overall lives.

From the first-person perspective, it seems plausible that, all things considered, we would prefer a life that includes contributing to the overthrow of a malign dictator to the same life without this contribution. Imagine that you are watching the video of your very early life and come to the point at which your parents are deciding whether to take you as an infant to the political rally or leave you safely at home with a relative. Imagine you know that those who went to the rally ended up playing a vital role in the dictator's downfall, and that even infants could make a difference, perhaps a significant difference. Given that knowledge, it seems likely that one would hope that one's parents take one along to the rally. All things being equal, one's life is better for making such a contribution. Or, imagine that Irmgard Hunt is watching a video of her younger self sitting on Hitler's lap while the official photographer snaps the picture. Or, Alex Kurzem is watching a video of the making of the Nazi propaganda film, with his younger self standing there in his crisp uniform. From what they tell us, it seems clear that it would be a great relief for them to notice that the camera is not working. Definitive proof that they did not make this passive contribution has implications for their lives, and for them.

From the second-person perspective, these conclusions seem plausible as well. Presumably, we would hope for the sake of those for whom we care that they contribute to the overthrow of a vicious dictator rather than not. And, from a third-person perspective, a life that includes such an important contribution seems preferable to the same life absent that contribution. Being part of the process that brings down the dictator becomes part of the narrative of the lives of only those who were present and enhances the lives of only those individuals (at least directly). That life is better, preferable, to the same life absent the contribution, even though the contribution must be made when the individual is an infant.

We have seen that contributions to valuable projects independent of our will can cast positive light on our lives, similar to the way in which contributions to negative projects independent of our will can cast a shadow over our lives. The value for the contributors' overall lives of making a contribution to overthrowing the dictator does not depend on its political nature. It depends on their making the contribution, on their being part of the causal process and on the project being a valuable one. The same point then can apply to valuable nonbeneficial pediatric research studies. This conclusion provides support for and helps to explain the intuitions regarding the children who contributed to the rotavirus vaccine studies.

These contributions in no way influenced the children as moral agents, how they acted or how they thought about themselves or their lives. Nonetheless, there is a sense in which the children's lives are better for having made this contribution, compared to the same lives absent the contribution. We could imagine, for instance, parents preferring, for their children's sakes, that their children make these contributions. This attitude reflects the fact that being part of the causal process that leads to a valuable outcome involves an individual making a contribution to that outcome. And making positive contributions to valuable projects has positive implications for the contributor's life; by influencing or changing the world, our lives are influenced and changed. The narrative of our lives now includes the fact of our having made a positive contribution, yielding a preferable life narrative overall.

The Calamitous Discovery

Even those willing to grant the individual steps in the argument to this point might object that we nonetheless have arrived at a counterintuitive and perhaps even implausible conclusion, namely, that making contributions, including passive ones, to valuable projects can be in one's overall interests, even when one does not experience the result and does not personally value it. This conclusion contradicts intuitions that put autonomous individuals in control of determining what is in their own interests. The fact that we have such intuitions does not, however, establish that the present claim is false. Our intuitions, including those regarding what is and is not in our interests, are the product of a complex process that includes our personal, social, cultural, and religious histories, our cognitive development, and the place in the world and the time in history at which we find ourselves.

This history does not imply that we should ignore our intuitions when evaluating the plausibility of various claims and theories regarding what is in our interests. It does, however, provide good reason to think that no general account will be consistent with every relevant intuition we have regarding our interests. Our histories are too complex and themselves include competing and conflicting guidance on how we should live our lives. It is unlikely, to say the least, that our intuitions, which are the product of this history, will all be consistent and neatly point to one unifying theory of our interests. Recognizing this problem, one approach to evaluating conclusions based on a series of arguments, each of which is defended in part by appeal to various intuitions, is to consider the general plausibility of the final view. To what does the view commit us?

We have come to the claim that making even passive contributions to valuable projects can be in individuals' interests in at least three ways. These contributions can be indirectly in individuals' interests to the extent that they later come to embrace the contributions and make them part of a better life narrative for themselves. These contributions also can represent valuable human achievements and provide one way for individuals to engage in meaningful relationships. This view seems implausible because purely passive contributions fail to satisfy some plausible conditions on what is required for it to be the case that an individual's making a contribution promotes her interests. Infants, to take the clearest example, do not understand the value of the project in question (e.g., overthrowing the dictator); they do not realize that they are making a contribution to the project, they do not value making the contribution at the time they make it, and their making the contribution does not affect them in any way.

To evaluate this concern, it is important to be clear on the relevance of these subjective factors, factors that concern the individual's relationship to the project in question, for determining whether a given contribution promotes an individual's interests. As we have seen, these factors do not influence whether the project itself is valuable. The fact that infants do not recognize the value of a given research project and are not in a position to embrace its value at the time has no bearing on whether the project itself is valuable. Similarly, these factors do not influence whether the infants are part of the causal process that leads to the study results. The infants in the rotavirus studies made a causal contribution to the study—determined by the fact that the infants were an important part of the causal antecedents to the results—even though they did not realize they were doing so, at least at the time.

Although these factors do not influence the value of the project or the fact that the infants made a causal contribution to it, they do seem relevant to determining whether, in effect, the infants get credit for making the contributions. Again, we need to be clear here. The infants do not get any credit at the level of moral agency or persons. We do not praise them for making these contributions. Instead, the question is whether the causal contributions make for a better life overall for the infants, and whether it is good *for them* to have a better life in this way. Given the causal facts, these contributions are part of a complete description of the infants' lives. A complete description would include the fact that they went to the rally or participated in the study, and their involvement contributed to the overthrow of the dictator or the development of a vaccine. Still, one might object that such contributions do not influence how we evaluate the infants' lives, given their lack of awareness and understanding, and the fact that the experience does not affect them or affects them in a negative way (the political rally does not affect them at all; undergoing procedures as part of a nonbeneficial pediatric research affects them in a negative way).

Two possibilities exist here. First, it might be correct that purely passive contributions say nothing about an individual's overall life. Second, it might be that purely passive contributions say very little about an individual's overall life, and the emphasis on autonomy leads us to essentially ignore such contributions when developing a philosophical account of a valuable life. With these options in mind, consider the following example.

THE CALAMITOUS DISCOVERY

Imagine we discover in the year 2100 that, for the previous 100 years, human beings have been a critical part of the causal antecedents that led to the deaths of millions of sentient, self-conscious, and autonomous beings whose interests are very much like our own (some might put this point by stating that the beings have moral status that is roughly equivalent to our own).

We could fill this example out in different ways that would have very different consequences for how we would judge ourselves and our lives in response to the discovery. If we knew we were having this impact and even were killing these beings intentionally for a minor and avoidable cause—perhaps we were unwilling to take the few steps necessary to avoid destroying them—the judgment on us and our lives would be harsh indeed. We did something horrific and our lives were, at least in that respect, horrific as well. As we alter the facts, this judgment would become progressively less harsh. Imagine that we did not know the beings were self-conscious; we could easily have done the requisite experiments to find out, but declined to do so for no very good reason. Here, the judgment would be harsh, but perhaps not so harsh as formerly.

If we continue to strip away the extent to which these actions went through our agency, we would come to the point at which they in no way reflected negatively on our agency, on us as moral agents. Imagine that we did not know we were stepping on any sentient beings at all; that given the state of technology at the time, we could not possibly have known—perhaps the beings are microscopic and there was no evidence that they existed (to make the example even more passive we might imagine that the beings died as the result of light reflecting off us when we wore a specific color clothing). Finally, imagine that we could not be faulted for the comparatively impoverished state of our technology. I take it that a possible description exists along these lines under which we would conclude that our involvement in the causal process leading to the deaths of all these beings in no way reflects badly on us as moral agents. It was a tragic and unfortunate accident.

The vital question, then, is whether the same description, the one which leads us to absolve ourselves morally, would lead us to conclude that the fact of our being causally involved in the deaths of millions of beings with interests much like our own says nothing about our lives overall. Or, that it does, but that fact is not relevant to us, to our own interests? Would we, for example, be indifferent, for our own sakes, between that life and the same life without being involved in so much death? Imagine that an insignificant change in our lives could have resulted in our avoiding being part of this process. Looking back, would we be indifferent, for our own sakes, between the imagined life versus the alternative of the same life with an insignificant alteration that would have taken us out of the causal process and saved all these beings?

We would likely disagree on the extent to which these facts color our overall lives. One might regard these facts as a terrible blight, others might regard them as unfortunate and tragic for the beings who died, but as merely a shadow rather than a blight as far as the evaluation of our own lives is concerned. Recognizing room for disagreement, it seems clear that we would prefer, *for ourselves,* the life that did not include being involved in bringing about the deaths of all these individuals with interests much like our own (or: significant moral status). Notice that this conclusion stands even though we did not know at the time and could not have known the contributions we were making. In this case, the causal facts, our being part of the causal process that led to these deaths, seems sufficient for it to be part of our lives and for it to reflect, to some extent, on a full and proper evaluation of our lives.

The calamitous discovery case offers a negative example of the fact that we have an interest in meaningful relationships. It is in the interests of adults at least to be involved in meaningful projects and to avoid being involved in projects with negative value, even when the involvement is limited to having an unknowing causal role in bringing about a negative outcome. To consider whether the same conclusion applies to children who participate in nonbeneficial pediatric research, we need to evaluate the relevance of at least two differences between the causal contributions made in the two cases. First, the calamitous discovery case involves contributing to a negative cause, whereas nonbeneficial pediatric research involves contributing to a valuable cause. Since we considered the normative asymmetry objection previously, I will not rehearse those arguments here. The fact that the project in question is positive or negative does not change the fact that one made a causal contribution to it that becomes part of one's life.

The normative difference between the two contributions does seem relevant to a second difference between the two cases. In the calamitous discovery case, we are simply going about our lives and, in effect, killing morally significant beings without any knowledge or intention. In the case of nonbeneficial pediatric research, the infants similarly are making the contributions without any knowledge or intention. However, in this case, others, the children's parents and the investigators, are deciding for the children that they will make this contribution. The adults here are acting with knowledge and intention.

Recognizing this difference, one might argue, consistent with Ramsey's view, that parents do not have the right to decide the causes to which their children contribute. Instead, to the extent possible, the parents should rear their children to be competent adults who can make these decisions for themselves. One might assume that the normative difference between making contributions to negative and valuable projects gains traction here. Presumably, parents should protect their children from making contributions as infants to negative, even horrific projects. Parents should prevent their young children from killing beings with interests like ours. Imagine parents caught in a philosopher's nightmare and faced with the choice of either their infant being part of the causal process that leads to the deaths of a number of persons, or the exact same number of deaths occurring as the result of a tornado. Parents who are indifferent between these options, *for the sake of their infants,* do not understand the nature of their infants' interests.

While this seems right, it might be the case because the contribution in question involves a relationship to a horrible project our outcome. One might assume that we would have a different view of whether the parents should prefer the option that involves the infants contributing to a positive project. Perhaps this is not a decision that parents should make. Or, perhaps, if the parents make the decision to have their infants contribute to a valuable project that decision promotes the parents' interests, but the resulting contribution does not advance the infants' interests. Individuals themselves, we might say, should write the narrative of their own lives. We will consider this view in the next two sections.

The Ubiquity of Competing Considerations

The fact that it is in individuals' interests in general to contribute to valuable projects does not imply that contributing to a particular valuable project necessarily will be in a given child's interests. Hence, this fact does not relieve parents and investigators of the obligation to make a reasonable assessment for the individual child in individual cases. The decision whether to enroll one's child in a valuable project that poses risks and burdens, whether it is an opera, a political rally, or a nonbeneficial pediatric research study, requires parents to make a risk–benefit assessment with respect to this child's interests. Do the potential benefits to the child justify the risks? This evaluation can be difficult because the potential benefits, like the risks, are uncertain.

We have seen that participation in nonbeneficial pediatric research offers at least three types of potential benefits to participating children. First, children may derive educational benefit from participating in a study. Second, children may come to embrace the contribution as an adult, and the fact of having made the contribution may influence the child's future behavior. Third, making contributions to valuable projects can be in individuals' interests by making for a better or preferable life overall, even when the children do not learn from the experience and do not come to embrace it as an adult. The fact of having made the contribution can be valuable for their lives and valuable for them because one of the things that is in their interests is having a better life overall.

The educational and embracing benefits are subjective in the sense that they depend on the attitude and responses of the individual child. Thus, it may be difficult for a parent to estimate whether their particular child will learn from the experience or will come to embrace it. Thus, absent reasons to think that their child in particular will experience these benefits, the potential that they will be realized can justify only very low risks. The benefit to be gained from contributing to a valuable project is not subjective in this sense; it does not depend, in most cases, on the attitudes of the child in question. The fact of making a contribution to a valuable project can be in the child's interests, even if the child does not learn from it or later come to embrace it (we will come to some possible exceptions in a moment).

For older, autonomous children, there can be value in the attempt to contribute to a valuable project. That attempt says something about the child as a person, even if the project ultimately is fruitless. Since younger children do not make an autonomous decision, the value of their contribution depends largely on the project being valuable. There is something of a risk, given that any given research project may end up having no value. For example, a study that is unable to enroll a sufficient number of subjects may never address the scientific question posed by the study. In addition, many studies end up showing that the intervention in question is not effective or is too toxic. However, even studies that are not successful in the sense of identifying a valuable or potentially valuable intervention nonetheless can have important value. Identifying which approaches do not work often is a vital step in determining which ones do. Thus, parents can be reasonably confident that a well-designed and well-run study will be valuable; hence, contributing to it can be valuable for their child.

The extent to which contributing to a valuable project will be in a child's interests depends on the factors that define the child's contribution. The more factors present and the greater the extent to which they are realized in a given case increases the extent to which making the contribution is in a child's interests. Participation in nonbeneficial research that goes through the child's agency to a greater extent, requires more effort or more skill, increases the extent to which it is in the child's interests, hence, increases the level of risks to which they can justifiably be exposed. Conversely, the fewer factors present, the less the contribution is in the child's interests, the lower the level of risks that can be justified. Passive participation as an infant says little about the child's life, hence, justifies only very low risks.

In addition to these general considerations, parents should have reason to believe that the contribution in question will be in the interests of their child in particular. At a minimum, the contribution should be consistent with a reasonable range of plausible life plans, and there should be no positive and compelling reason to think that this child in particular will not inhabit one of the life plans within that range. The point here is that the (more) objective value of contributing to a valuable project or cause can be negated by the specific values of the individual in question. We saw this possibility previously with respect to the value of close relationships. Having (some) close relationships is objectively part of a (more) valuable human life. The value of these relationships does not require that the individual in question value them. At the same time, this value may be negated by certain goals or life plans. Close relationships may not be in the overall interests of an individual who pursues the life of a cloistered monk.

Parents should not place their child in the opera if they have good reason (*per impossible?*) to believe that the child will grow up to eschew the arts and contributions to them. Parents also must make tradeoffs and recognize opportunity costs. Participating in the opera precludes the child from playing or attending a school event at the time. Thus, it is not enough that the opera is in the child's interests. At a minimum no alternative and mutually exclusive course should be available to the child that would clearly further his interests to a greater degree.

The life plan that the child comes to adopt will be greatly influenced by the culture and society in which he lives. This is not to say that some do not come to reject the values and views of their own society, only that those values and views will shape the child. These values and views can provide the parent with reason for thinking that some life plans are extremely unlikely for the child to inhabit. A possible example here might be reproductive cloning. The fact that many in a given society oppose it provides some reason to think that a given child raised in that society will come to oppose it, and that fact provides reason not to enroll the child in research aimed at developing improved techniques of reproductive cloning.

Finally, parents needs to make the decision not for the average child, but for *their* child, evaluating the likely impact of the experience itself on the child, and evaluating the risks and potential benefits given what they know about their child. Parents who put their morbidly shy children in an opera should not be commended on the grounds that it is in the child's long-term interests. But, here too, complications arise. The parents may reasonably make the determination that this experience will not scare the child, but will help him to overcome his shyness. Reason to believe that this child will eschew the arts provides reason not to enroll him in a valuable opera, yet evidence that participation in the opera may result in the child coming to recognize the value of the arts may provide reason to give it a try.

The courts endorse the need to make a particular evaluation for the child in question in the claim that parents are not free to make martyrs of their children. This suggests that the risks cannot be too great to the child, and parents should not expose the child to risks purely for causes that the parent deems good. Imagine that the political rally involves a project that is particularly important given the values and beliefs of the parents, such that they are willing to face great and grave risks to make this contribution. In this case, it may be that the parents can make the decision to participate themselves (imagine aunts and uncles are ready and willing and able to care for the child), but they cannot take the child to this march, they cannot place the child at serious risk. There may not be other marches, but there will be other important causes, and the parents cannot place the child at serious risk and jeopardize to a serious degree the child's opportunity to make contributions to those projects later in life.

Critics might respond that even a careful evaluation along these lines does not give parents the right to make these decisions for the child. Parents, of course, have the right to make decisions that will further their children's education. However, parents do not have the right to enroll the child in nonbeneficial research on the grounds that contributing to a valuable project with the potential to help others is in the child's interests. Whether one helps others is the sole purview of the individuals themselves, when they become competent adults and can decide for themselves the charitable projects to which they will contribute.

Making Decisions for Children

The fact that participation in nonbeneficial research can be in a child's interests represents a necessary but not a sufficient condition on its acceptability. In addition, it needs to be the case, at least, that parents may enroll their children in such research and that it is appropriate for third parties to be involved in it. A number of commentators argue specifically that it is inappropriate for parents to enroll their children in nonbeneficial research. Paul Ramsey writes:

> When the child is grown he may put away childish things and become a true volunteer. This is the meaning of being a volunteer: that a man enter and establish a consensual relation in some joint venture for medical progress—where before he could not, nor could anyone else, "volunteer" him for submission to unknown possible hazards for the sake of good to come.[17]

And Leonard Glantz has argued:

> When a researcher asks a person to be a research subject, the researcher is asking for a gift. Gifts are made knowingly and voluntarily by one person to another. If the transaction is not knowing and voluntary, it is not a gift. In general, gifts may not be made by surrogates. Faced with the possibility of removing a kidney from an incompetent person to "donate" it to a family member, the court ruled that since guardians cannot make gifts of money or property, they certainly could not make gifts of an organ.[18]

Ramsey is surely correct that, when we choose for someone else, as a parent chooses for a child that he will participate in a clinical research study, that individual is not a volunteer. The infants enrolled in the rotavirus vaccine study did not and could not understand, much less endorse the goals of the study. They did not volunteer, and their contributions cannot be described accurately as gifts they offer others. As we have seen, parents may decide to enroll their children in nonbeneficial research when it offers sufficient potential for educational benefit. We have also seen that this justification likely applies to only a small percentage of all nonbeneficial pediatric research. This fact places greater weight on the possibility that participating in nonbeneficial research can be in children's interests because they may later embrace the contribution and it involves their contributing to a valuable project. However, critics argue that it is inappropriate for parents to make decisions for their children on these grounds. If this argument is correct, it would greatly undermine the present justification for nonbeneficial pediatric research.

Ramsey's and Glantz's objections to nonbeneficial pediatric research seem clear implications of the standard analysis of nonbeneficial research with adults. Leaving aside those types of studies where informed consent might be waived, such as research on medical records, why is it acceptable for investigators to involve competent adults in clinical research studies that conflict with the adults' clinical interests? The standard and, I take it, correct response, is that we allow competent adults to make decisions that affect themselves in this way. Respect for competence has two sides. It requires that we do not force choices on competent individuals against their will, and also that we respect their choices for themselves even when those choices conflict with their own interests, at least to some extent. In these cases, we allow adults to volunteer to help others or make a gift to others. It seems to follow that nonbeneficial research is acceptable provided the individuals volunteer or give their participation as a gift. This analysis seems to imply that nonbeneficial pediatric research is unacceptable, at least to the extent that it involves children who are unable to volunteer or provide gifts of this kind. And if it is clearly unacceptable for the children to be enrolled, it is plausible to assume that it is unacceptable for their parents to enroll them.

This analysis is based on the widespread assumption that the ethical justification for enrolling competent adults will be the same as the ethical justification for enrolling children. Thus, making a gift of one's contribution is not merely one way to justify nonbeneficial clinical research, it is the only way. Again, we need to consider the possibility that children's lack of autonomy renders them unable to give consent and also changes the relevant moral considerations. This assumption is tied to a similar one regarding the decision-making of parents.

In medicine, individuals who make decisions for those who are unable to consent are called surrogates. And it is widely argued that surrogates should make decisions based on the *substituted judgment standard*. Essentially this standard envisions surrogates as a kind of medium or channel for the preferences and values of the patient, making the decision that the patient would have made, or the decision that is best supported by the patient's preferences and values.[19] This raises concern with respect to nonbeneficial pediatric research because, by standing in the child's position, it seems that the parent cannot volunteer the child or make a gift on behalf of another, and the child does not have competent preferences and values on which the parent might base a substituted judgment.

Leaving aside the extent to which this common view offers an accurate description of the role of surrogates for adults who have lost the ability to provide informed consent, the role of parents in making decisions for their children is very different. Consider the extent to which furthering one's interests properly figures as a reason for doing the right thing. We typically do not regard the fact that it is in one's interests, to the extent that it is, to contribute to a project to help others as the reason for autonomous adults to make the contribution. The potential to further one's own interests should not, at a minimum, be the primary reason that one helps others.

Imagine someone who contributes to Oxfam and walks little old ladies across the street. When asked why she does these things, the individual replies that doing so is the ethically proper thing to do and she does the ethically proper thing because it redounds to her interests, it implies that she is a better person and has a better life overall. This seems a bad reason and may well be thought to detract from the credit of the contribution. One should contribute to Oxfam because it is the right thing to do or, in a less Kantian state of mind, because others need assistance. One should help little old ladies cross the street because they need to get to the other side and are unable to get there safely on their own.

This feature of practical reason traces to the close connection in most cases between agency and the value of making a contribution for an individual. Because so much of the value of making a contribution ties to individuals' agency we tend to evaluate practical reasons assuming the perspective of an autonomous agent. From this perspective, most of the value of doing the right thing for the agent involves the extent to which it reflects on the individual as a moral agent. When it comes to autonomous agents, there is something unseemly about making valuable contributions because doing so is in one's own interests. At least a good deal of the concern in this case traces to the fact that autonomous agents have available to them and, we hope, recognize the other directed reasons to provide assistance. The focus on their own interests suggests they do not recognize or perhaps do not care about these reasons, thereby turning charity into a kind of enlightened selfishness.

These examples illustrate the complex relationship between the different factors that influence the extent to which a given contribution has implications for an individual's life overall. Exerting more effort when making a contribution to a valuable project typically implies that the contribution has greater value for one's life. However, imagine that the individual makes this contribution only to impress someone in an unseemly way. The greater the effort in that case, the more the individual works at impressing others in an unseemly way, the more we tend to judge them negatively.

Parents are in a very different position with respect to their children. Although an autonomous individual should not decide to help others primarily in order to improve his own life, parents can and should make decisions for their children based on which options will improve the child's life overall. This clarifies one way in which parents do not simply stand in their children's shoes when making decisions for them. The fact that parents are making decisions for someone else, for their child in particular, changes the considerations relevant to making those decisions. Unlike autonomous agents, it is entirely proper for parents to decide whether their child will contribute to a given project based on whether doing so is in the child's interests, including the interest they have in helping others. Thus, parents can make this decision because it promotes the child's biological needs, results in pleasant experiences for the child, or teaches the child a valuable lesson that will help him in the future. The parent also can make this decision because it has the potential to make for a better life for the child, in a way that promotes the child's interest in living a better life overall.

Granting that parents should make decisions for their children based (largely) on their children's interests, one might argue, to recall a previous claim, that parental decision making is restricted in this sense. The obligations of a parent are to protect the child from harm and to help develop in the child those abilities he needs to lead a valuable life overall and decide *for himself* what kind of life he will lead. The parent does not have the right to make positive decisions regarding the kinds of contributions the child will or will not make. That is a decision for the individual to make when he becomes an adult, able to make such decisions for himself. Parental decision making should be limited to furthering the more basic interests of the child.

Against this view, it seems clear that parents are empowered to make decisions to further their children's broader interests, at least until the children can make these decisions for themselves. One reason for this is that having certain experiences and making certain contributions that are valuable for the individual are time sensitive. Some experiences can be had, some contributions can be made, only when the individual is not able to decide for himself. This broader role is evident in parental decisions to introduce their infants to important and famous persons. Parents often go to great lengths to have the infant or toddler meet the president or a movie star. It might be that the parent thinks meeting famous people will bring the child some good luck and in that sense might be in the infant's long-term interests. But parents need not make this assumption to justify so acting. The parent may take the view that a life that includes meeting the president is to be preferred for the child to a life which does not include this experience. We might debate whether the experience of meeting the president as an infant is in an individual's interests in the sense of leading to a preferable life for him. But, leaving aside what one would recommend in this example, it seems clear that this is an appropriate basis for parental decisions; the betterment of a child's overall life provides a reason for parents to choose certain options for their children.

Despite the present argument, it seems counterintuitive to some extent to claim that it is good for children to be enrolled in clinical research that conflicts with their clinical interests. Part of the concern traces to the fact that, in making this claim, one seems to be making a claim about the reasons to enroll children in such research, or even the reasons to conduct such research in the first place. To see this, contrast the present claim regarding children's interests with a claim that it is in children's interests to play on the playground. In that case, the goodness for the children provides a reason to build playgrounds and a reason to take children to them. In contrast, the reason to conduct nonbeneficial pediatric research, and the reason to enroll specific children in such research, is that it offers the potential to improve health and well-being for other, typically future children. If this potential were not present, we should not conduct such research.

The sense in which it is in the interests of individual children to participate in such research depends on its having this potential to benefit other children. This potential makes the research an important project and offers participating children the opportunity to contribute to an important project (an opportunity that is rare for very young children). The point here is that one can ask from different perspectives for the justification of conducting nonbeneficial research with children. From the perspective of society and the perspective of individual investigators, the reason to conduct the research is the potential to benefit other children. At the same time, this potential makes it possible that participation is in children's interests and, thereby, provides parents with a reason to enroll them.

The Value of Making a Contribution

The present chapter has focused on the extent to which the contributions children make to valuable research projects can be in their interests in the sense that a life which includes the contribution is to be preferred, not just in some objective, abstract way, but is to be preferred for the sake of the individual whose life it is. We have seen that this claim is consistent with the judgments we make regarding the rearing and treatment of children in other contexts in which the possibility of making a contribution to worthwhile causes can justify parents exposing young children, even infants, to some risks and burdens.

This consistency supports the claim that the value of contributing to important projects can justify enrolling children in nonbeneficial research;

this is not an ad hoc justification of nonbeneficial pediatric research alone. Rather, this justification follows from the application of a more general view on the acceptable treatment of children in this specific context. Recognizing this support, an argument implying that causal contributions that do not go through one's agency can possibly promote one's interests only if one is a child would cast some doubt on the view in general, raising suspicion that this justification serves as more of a rationale for how adults want to treat children than an account of how children ought to be treated. A finding that this type of contribution can also influence our evaluation of the lives of competent adults would, in contrast, lend further support to this account.

To consider an example from clinical research, one methodology for studying drug abuse and drug treatment involves individuals being randomized, in a double-blind design, to receive injections of a drug or placebo, for instance, alcohol or saline solution. The individuals are then asked to perform a series of motor tasks, such as responding to cues on a computer. This research paradigm can be exploited to conduct other types of research that rely on the presence of individuals who have been exposed to drugs. For example, this research paradigm can be of interest to employers who want to improve their ability to detect employees who are under the influence of alcohol. Imagine investigators place a one-way mirror in the side of the clinic where the alcohol testing is being conducted. While the motor response tests are ongoing, security guards from the company are placed on the other side of the mirror and given the opportunity to test and practice their ability to identify individuals who are under the influence of alcohol by learning to distinguish the individuals in the experimental clinic who were randomized to alcohol from those randomized to placebo.

One might assume that no reason exists to obtain adult subjects' informed consent for these supplementary detection studies. The security guards are not interacting with the research subjects, and the presence of the guards and the secondary study does not in any way influence the research subjects; it does not change what they are asked to do, and it does not increase the risks of what they are doing. Indeed, the secondary study is set up in such a way that the research subjects will never even know that it occurred. To make this clear, imagine that the investigators agree that the secondary study will never be written up or reported. It will only be used by the company for training purposes (perhaps employment in the company requires background training unavailable to the research participants, such that there is no chance they could work for the company). These cases are effectively observational studies in which the individuals are not making an active contribution to the secondary study. Their actions are the same whether the secondary study takes place or not.

Thus, if one takes the view that research contributions are relevant to an individual only when they have some experiential impact on her or goes through her will it seems to follow that no reason exists to ask for consent in these cases. Is this the right conclusion?

With the secondary study in place, the research subjects are contributing to training industry employees to be better able to detect individuals at work who are under the influence of alcohol. They are making this contribution in a causal sense, even though the study does not affect them personally and they may never know that it occurs. This factor provides a reason to ask them whether they want to make this contribution. The individuals may not want to be part of this study and may even object to the premise of improving the ability of employers to detect employees who are using alcohol.

This is not enough of an argument to establish that the individuals' consent *should* be solicited and conclude that the study would be unethical without specific consent for this secondary study. Making that argument would require further analysis regarding how important it is for individuals to control whether they make this contribution. How much of an impact does this study have on the individuals' interests? For present purposes, we need not answer that question. Rather, the point is that it makes sense to ask this question and at least one reason exists to solicit their consent, despite the absence of impact on, or risks to them. They are making this contribution in a causal sense, and that sense alone has some implications for their lives. The fact that this is a relevant consideration highlights the relevance of physical contributions to research projects in cases other than those with children.

One might try to resist this conclusion by arguing that the reasons why we should solicit consent for the secondary study do not trace to the possibility that these individuals are making a contribution to it that is relevant to their own interests. One might instead claim that it is just a matter of respect for these individuals. They are able to decide, so they should be allowed to decide. The problem with this response is that it provides no reason to think that we should solicit individuals' consent for this study in particular. To take an extreme example, we do not ask the consent of some individuals to conduct a study that enrolls others and has nothing to do with them. We solicit individuals' consent for studies relevant to them, in particular, studies that may have an impact on their interests. In this way, the plausibility of the claim that we have reason to solicit the consent of these individuals provides support for the current thesis that making such contributions can have an impact on individuals' interests.

Another situation in which individuals make purely causal contributions to a research study involves research with stored biological samples. Empirical data on individuals' views on research using stored biological samples suggests that individuals themselves care about these types of causal contributions. Over the past 20 years, a dramatic increase has occurred in the scientific interest in human biological samples, including blood, tissue, and DNA. Many research studies now routinely obtain biological samples from individuals and store them for future research purposes. For a long time, hospitals also have routinely stored leftover biological samples. For example, hospitals routinely store leftover surgical samples obtained from individuals with cancer. Historically, these samples have been stored for reasons related to the individual's medical care. They can be useful if questions arise about an individual's diagnosis, or in cases where the original sample sent for analysis is lost.

With the development of advanced genetic and biological techniques, these samples have gained enormous scientific value, and researchers have been asking the institutions where the samples are stored to make them available for research purposes. One could argue and, indeed, a number of commentators and organizations have argued, that there is no need to consider or appeal to the preferences of the individuals from whom the samples were obtained, and this is thought to be especially clear in cases in which the samples were simply leftover after a clinically indicated procedure. This analysis makes sense. Imagine that an individual comes in for a clinically indicated procedure to remove a tumor. The tumor is removed, part of it is sent for clinical analysis to determine the type of tumor, and the remainder is stored in the hospital freezers. A year later, an investigator with an interest in the nature of such tumors comes along and requests access to this individual's tumor sample, but agrees that the sample will be stripped of any personal identifiers before it is handed over. Any subsequent research done on this sample will pose no risks at all to the source individual. For example, the investigator will leave plenty of tissue behind for any future clinical needs.

The sample is out of the patient's body and stored, and it will be stripped of any identifiers, so there is no possibility of confidentiality risks or of the researcher even learning the identity of the source of the sample. Finally, imagine that the research does not even pose a chance of harm (e.g., risk of stigma) to any groups to which the individual belongs. Granting all of this, the individuals nonetheless are (minimally) causally contributing to this future research and that fact seems to provide at least one reason (although not necessarily a determinative reason) to allow them to decide whether they make this contribution. The reason again is not that the research poses any risks to these individuals or even asks anything additional of them, but simply that the proposed research involves these individuals contributing to the research in question.

The claim that these causal contributions have relevance for an individual's life is supported by empirical data.[20] The vast majority of individuals surveyed are willing to have their biological samples used for research purposes. At the same time, the vast majority feel strongly that they should be asked and be able to decide whether their samples are used for research purposes, and a small minority do not want their samples to be so used. These views are relatively constant even when one removes many of the facts that might be thought relevant to the individuals' interests. For example, these views are consistent even when the research involves leftover samples and samples that have been stripped of the individual's personal identifiers to the extent that there is no way to trace back from the sample to the individual's identity. Despite these measures, many individuals still want to control the use of their samples and want to be able to decide the purposes for which they are used.

These data suggest that individuals do not regard the use of their leftover samples as completely foreign to them. Instead, they want to have a say in whether the samples are used for research, and many of them do not want the samples used for projects to which they are opposed, such as cloning. The claim here is not simply that they do not want any samples taken from anyone used for such research. They may have that view as well. But here they feel they are making a contribution to the research when it is their samples that are being used. These data suggest two points of relevance. First, individuals do feel that the projects to which they contribute have implications for them. Second, at least for many individuals, the sense of what counts as their making a contribution is very broad, covering not only the things that they do as autonomous agents, but also the purely causal relationships into which they enter or are entered. This includes the causal impact that they have on the world via biological samples taken from them.

These examples and attitudes support the present claim that the causal relationships into which an individual enters as part of a research project are relevant to that individual's overall life, even when they do not affect the individual at all, nor go through the individual's agency in any meaningful sense, such that what remains is the bare fact of making a causal contribution. This possibility highlights in a particular way the relevance of the physical body to research. Often, the fact that clinical research impinges on and violates the body is taken as a cardinal sign of its wrongness, especially with respect to nonbeneficial research with children who cannot consent. In the words of Leonard Glantz, one of the more astute skeptics of nonbeneficial pediatric research: "It is the class of [nonbeneficial] research that involves children's bodies being invaded with drugs or devices that is the true cause of concern."[21]

Invasions of the body do have special significance and raise the level of concern around nonbeneficial pediatric research. At the same time, the interactions with an individual's body, even viewing him through a one-way mirror or using his leftover, anonymous tissue samples, brings the individual into the causal nexus of the research project and, in that way, potentially has implications for the individual's life overall. This factor goes beyond what are properly thought of as bodily invasions, such as needle sticks, and reveals that this role of the body can be both problematic and also beneficial, depending on the nature of the study and the nature of the individuals who make contributions to the study. Interacting with children as physical beings in the research setting can lead to exploitation, but it also can lead to promotion of their interests given the interest they have in contributing to worthwhile projects.

One might object that the present argument relies on data from individuals who are simply confused regarding what is in their interests. The use of biological samples can pose risks to individuals in a number of ways. It can possibly lead to information about them that they are better off not knowing. It can lead to others having information about the individuals (e.g., they have a gene that puts them at risk for Alzheimer disease) that could undermine their ability to get a job or obtain health care insurance. In contrast, the mere use of the samples, when it does not affect these individuals personally, is not relevant to their interests. Merely making this kind of contribution says nothing about these individuals' interests.

It is important here to recognize the limitations of any arguments regarding what is, and what is not in our interests. There are no knockdown arguments here, but only arguments that rely on plausibility, given what we know about ourselves and our lives, and what we regard as important for us. This point is underscored by the fact that one can always question claims regarding what is in our interests by asking why we should care about the thing in question. Why, for example, should we care about our own experiences? Or, why should we care about achieving our own ends or satisfying our own experiences? The fact that these questions make sense does not imply that the view of our interests thereby questioned is problematic. At some point, the proper response to the skeptic is to ignore rather than engage him. Another way to put this point is in terms of the limitations of "open question" type arguments with regard to our interests. It is to some extent an open question whether individuals do and should care about their experiences. But this is not a reason to think that we should stop caring about our experiences or the experiences of others. The best we can do in trying to determine what is in our interests is to develop the account of what matters for us based on what makes the most sense to us.

Data that many individuals regard something, say contributing to a given research study through the provision of biological samples, as relevant to their interests does not imply that it is relevant. But, we have no other sources for determining our interests than what we think is in our interests. Absent some reason to think the individuals from whom the data were obtained are mistaken or confused, or some reason to think that we simply know better than they do, the fact that they have these views provides some reason to think that these things can be relevant to our interests. This is especially relevant when the view is widely held across many people, in many places and different times. The fact that their views conflict with the account of interests that we accept shows only that they or our account is wrong. We need some reason independent of that conflict to reject their views and what they imply regarding the nature of our interests.

The claim that purely physical contributions that do not go through an individual's will can nonetheless have implications for the individual's life is consistent with a broader perspective on the relevance of causal contributions to our lives. The causal contributions we make can have implications, good or ill, for our lives, and in turn for us, even when we do not know they are occurring and are not in any way responsible for their occurring. This finding is consistent with our views on contributions made by adults and is supported by empirical data on competent adults' own views of the causal contributions they make. To this point, we have seen that this possibility provides a general justification for nonbeneficial pediatric research, one that is not dependent on the children being of an age at which they can learn from their participation or the possibility that the children will later come to embrace their contribution. The risks of nonbeneficial pediatric research can be justified by the fact that contributing to worthwhile projects is in the interests of the children who participate. The next chapter considers in more detail the implications of this justification for nonbeneficial pediatric research and how it ought to be conducted.

EIGHT | Implications

Limits on the Personal Value of Passive Contributions

In standard cases, making a contribution to at least some valuable projects is in the overall interests of the individual who makes the contribution. This is suggested by the fact that we regard as preferable and prefer for those for whom we care, a life that includes making contributions to valuable projects. Of course, our evaluation of the contributions individuals make, what they imply about them and their lives, and the significance of these implications, is strongly influenced by how the contribution fits into their overall life, into their goals, plans, and projects, not to mention the manner in which they contributed to the project or relationship in question. Autonomous adults typically are in a position to make *active* contributions to valuable projects. They are in a position to recognize the importance of the project and to contribute to it intentionally and diligently. Given this possibility, we tend not to regard as valuable passive contributions made by competent adults, and we may even regard these contributions in a negative light, implying that the individual could have, but did not actively embrace the cause or the contribution in question. Here, as elsewhere, our normative evaluations depend on the options available to the agent in question. A full evaluation of the normative status of what an agent did often depends on knowing what the agent could have done otherwise.

Part of taking seriously the fact that children are not autonomous involves refraining from evaluating the contributions they make against the same background or contrast class. Infants and young children do not have available to them the option of making an autonomous decision to contribute to important causes and projects. For them, the challenge is not to determine the value of making a passive contribution as opposed to an active one; the challenge is to determine the value of making a passive contribution as opposed to making no contribution at all. This is the challenge posed by nonbeneficial pediatric research with infants and young children. I have argued that making a contribution to an important pediatric study can be in the interests of infants and young children, in at least two ways. A life that includes contributing to the development of a rotavirus vaccine is preferable to the same life absent that contribution. This is true even though active contributions tend to be preferable to passive ones. When one cannot make an active contribution to a worthwhile cause, end, or relationship, a passive one may be better than no contribution at all.

Individuals who make passive contributions to valuable causes also may come to embrace those contributions as adults. They may come to regard the contribution as a valuable, even if minor aspect of their lives. Passive contributions so embraced may then amplify in personal significance in a number of ways. The individual may come to regard the passive contribution as an important chapter in their lives, and this attitude may in turn influence in positive ways the future course of the individual's life. This possibility involves an implicit rejection of Parfit's advice to regard the psychologically distant and disconnected parts of our lives as effectively those of a different person. As we have seen, one can be inspired by the doings and examples of others, including the first grade teacher, Ann, who inspires her students to do good things with their lives. But one can embrace only those contributions that one made personally.

This conclusion highlights an important limitation of Parfit's account. That account of our lives and our interests can be understood as being motivated by the desire to minimize the prudential reasons for an excessive regard for the interests of oneself to the exclusion of others. The view that one effectively will not be the same person in 20 years decreases the prudential reasons to focus on one's own future interests (e.g. by hoarding one's money for one's future self) and, hopefully, increases the extent to which one is motivated to help others in the here and now. This view may decrease selfishness by decreasing the extent to which we assume that furthering our own interests involving improving our personal lot over time to the exclusion of others.

The present analysis suggests an alternative possibility. Concern about the nature of our lives over time may reduce the prudential force of selfish concerns by increasing the extent to which we attempt to lead a better life, one that includes contributions to worthwhile causes and relationships. While this possibility alone does not provide a conclusive response to Parfit's challenge, it does underscore the point made previously that the metaphysical facts cited by Parfit, even if one accepts them, do not necessarily lead to the normative conclusions he endorses.

The extent to which contributions to a valuable project are in an individual's interests depends on the nature of the contribution in question. It depends on at least the magnitude of the individual's contribution relative to the valuable outcome, the extent to which the contribution engages or goes through the individual's agency, the level of skill involved in making the contribution, the degree of effort, and the extent to which the contribution is unique to the individual. We also saw that the value of the project itself influences the extent to which the contribution has personal significance for the contributor; all things being equal, better to contribute to a more valuable project than a less valuable one.

Passive contributions *are* contributions and, as such, can have implications for how we evaluate the contributor's life. At the same time, purely passive contributions alone have only minor implications for an individual's overall life; they contribute only a very minor thread to the narrative of the contributor's life.[1] In addition, it seems plausible to assume that the possibility of one's embracing a previous contribution and the significance that doing so plays in an individual's life will track the same factors which determine the personal significance of a given contribution for one's overall interests. One is more likely to later embrace a contribution of greater magnitude, as well as contributions that involved greater skill and a higher degree of personal uniqueness.

To appreciate the implications of this analysis for nonbeneficial pediatric research it is important to note that passive contributions say little about the contributor's life even when she contributes to a project of tremendous value. The lives of the infants who were involved in the rotavirus vaccine studies are somewhat better overall because they contributed to this important project. In effect, the fact that the contribution was passive places a significant discount rate on the extent to which making the contribution has implications for the children's lives. It is for this reason that even contributions to valuable projects say very little about the contributor's lives, although they have some implications and greater implications than contributions to lesser projects. These implications may be increased if the individual later comes to embrace the contribution in question. And this possibility, factored by the likelihood of its being realized, provides additional reason for parents to have their young children contribute to valuable projects, including nonbeneficial research studies.

Parents have very little, if any, evidence regarding whether their young children will later come to embrace a contribution. At the time the decision must be made, the child's nature will be insufficiently developed to provide the basis for confident predictions in this regard. This is one aspect of the present analysis that would benefit from empirical research. Follow-up of individuals who participated in clinical research studies as young children could provide data on whether these contributions in fact are embraced later in life, as well as data on the aspects of the study and the contribution that influence this, or influence how strongly the contributions are embraced.

The magnitude, uniqueness, and amount of effort that characterizes children's contributions to a given nonbeneficial pediatric research are largely fixed by the scientific needs and goals of the study. The nature of the study as described in the study plan or protocol, determines how much effort is required from a given child, how much others contribute, and the extent to which the child's contribution could have been made by others. The extent to which the involvement engages the participants' agency, in contrast, can be influenced, in some cases at least, by means of subject selection, by altering who is enrolled in the study. Investigators can increase the personal significance of the contributions children make to a given research study by enrolling older children who can understand and perhaps even make their own decisions, as opposed to enrolling younger children. A study that enrolls very young children does not allow for the contributions they make to the study to go through their agency. The same study conducted with teenagers will involve contributions that can go through the participants' agency and, thereby, represent contributions of greater personal significance (assuming the children understand and agree to enroll). In addition, investigators can increase the extent to which the contribution engages teenager's agency by involving them to a greater degree in the study, helping them to understand and become active contributors.

A number of commentators have argued that involving children in the research decision-making process offers a way to respect them as individuals.[2] Here we see that enrolling children who can make their own decisions, rather than younger children who cannot, also offers a way to increase the benefits of the research by increasing the personal significance for the children who participate in it. This argument for preferring the enrollment of children who are able to understand and make their own decisions is consistent with the widely accepted principle that it is better to enroll adults in research than older children, and better to enroll older children than younger children. In the words of the Belmont Report: "there is an order of preference in the selection of classes of subjects (e.g., adults before children)."[3] Older children are to be preferred because their increased ability to understand and make decisions allows them to accept the risks and burdens of research participation in a way that is not available to younger children.[4]

As Bartholome notes, the potential for children to benefit from their participation in nonbeneficial research provides a further reason to prefer older to younger children. Bartholome focused on the possibility that children might gain educational benefit, learning to develop a "disposition toward choosing that which is good."[5] Bartholome, in effect, is taking seriously the claim made by the National Commission that the "scope of parental authority includes the right to choose activities and define a manner of life for their children."[6] Bartholome recognizes that children need certain capacities, including the relevant concepts, to be in a position to gain educational benefit from their participation in nonbeneficial research. They need to recognize that they are participating in research and that the research is designed to benefit others.

Expanding our consideration of the ways in which children can benefit to include the significance of making contributions to valuable projects provides a further argument for preferring older children. They can make more active contributions than younger children. Although an individual should not decide to contribute to important projects primarily to gain educational benefit for himself or to thereby have led a better life overall, parents can and should make decisions for their children because they will improve their children's lives overall. This includes the projects to which the child will contribute as a child. Ramsey argues that a "parent's decisive concern is for the care and protection of the child, to whom he owes the highest fiduciary loyalty."[7] However, as we saw previously, the precept that parents should help their children by first protecting them from all risk is counterproductive at best and likely impossible.

Parents should raise their children to have and to lead productive, satisfying, flourishing, and valuable lives and, to that end, parents have to take some risks with their children and allow their children to take risks by being involved in practices and projects that pose risks. The importance of parents providing their children with positive opportunities for growth and development is reflected in the fact that being overly protective of one's children is itself risky. One runs the risk of the children failing to have the experiences, and failing to develop the capacities and abilities, they need for a flourishing life. To learn to walk, children have to run the risk of falling. It is for this reason that trying to protect one's children from all risks is counterproductive.

The present analysis provides two justifications for nonbeneficial pediatric research: contributing to such research can be in the child's interests to the extent that it involves the child making a (passive) contribution to a valuable project, and the child may come to embrace the contribution as an adult. These two possibilities provide sufficient conditions on the ethical acceptability of exposing children to some research risks for the benefit of others, a claim that should not be confused with the very different project of attempting to define the necessary conditions on the acceptability of such research. It may be that alternative accounts also justify the same projects justified here, and these or other accounts may justify some nonbeneficial pediatric research that remains unjustified on the present account. To take one example, I have not and will not consider here the possibility that purely Utilitarian arguments may justify at least some nonbeneficial pediatric research. I also will not consider the possibility that one might justify some nonbeneficial pediatric research by paying the children who participate in it. This leaves open the question of whether there are and, if so, whether one might be able to justify on other grounds, nonbeneficial pediatric research studies in which participation does not contribute to, and might well detract from, the overall lives of the participating children.[8]

As mentioned briefly at the beginning, the present argument may seem ironic to the extent that it relies on the claim that nonbeneficial pediatric research studies can be ethically acceptable because they can be in the interests of the participating children. If this argument is right, it seems to imply that what I have been describing as nonbeneficial research is not nonbeneficial at all. It is in fact beneficial research, at least as far as the children's overall interests are concerned. The apparent inconsistency arises if one regards nonbeneficial research as research that is inconsistent with participating children's interests, all things considered. This inconsistency is resolved once we recognize that the conflicting judgments depend on different interests. Nonbeneficial studies are those that do not provide a compensating potential for clinical benefit. Such studies are not in individuals' medical or clinical interests. But, participation in these studies can promote other interests children have and if the conflict with their clinical interests is not too great, participation can be in their overall interests.[9]

Moral Claims on Third Parties

The claim that it can be within parents' purview to enroll their children in nonbeneficial pediatric research does not imply necessarily that it is acceptable for others to be involved in the research. This does not follow immediately for several reasons. First, the moral claims on third parties, those who are not party to the family relationship in question, may be different. Parents may not be able to make martyrs of their children, as the courts remind us, but parents certainly are allowed to sacrifice in small ways at least the interests of one child for the interests of others, at least others in the same family. In addition, we allow parents, free from state interference (although perhaps not free of state persuasion) to treat their children in ways that are contrary to the child's interests, provided the conflict is not too great. Individuals other than parents have significantly less leeway in how they treat children.

The claims on third parties in the case of clinical research also can be different because these parties play a very different role in the research. The parents decide whether the child can participate in the research, but clinicians expose the children to any risks, administer the drugs, insert the needles.[10] In this way, the clinicians, not the parents, are the proximate causes of the (conditions that pose the) risks the children face. Also, in the cases we are considering, nonbeneficial pediatric research is conducted for the good of society, in the name of others (reminder: we are leaving to the side ethical issues raised by pediatric research conducted for financial benefit). These very different roles place moral claims on the clinicians and society as well. It is not sufficient for these parties to simply defer to the parents on the grounds that if the parents can choose to enroll their children in a given nonbeneficial pediatric research study, the clinicians and society have no additional duties to discharge toward the children.

Because the research is being conducted by clinicians, in the name of society, an obligation exists to evaluate whether the research is appropriate for children; both that nonbeneficial pediatric research in general is appropriate and that a particular study is appropriate before it is conducted and children are exposed to its risks. Although participation in nonbeneficial pediatric research says something about the participants' lives, it says very little about an individual's overall life when the contribution is a relatively passive or purely passive one of the type available to young children and infants. In these cases, the children's interests may justify exposing them to risks and thus justify the involvement of clinicians and society, but the obligation on these parties to ensure that their role is appropriate places on them obligations to exercise due diligence in ensuring that the appropriate requirements have been satisfied and the relevant safeguards are in place, especially an obligation to evaluate whether the study is valuable and the risks sufficiently low. The requirements for independent review and risk limits are almost universally endorsed in writings on and guidelines for pediatric research. The fact that the present analysis is consistent with, and provides theoretical justification for these requirements offers support for it.

The Necessity of Value

Existing regulations on pediatric research focus, quite rightly, on the risks to which children are exposed, especially in the context of nonbeneficial research. One stipulation, which applies to all clinical research, emphasizes the importance of minimizing the risks to which children are exposed. This can be accomplished in a number of ways. Procedures proposed in the research setting sometimes can be replaced by clinical procedures the children are scheduled to or already have undergone. Rather than expose children to a series of extra needle sticks for research purposes, researchers may be able to obtain the blood they need during a clinically indicated needle stick. Rather than expose children to another kidney biopsy, investigators may be able to gather the information they need from a previously, especially if recently performed, clinical biopsy. Even required procedures can be altered to reduce their risks. When possible, researchers should consider a topical anesthetic, such as EMLA cream, to minimize the distress and discomfort of research injections.[11]

Some data suggest that parents are not always reliable guides of what procedures will prove distressing to their children, making it imperative to evaluate the children's own prospective views and actual experiences. One study found that children were much more concerned by evaluation of their sexual maturation (i.e., Tanner staging), which requires undressing in front of research staff, than by invasive procedures; the parents were concerned by the invasive procedures and regarded the evaluation as innocuous.[12] Parents can get things wrong in the other direction as well. My experience has been that children with life-threatening illnesses often enjoy and gain benefit from participating in survey research that involves answering questions about their disease, whereas parents tend to worry that these surveys will frighten or depress their children.

The task of minimizing risks and ensuring that any remaining risks are sufficiently low is so important that one might easily come to the conclusion that it is essentially all that matters from the point of view of protecting children in the context of nonbeneficial pediatric research. If the children are not going to benefit, there is no sense in which one might be able to make the study more beneficial for them, hence, one should focus on minimizing the risks to the greatest extent possible, thus rendering the risk–benefit ratio as least unfavorable as possible. Although this task is obviously important, it is not the only consideration relevant to protecting children in the context of nonbeneficial pediatric research.

Nonbeneficial pediatric research by definition does not offer a compensating potential for clinical benefit. The justification for exposing children to risks comes from the social value of the research or the research procedure. However, those who are involved in nonbeneficial pediatric research typically have been trained to do what is in the child's best interests; many of them are pediatricians and the rest are adults who are subject to a general obligation to protect children and act in their best interests. Given this perspective, an embarrassment often arises due to the fact that the research will benefit others. It is this very feature that raises the potential or, in the views of many, the reality of the exploitation of those children who participate in nonbeneficial pediatric research.[13] One cannot change this reality, but one can try to ignore it, and this, in my experience, is often what occurs in nonbeneficial pediatric research. The fact that a procedure involves research is ignored or downplayed in communication with the child and parents, and the clinicians themselves often push this fact to the back of their minds.

This situation, which has been described as a "collusion of misunderstanding," is not unique to pediatric research.[14] It can arise whenever investigators enroll patients, especially when the patients have live-threatening conditions and the investigators are also physicians who have been trained to treat patients with the very conditions they are studying. Although this reaction is understandable, it has the detrimental consequence of obscuring the social value of the research. Yet, what makes it acceptable to enroll children in nonbeneficial research is its very social value. Contributing to valuable projects is in children's interests because doing so contributes to the children's lives overall, and may represent a contribution which the children later embrace. This suggests that an emphasis on ensuring the social value of the research and increasing it where possible is not in conflict with the interests of the participating children but, in fact, is at the heart of promoting their interests. Ensuring and increasing the social value of the research is a necessary condition on it being acceptable to enroll children. This requirement can be realized in several ways.

First, for it to be acceptable to enroll children in nonbeneficial research it must be the case that the research is valuable. Thus, it is crucial to have in place sufficient mechanisms to ensure that this condition is realized in practice. This is not some secondary or supererogatory moral demand; this requirement is vital to making the research ethical. The determination that the research is ethical, however, does not end the need to be cognizant of its value. Often the conduct of nonbeneficial pediatric research involves a reluctance to make the value explicit, and data reveal that individuals often confuse clinical research with clinical care and even can be unaware that they are participating in research at all.[15] This is problematic for several reasons.

The value for a given individual of making a contribution to a valuable project depends, in part, on the extent to which the contribution is an active one, the individual recognizes the contribution, embraces it, and intentionally works to advance the project in question. Second, the possibility that later in life participants will embrace the contributions they make to clinical research as children—the possibility that this contribution will come to be regarded as a valuable part of their lives and shape their future behavior—requires that the individuals are aware at some point of having made the contribution. Older children cannot become actively involved in a contribution they do not realize they are making. And an individual cannot embrace later in life a contribution he is unaware of having made as a young child. Calling attention to the research aspect of the child's involvement also offers the chance, when possible, for the child to benefit by gaining educational benefit from his research participation. It is essential therefore to minimize risks, but also to ensure and enhance the social value of the research as a way of furthering the interests of the children who participate in it.

The claim that making contributions to valuable projects can be in individuals' interests provides a justification for research that otherwise might seem unethical, such as nonbeneficial research with infants. At the same time, it is important to recognize that this account also may imply that some research that otherwise seems innocuous is unacceptable. In particular, an exclusive focus on the personal goals and experiential interests of the participating children implies that no reason exists to be concerned with research that has little or no effect on the children, especially research that poses essentially no risks to them. On the present view, the absence of physical risks, while important, does not exhaust the normative evaluation of nonbeneficial pediatric research (or research in general for that matter). One needs to ask the further question of whether making the contribution in question is consistent with the individual's interests.

We considered the fact that many individuals oppose efforts to clone human beings and regard such efforts as unethical. If these individuals are correct, and cloning human beings is unethical, contributing to research aimed at developing techniques for human cloning would be contrary to children's interests, even when the research does not pose any risks of physical harm to them. In addition, the fact that many individuals oppose this type of research provides some reason to believe that a given child will come to oppose such research, that contributing to it will be counter to the goals and values the individual develops as an adult, providing further reason not to enroll them in such research as a child.

Minimal Risks and Sliding Scales

It is widely agreed that nonbeneficial pediatric research is acceptable only when the risks are sufficiently low. What is in dispute is the standard that should be used to determine (or what definition should be used to define) what constitutes sufficiently low risks in this context. Many guidelines define acceptably low risks based on the level of risks children face in daily life. Australia's guidelines allow research interventions when "the probability and magnitude of harm or discomfort anticipated in the research are not greater in and of themselves than those ordinarily encountered in daily life."[16] Guidelines from Nepal and the United States combine this definition with the routine examinations standard, defining "minimal" risks as "not greater in and of themselves than those ordinarily encountered in daily life or during the performance of routine physical or psychological examinations or tests."[17–19]

The "risks of daily life" standard suffers, as described in Chapter 3, several, at least theoretical, shortcomings.[20] Many of the activities of daily life are permitted, and their risks accepted, because they offer children the potential for personal benefit. Parents do not allow their children to play basketball because they regard the risks as somehow inherently acceptable; parents accept these risks because they assume their children will benefit from playing and the only way to realize that benefit is to run the attendant risks. It follows that the level of risk we accept in daily life may be inappropriate in the setting of nonbeneficial research. Moreover, the fact that children happen to face a given level of risk in daily life does not mean it is acceptable to expose them to those risks.[21] A prominent article cited earlier claims that the risks of daily life are not just accepted, but are acceptable. However, as Ross and Nelson note, one cannot justify exposing children to risks equivalent to those they face in daily life "simply because these risks are ordinarily encountered."[22] The appropriateness of a given level of risk is not implied by its presence in children's lives. Infants face approximately a 140 in 1 million risk of suffocation per year, which represents almost a 30 times greater risk compared to older children.[23] It does not follow that infants may be enrolled in nonbeneficial pediatric research that poses a similar risk of suffocation and certainly there is no reason to think that it is acceptable to expose infants to a 30 times greater risk of death in nonbeneficial pediatric research compared to older children.

We have seen that enrolling children in nonbeneficial pediatric research can be justified on the grounds that participating in research can be in children's overall interests, in the sense of saying something positive about their overall lives. In principle at least, this view provides a straightforward way to define what counts as acceptable risks in this regard. Risks are justified by the extent to which contributing to the research is in the children's overall interests. This approach will be difficult to implement given the difficulty of determining how much it is an individual's interests to contribute to a given valuable project. How much a given contribution contributes to an individual's interests depends on the five factors of one's engagement with a contribution. These factors, then, provide a rough guide for estimating to what extent a given contribution is in an individual's interests. What is the magnitude of the child's contribution? To what extent, if any, did the contribution go through the child's agency? How much effort did it require? In theory, this variation supports a sliding scale for what constitutes acceptable risks in nonbeneficial pediatric research. The greater participation in a given nonbeneficial pediatric research intervention or study will realize these five factors, the greater the risks that can be justified. This conclusion is consistent with the argument made by a number of commentators to the effect that children who understand more should be allowed to face greater research risks.[24] Ackerman argues that allowing somewhat greater research risks can be "appropriate for older children with mature decision-making capacities."[25]

These claims need to be distinguished from a related claim regarding the relationship between age and risk in pediatric research. Here the claim is that a greater level of risk can be acceptable (e.g., regarded as minimal) in older children who are able to understand and make their own decisions. This view implies that a given level of risk might be acceptable for older children, but unacceptable for infants and toddlers. A different possibility arises because the same procedure may pose different levels of risk in older children versus younger children. For example, some procedures, such as MRI, might cause anxiety in younger children, but not older children who are less liable to be frightened by it.

Consistent with the arguments of a number of commentators, including Ackerman and Nelson cited previously, the present analysis points to at least two standards, roughly corresponding to whether the contributions the children are making are more passive or more active. Infants and very young children are not in a position to understand and endorse their research participation, and therefore make only passive contributions to nonbeneficial pediatric research. Because these passive contributions say very little about the children's overall lives, and assuming that there is a low chance that the individuals will come to regard them as significant parts of their lives, they justify only very low risks. Teenagers, in contrast, are able to understand a good deal about their research participation, and their contributions can be much more active, hence, say more about their overall lives. In addition, it seems plausible to assume that individuals will be more apt to embrace as adults contributions made as children when the contributions were more active ones. It follows that it can be acceptable to expose these children to somewhat greater risks than younger children, yielding two risk standards for nonbeneficial pediatric research.[26]

Exceptional Cases

The U.S. regulations allow institutional review boards (IRBs) to approve nonbeneficial pediatric research when the risks are minimal or only a minor increase over minimal and the research satisfies several additional requirements. In principle, the U.S. regulations also allow children to be enrolled in nonbeneficial research that poses more than a minor increase over minimal risk provided it is approved by the Secretary of the Department of Health and Human Services (45CFR46.407). Specifically, the regulations require that: a) the IRB finds that the research presents a reasonable opportunity to further the understanding, prevention, or alleviation of a serious problem affecting the health or welfare of children; and b) the Secretary, after consultation with a panel of experts in pertinent disciplines and following opportunity for public review and comment, has determined that the research presents a reasonable opportunity to further the understanding, prevention, or alleviation of a serious problem affecting the health or welfare of children, and the research will be conducted in accordance with sound ethical principles.[27]

This 407 category has been used rarely, and little data are available on it, although an effort has been made to make the process more user-friendly.[28] It appears, in practice, that the studies reviewed and approved under this mechanism pose very low risks to the participating children.[29] However, in principle, this category allows the possibility of approving nonbeneficial pediatric research that poses risks greater than a minor increase over minimal, with no explicit limit on the extent of the research risks, thus raising the question of whether nonbeneficial pediatric research that poses high risks might be approved in this category.[30]

One possibility would be to argue that the standards used to regulate the risks of pediatric research (i.e., minimal risk and a minor increase over minimal risk) are not those that strictly define when such research is acceptable. Rather, these standards might represent the kind of necessary compromise between the pertinent ethical principles and applicable practical standards required when developing policies to regulate social practice. Put differently, it might be the case that nonbeneficial pediatric research that poses greater risks can, in principle, be justified. However, adopting standards that explicitly allow such research might run too great a risk of inappropriate studies being approved. The existing risk standards might address this possibility by being defined in such a way as to block the inappropriate studies, recognizing that the same standards will pose an obstacle to some appropriate exceptions. To determine whether or not this might be the case, we need to consider whether exceptional cases exist that do not satisfy the existing risk standards on nonbeneficial pediatric research, yet might be acceptable in some circumstances.

The present analysis suggests at least two possible exceptions. First, it might be acceptable in some cases to allow older children who can understand and make their own decisions to be exposed to greater research risks for the benefit of others compared to younger children who cannot understand. We have considered the possibility of accommodating this difference within the regulatory structure by adopting two different thresholds for what constitutes minimal risk, one threshold for younger children who cannot understand and a somewhat higher threshold for research with older children able to understand. While adoption of two risk thresholds for nonbeneficial pediatric research is supported by the relevant normative considerations, it may be too confusing for review committees to implement in practice. Data, supported by a wealth of anecdotal experience, reveal that review committees often have difficulty implementing one minimal risk standard.[31] Adoption of two minimal risk standards may make things worse, rather than better. An alternative approach would be to use only one minimal risk standard for nonbeneficial pediatric research, but then allow somewhat greater risks in older children who can understand and make their own decisions as exceptional cases, with implementation of this second minimal risk standard taking place at the level of the 407 approval process.

A second possible exception traces to variability in the value of different pediatric research studies. Contributing to a more valuable study can say more about one's overall life and, on those grounds, could justify somewhat greater risks. In principle, this could provide a second factor for the panel to consider, whether the study is an especially valuable one. Here, again, it is important to emphasize that purely passive contributions say little about an overall life, even when the project is very valuable. Thus, even very valuable projects such as the rotavirus vaccine studies might justify greater, but still only relatively low risks. A further complication in this regard is that evaluating the social value of a given study prospectively can be very difficult. Often what social value a study has depends a good deal on the findings of the study. This is determined at the end of the study, but whether the risks are acceptable for children must be determined at the outset. The uncertainty of the ultimate value of any given study places further limitations on the extent to which the opportunity to contribute to it, including studies that might have significant value, can justify higher-risk nonbeneficial pediatric research. Bracketing these complications, it appears that exceptional cases can be justified in which children face somewhat greater risks than those allowed under the risk standards by which IRBs can approve nonbeneficial pediatric research.

Adults and Older Children First

Many guidelines, perhaps most notably the Belmont report in the United States, state that all things being equal it is better to conduct nonbeneficial research with adults than children, and with older children rather than younger children.[32] The primary reason for this in the case of adults and older teenagers is that they are able to understand the research and make their own autonomous decision to enroll, in a way that is not possible for younger children. For the most part, the present account is consistent with this view and provides an additional reason to endorse it.

Making an active contribution says more about an individual's overall life, and making a more active contribution says more than making a less active one. This implies that, all things being equal, it is better to enroll those who are able to make a more active contribution. Since the extent to which a contribution is active traces largely to the extent to which it goes through the individual's agency, the present consideration provides a further reason for preferring adults who can make fully active contributions and teenagers rather than younger children. With that said, the present account also provides a tempering consideration on this preference that becomes clear when one asks how strong the preference for adults over children should be. In other words, what counts as an adequate justification for enrolling children in clinical research?

One might assume that this preference should be a strict one: the enrollment of adults and older children who can give consent should always be preferred to the enrollment of younger children, at least when it comes to nonbeneficial research. On this view, investigators should be allowed to enroll children in nonbeneficial research only when the scientific question posed by the study cannot be answered by enrolling those who can consent. This approach has been endorsed by many commentators and adopted by a number of regulations. Canadian research regulations stipulate that "individuals who are not legally competent shall only be asked to become research subjects when the research question can only be addressed using individuals within the identified group(s)."[33] The Council for International Organizations of Medical Sciences (CIOMS) guidelines state: "Before undertaking research involving children, the investigator must ensure that the research might not equally well be carried out with adults."[34]

These versions of the requirement raise the question of when it is the case that research cannot be *equally well* carried out with adults. Are these reasons limited to scientific considerations or might they include others, for example, the fact that the study would be less risky to children compared to adults? Given the importance of obtaining informed consent for clinical research, the requirement for enrolling children only when the research cannot be conducted with competent individuals makes sense. This conclusion is further strengthened if one assumes that enrollment in nonbeneficial research is always inconsistent with younger children's overall interests, in which case investigators always should prefer enrolling those who can give their own consent over enrolling a younger child who cannot consent. At least two different arguments can be used to support this strict preference.

First, one might argue that participation in nonbeneficial research is always contrary to the participants' interests, and that the conduct of such research is acceptable only when the individuals recognize this conflict and agree to participate, presumably on altruistic grounds. Certainly we allow competent adults to make decisions contrary to their own interests, particularly when their actions are supported by moral considerations. One might make this argument even stronger by endorsing the view that informed consent is morally transformative in the sense that actions performed on consenting adults necessarily raise no normative concerns. If this were the case there would seem to be no normative reason to prefer an alternative approach to conducting a given nonbeneficial study with consent adults.

A second possibility would be to grant the present argument, but only to the extent that it applies to competent adults. That is, one might hold the view that contributing to valuable projects, including nonbeneficial clinical research studies, can be in individuals' interests to the extent that they autonomously agree to make the contribution in question and, perhaps, only when that contribution furthers the individuals' own projects and goals. This view might support a strict preference for enrolling adults over children, particularly children who are not able to provide informed consent.

I have argued that enrollment in nonbeneficial research can be in the interests of even very young children who are unable to understand and make their own decisions. If this is right, it creates at least the possibility that, in some cases, it may be preferable to enroll in nonbeneficial research younger children who cannot understand rather than adults or older children, even when it would be possible to answer the scientific hypothesis in question by enrolling adults or older children. This conclusion suggests that there may be sufficiently compelling justifications to enroll children rather than individuals who can consent beyond the fact that, for scientific reasons, it is not possible to answer the question posed by enrolling those who can consent.

One possibility arises in the case of research that poses very different risks to adults versus young children. Imagine a study that poses serious risks to adults and teenagers but very low risks to young children. This possibility may arise in a number of contexts. For example, the relatively immature immune system of very young children can place them at lower risk for serious immune reactions to certain drugs. Further imagine that the research would be of the same value whether it is conducted with adults or young children. The view that nonbeneficial research is always inconsistent with children's overall interests, especially when combined with the claim that informed consent is maximally transformative, might imply a strict preference for enrolling adults over children, even when the risks to the children are minor and those to the adults significant. This view suggests that investigators should prefer the enrollment of competent adults even when the risk of death they would face is three or even four orders of magnitude greater than the risk of death posed to very young children.

The present analysis that contributing to nonbeneficial research can be in children's overall interests, that such contributions have positive implications for the children's lives, suggests an alternative response to such cases. This view would not justify enrolling young children rather than adults when a significant difference in risks is present, but the risks to young children are nonetheless significant. It would, however, provide a justification for enrolling younger children when a significant difference in risks is present and the risks posed to the young are low. Very low risks to young children can be justified by the extent to which their making a contribution to a valuable study contributes to their overall interests. Estimation of the risks to which younger children can be appropriately exposed depends on a determination of the prospective value of the study and what level of risks contributing to that end justifies. When this condition is satisfied, it can be appropriate to enroll younger children on the grounds that participation is not contrary to their interests.

Children Helping Adults

The extent to which it can be in children's overall interests to participate in nonbeneficial research depends on the extent to which the research has the potential to benefit others. Importantly, this argument does not require that the research in question benefits other *children*, raising the possibility that it may be acceptable to enroll children in nonbeneficial research to benefit adults. This view conflicts with the views of some commentators and guidelines which stipulate that children should be enrolled in nonbeneficial research only when the research has the potential to benefit other children. The U.S. regulations allow the approval of nonbeneficial pediatric research that poses more than a minor increase over minimal risk only when the "research presents a reasonable opportunity to further the understanding, prevention, or alleviation of a serious problem affecting the health or welfare of children" (45CFR46.407). Similarly, a working group of European pediatricians concluded that nonbeneficial pediatric research is acceptable only when "it is necessary to promote the health of the population represented and cannot be performed on legally competent persons instead."[35] The Indian Council for Medical Research guidelines stipulate that before conducting research in children "the investigator must ensure that the purpose of the research is to obtain knowledge relevant to health needs of children."[36]

The claim that children should be enrolled in nonbeneficial research only when it has the potential to benefit children as a group might be proxy for the distinct requirement, just discussed, that those who cannot consent, including children, should be enrolled in nonbeneficial research only when a compelling reason exists to enroll them rather than individuals who can consent. One might assume that a compelling reason can exist to enroll children only when the research concerns the health of children; otherwise, the investigators could just as well enroll those who can consent. This line of reasoning appears to underpin the current U.S. stipulation that children may be enrolled in nonbeneficial research that poses a minor increase over minimal risk only when it is likely to yield generalizable knowledge about their disorder or condition (45CFR46.406).

At the time this requirement was proposed by the National Commission, one of its members argued in dissent that endorsement of it implies that it is acceptable in the context of nonbeneficial research to expose already sick children to greater risks than healthy children.[37] Several commentators have echoed this criticism in recent years, arguing either that research of this level of risk should not be allowed or, if allowed, should not be limited to children who have a condition or illness.[38] The chairman of the Commission, Kenneth Ryan, took the unusual step of explicitly responding to this dissent. He argued that the requirement had been misunderstood in the dissent and that it was intended to ensure that children are enrolled in this category of research only when they are the only suitable candidates. Ryan's response suggested that at least a majority of the members of The National Commission endorsed the requirement because they assumed that investigators would need to enroll children in this category of research only when the research focused on a condition from which the children suffered.

The first problem with this view is that it is sometimes necessary to enroll in nonbeneficial research children who do not suffer from the condition under study. Studies with healthy children to establish a normal baseline are examples, and establish that the requirement that the research must yield information concerning the participants' condition or illness is not functionally equivalent to the requirement that children should be enrolled only when a compelling scientific reason exists to enroll them. Similarly, there might be cases in which children are needed to study diseases that affect adults only. For example, there is some reason to believe that the first manifestations of Alzheimer disease occur very early in life.[39] If these signs occur early enough, studies of individuals who definitively do not have the disease may need to enroll children.

Alternatively, one might argue that whether contributing to a valuable project is in some children's overall interests depends on specifically who will benefit, that children do not gain from helping people in general, but only from aiding particular classes of individuals. This position recalls Hans Jonas's claim that nonbeneficial research is ethical only when the subjects identify with the goals of the research.[40] One might think that the goals with which different individuals identify would be an empirical question; one would have to survey and study individuals to determine what their personal goals were. Jonas, however, considered the question at least to a certain extent to be tractable to conceptual analysis. His general view seems to be that nonbeneficial research would be ethical when the scientific goals of the research were endorsed by the competent adults who were enrolled in the research.

At times, Jonas seems to have held even a stronger view, according to which nonbeneficial research can be ethical only when it involves a disease from which the individuals suffer. For Jonas, it seems that this is the only case in which individuals can identify with the scientific goals of a study. One could sufficiently embrace the cause of curing or at least finding treatments for Alzheimer disease only if one suffers from the disease oneself. Although this seems an overly restrictive account of the extent to which autonomous individuals can adopt goals as their own, and these goals can become important, even central to these individuals' sense of self, we need not consider that question here.

The claim that nonbeneficial research can be acceptable only when apparently autonomous adults share its goals implies that nonbeneficial research with children is necessarily unethical. This view appears to be based on assumptions about the extent to which individuals decide for themselves what is in their interests and what their goals are. In other words, it seems that Jonas assumes that no objective account exists of what is in an individual's interests independent of the goals and values of the individual in question. Jonas may have thought that these limits followed from an analysis of human psychology, not from a normative analysis of what constitutes an individual's interests. However, since autonomous adults do not fully determine what is in their own interests, some contributions may be in their interests as a matter of more objective fact, and this may apply to them in virtue of the kinds of individuals they are, not in virtue of their endorsing the ends in question.

This is the argument of the present analysis. Contributing to valuable projects can be in an individual's overall interests, independent of whether the individual in question personally has the goal of promoting that cause (here I am bracketing the possibility that contributing to the cause may be contrary to the individual's own projects and goals, in which case the contribution may be counter to his overall interests). For very young children, it is not clear that any way exists in which contributing to the health of other young children promotes their interests more than contributing to the health of teenagers or adults. With that said, there may be an important pragmatic reason to limit the participation of children to research on illnesses of children.[41]

One might worry that a policy of allowing children to be enrolled in clinical research designed to benefit adults is prone to abuse, with review committees allowing children to be enrolled even in research that could just as well be conducted with adults. This potential may be increased by the fact that adults will decide who gets enrolled, and young children are unable to have a say in these decisions. Policies on clinical research should allow the enrollment of those who cannot consent only when a compelling reason exists to enroll them rather than individuals who can consent. This policy is needed even if one does not allow children to be enrolled in research to benefit adults. Thus, rather than limit children to research on pediatric diseases, it may be better to focus on ensuring proper implementation of this compelling justification requirement.

NINE | Objections and the Potential for Abuse

You Will Eat Your Spinach

The conclusion that making causal contributions to valuable projects can be in an individual's interests, even when the contribution is a passive one in the sense of not going through the individual's agency, seems to justify forcing individuals to contribute to valuable projects. If passive contributions redound to one's credit, then so too it seems do forced contributions. If the fact of making a causal contribution alone renders the contribution in one's overall interests, the importance of respecting autonomous adults seems lost. Moreover, it seems that investigators could justify forcing children to participate in nonbeneficial research, thus violating the widely endorsed standards that children who express sustained dissent should be removed from research that does not offer a compensating potential for clinical benefit.

Typically, it is thought that competent adults should decide for themselves whether they contribute to a given project. Or, if it is determined in a particular case that respect for the individual is overridden by competing, perhaps social value considerations, then we may be able to justify forcing the individual to contribute. Thus, individuals can be forced to make contributions to projects that they oppose through the social control of their tax dollars. In times of military conscription, individuals may even be forced to put their lives at stake for the good of society. However, we tend to regard these cases as those in which competing interests override the individuals' own claims for how we should treat them and the control they typically exercise over the contributions they make.

This approach has two important virtues. First, the claim of the individual not to be forced to contribute to projects deemed valuable by others, or by society in general, provides an important protection. Although society may win out in some cases, the fact that prima facie there exists a strong claim that we should not force individuals and that doing so is contrary to their interests places a brake on our doing so. Second, even when the individual is forced, he has remaining to him the dignity that comes from the claim that he was forced to do so, that doing so was against his interests, but overridden by the interests of others. On the present account, both virtues appear lost.

Contributing to valuable projects is seen as being in individuals' interests, even when the contribution does not go through their agency, even when they do not choose to make the contribution. This implication seems to eliminate the individual's own interests as a protection, one which pushes back on the extent to which we can use him for the benefit of others. Instead, we can use others as much as we want; that brake is gone, and with it the consolation that comes from recognizing when individuals are forced that it is for the interests of others, not for their own sake. Now it seems that we have arrived at the claim that we are forcing the individual for their own good, so that their own interests become complicit in the attempt to force them to do what they prefer not to do.

To evaluate this concern it is important to distinguish reasons from determinative reasons. In general, contributing to a valuable cause or project promotes a person's interests. The conclusion that we can on these grounds force competent adults to contribute to the overall good against their will assumes that this reason qualifies as a determinative reason. Yet, this is only one consideration that goes into determining how we should treat individuals. It would follow that we can force competent adults to contribute to valuable projects for their own good only if there exists some range of cases that lack any countervailing considerations of greater significance.

In the case of competent adults a countervailing consideration is essentially always present; namely, the moral importance of allowing competent adults to decide for themselves how their lives will go. The importance of treating competent individuals with respect in this sense is of great moral significance. In contrast, purely passive contributions promote individuals' own interests only to a very small extent. It follows that the value for an individual of contributing to valuable projects provides at best a minor reason to force her to contribute to valuable projects against her will. However, all things considered, this reason alone will not yield a determinative reason for so acting, given the greater significance for an individual of respecting her autonomy.[1] Although the value for the individual of contributing to valuable projects will not provide sufficient reason to force her for her own good, it often will provide reason to appeal to competent adults to agree to contribute. Appeals, even imploring appeals, are consistent with respect for individuals' autonomy.

To consider an analogous, but very different case, many studies have shown that consuming vegetables is in an individual's interests. Moreover, these studies are widely regarded as providing some reason for parents to feed their children vegetables. Yet, no one objects to these studies and their findings on the grounds that they might promote a practice of forcing competent adults to eat spinach.[2] The benefits to be gained are too low compared to the indignity of a competent adult being forced, and doing so conflicts with the general importance of respecting those who are able to make their own decisions. In addition, although we need not consider it in detail, there are compelling public policy reasons not to adopt a practice of forcing competent adults to make contributions for their own good. Such a practice likely would have negative consequences on a social scale that dramatically outweigh the benefits of adopting it in the first place.

My reliance on the indignity of forcing competent adults in this argument may be thought to imply that it can be acceptable to force adults who are no longer competent, such as individuals in a coma or individuals with severe Alzheimer disease. In these cases, the possibility of violating the individual's current autonomy is absent. To address this objection fully we would need to consider in some depth what constitutes adequate respect for adults who have lost the ability to make their own decisions.[3] Although this topic is beyond the scope of the present work, a response would begin with the fact that respect for these individuals includes respect for their competent preferences and values, even if they are no longer in a position to state, communicate, or defend them. Thus, there is, as with competent individuals, reason to respect their preferences and values.

This is the approach endorsed in current medical practice. We do not treat incompetent adults based simply on what is in the interests of society; for example, saving money by uniformly denying them medical care they are not capable of paying for. Instead, we appeal to evidence, when available, of their competent preferences and values, as expressed perhaps in a living will document. Although I will not defend the claim here, there also is reason to respect the objections of adults, even those who are no longer competent. It is a mistake, although a relatively common one, to assume that the value of respect for what individuals want is exhausted by the extent to which it respects their autonomy or puts the individual in a position to act consistently with their preferences and values. Respect for the choices of others also allows them to be in control of their lives. This control typically has value for individuals even when they are no longer competent.[4]

The extent to which we should be guided by the competent preferences and values of adults who are no longer competent is also central to determining the implications of the present analysis for research with these individuals. The fact that contributing to valuable projects is in the interests of those who make the contributions applies to everyone, offering a justification for enrolling adults who cannot consent in valuable research. To determine the practical implications of this fact requires an analysis of how to balance this value with the importance of respecting their competent and current preferences and values.

The claim that contributing to nonbeneficial pediatric research typically is in children's interests similarly provides one reason to enroll them in such research. However, to determine whether it follows that parents may force their children to participate in such research, one first must evaluate whether countervailing reasons exist against enrolling them in general or forcing them in particular. Since purely passive contributions have some implications for an individual's life, but not much, the opportunity to make a passive contribution, even to a very important research study, will provide a determinative reason to force a child to enroll only when no important counter reasons exist.[5] One obvious counter reason would be that the involvement in the study causes the child distress or pain. These factors would provide compelling reason to take a child out of a study, even though contributing to it passively may otherwise be in her interests. Sustained dissent of children that reflects anything beyond minor distress or pain should be regarded as reason to remove them from the study. The opportunity to contribute passively to an important project does not provide a reason to override this consideration. Even when the research itself will not be stressful for the child overriding their expressed dissent may well be. The desire to make one's own decisions tends to develop long before the ability to make wise decisions for onself.

The Unfairness of It All

By divorcing, to some extent, what constitutes a better life for an individual from those things that are within the individual's control, the present account invites a charge of unfairness. Individuals' lives are being judged based on decisions their parents made for them at the time they were children, taking them to a political rally or not, placing them on Hitler's lap. In this way, the present view seems to conflict with a strong intuition that the scope of individuals' control does, or at least should, determine the boundaries on appropriate judgments of them and their lives.

The quality of our lives is strongly influenced by events beyond our control in a number of ways.[6] Much of this dependence results from the fact that how well our lives go depends, in large part, on what we do with them, the accomplishments we realize, the benefits we bestow, the harms we cause. Our ability to do good or ill depends on the circumstances in which we find ourselves and the nature of our abilities. Although it is often said that one makes one's own opportunities, this is true only within the scope of one's capacities and in response to the range of opportunities one's society and the world, and one's time and place in it, makes available. A child born today in the developing world with HIV infection and without access to treatment, or a woman born in a sexist culture that denies many opportunities to woman, will end up with limited capacities, as well as limited opportunities. Through no fault of their own, many individuals are not afforded the opportunity for greatness.

Living in interesting and uncertain times poses many obstacles and evils, but often offers compensating opportunities for great accomplishments. One's life likely will be less calm and orderly, and opportunities for ordinary achievement—getting a higher degree, having a stable and successful career—may not be available. But the opportunities for greatness also may be comparatively increased. To help address a social evil or come to the aid of one's country in time of civil war, one has to live at a time and place where these opportunities arise. Jackie Robinson did not have available the opportunities open to African-American baseball players today: enormous salaries, widespread recognition and adulation, and the sense of self-worth and respect that comes with them. But, living in a time of segregation and casual acceptance of racism did provide him the opportunity for greatness: to be the first player to break the color barrier in professional baseball in the United States. This opportunity is unavailable to players today (although their sometimes enormous salaries provide them the opportunity for accomplishments of far greater significance and value than buying expensive clothes and building enormous houses).

The role of chance in the overall evaluation of our lives is ameliorated somewhat by the fact that we judge a life based largely on what an individual makes of it given his accidental opportunities and capacities. A tendency exists to want to drive out chance altogether and argue that only those things within our control have implications for us and our lives. One way to take this line of reasoning is to emphasize the importance of moral agency and voluntary action. Yet, the only way that we can affect change in the world, the only way that we can act on our good intentions, is through physical engagement with the world. But, once we engage with the world, once we do something, we necessarily create the possibility of influences and effects beyond our control. The casual ripples that extend out from our voluntary actions are not themselves within our control; yet, as consequences of what we have done, they can have implications for our lives.[7]

The Stoics were influenced by the first-person perspective on this present concern. They realized that a good deal of life is beyond our control. To increase the chances for a contented life, they argued that we should care about and value only those things within our control. Pushing this approach to its logical conclusion, some adopted and promoted the view that it is only our reactions to the world that matter. We should remain unconcerned with what happens in the world and focus on how we react to those happenings. This, it was argued, is all that we can control. The first problem with this view is that it is not clear to what extent we control even the reactions we have to the world. Often we exercise little control over feelings of anger in response to being taken advantage of or periods of depression following personal loss. More importantly, limiting the scope of value to the ambit of individual control omits much of what makes our lives valuable. In large part, many of the most important things in our lives involve others and our relationships with them; being loved, befriended, and cared for are crucial elements of a valuable life and to a large extent are beyond our control. We can influence but never control whether others care about or love us.

In the *Fragility of Goodness*, Martha Nussbaum elegantly canvasses what we should make of this fact and how we should react to it in deciding how to live our lives.[8] She traces Plato's endorsement of the philosophical life of contemplation and solitary reflection as the highest form of life in part to the desire to provide an account of the good life that is insulated from the vagaries of a life lived in the world: "I shall argue that the Platonic conception of the life of reason, including its emphasis upon stable and highly abstract objects, is itself a direct continuation of an aspiration to rational self-sufficiency."[9] Nussbaum is sympathetic to this attempt and recognizes its value. Nonetheless, she ultimately endorses what she describes as a more Aristotelian view of the good life. She grants the danger, the fragility, of a life that recognizes and emphasizes the importance of friends, relationships, and love, but ultimately argues that such a life is a more human and flourishing one.

The response to the charge of unfairness, then, is twofold. First, a good deal of how we are judged depends on what we do with our lives, and this is more or less under our control. Second, the fact that the universe of value contains things over which we have little or no control is simply a fact of our existence. In a sense, the lesson to be drawn from this fact is the opposite of the lesson preached by the Stoics. For them, the goal of an individual life was to focus on only those things within one's control. This view has the implication of driving individuals into themselves and away from others and their community. In this way, the Stoic philosophy has profoundly antipolitical implications. If all that matters is what goes on inside our heads, there is no reason for us or anyone else who adopts this philosophy to care about the structure of our social or political institutions. Fairness and justice lose their pull in such a place. If one is fated to be a slave, it may make sense to adopt this view. But, if one hopes to avoid slavery for oneself and others, one should be very concerned with the nature of social and political institutions.

The fact that the way our lives go depends in part of the behavior of others and the political and social structures in which we find ourselves provides incentive based on our own interests to care about others, about our social and political structures. Once we realize that our lives may end up being less valuable due to factors beyond our control, we have personal reasons for caring about those factors. If a social structure that allows children to be used for evil purposes can result in those children having a less valuable life through no fault of their own, we, all of us, have an additional reason for eliminating such practices and structures. If the way our society is structured shapes the consequences of our actions and, thereby, influences the value of our lives overall, we have a prudential reason to care about the structure of our society beyond what impact it has on our personal experience.

The consequences of our actions, not just our intentions in acting or our emotional reactions, have implications for our lives. This fact undermines the project of limiting all that we value to what we control, and raises legitimate concerns of unfairness. Yet, this same fact is vital to the opportunity for self-transcendence, the opportunity to go beyond our own personal desires and preferences to be part of a larger community, to transcend ourselves, our lives, and our deaths, to have meaning and importance that goes beyond ourselves. This impulse underscores how cramped and narrow the life of the Stoic would be. There would be some tranquility and reassurance in the fact that all one cared about was within one's control. But those benefits would be realized by limiting the scope of one's values to the point that life becomes very narrow, a kind of imprisonment to one's own feeling and preferences. And because one's feelings and reactions to the world are extinguished with one's life, this view would effectively eliminate the possibility of transcending our own lives and our own deaths in any meaningful way.

What Happened to Autonomy?

It is worth considering why the claim that making purely passive contributions can be in individuals' overall interest seems counterintuitive and inconsistent with a good deal of philosophical analysis in this area. There are two general ways to think about the philosophical project of providing a theory of value. The first is to provide a general theory of value: what is valuable in our lives, what makes our lives go better or worse, what constitutes a better overall life for us. A second project is to provide a theory of prudential value or practical reason: how we should try to live our lives to maximize the chances that our lives go well, that we realize the things cited by the general theory of value.

A great deal of our most important accomplishments flow from our agency, from taking on valuable projects and seeing them through. The fact that how we live as moral agents is so important to our lives overall provides good reason to focus one's analysis on this aspect. This focus is reinforced by the extent to which, in developing a philosophical analysis, one hopes to provide guidance, or a kind of instruction manual, for how persons ought to live their lives, how we ought to act. One of the more perspicacious proponents of this approach is Joseph Raz:

> Evaluation of people's well-being involves judgments about their lives, or periods of their lives, and the degree to which they do or did do well, were good or successful. In large measure our well-being consists in the whole-hearted and successful pursuit of valuable activity.[10]

Raz goes on to provide a compelling account of the prominent role activity plays in the judgment of valuable lives. For this project, there seems no point in considering the potential value for individuals of making purely passive contributions. These contributions say, as we have seen, little about one's life overall. Moreover, one cannot do much about them, at least directly. The philosophical project, to the extent that it is intended as an account of practical reason or prudential value, thus ignores purely passive contributions and seems to imply that they do not have any significance for the individual at all. Raz, for example, follows the previous quote one page later by stating: "The core idea is controlling one's conduct, being in charge. The definition of well-being... insists that activity is the key to well-being."[11] The qualification, in the previous quote, that activity "in large measure" determines our well-being seems almost forgotten here, and one begins to get the impression that all that matters for a valuable life is valuable activity and being in control, that nothing else matters, nothing else is relevant to how well our lives go overall. This perspective is consistent with Raz's claim, considered previously, that passive contributions to valuable projects—Mary (unknowingly) serving as the subject for a great work of art—do not enhance our lives at all.

Clear reasons exist why the philosophical project downplays the importance of those things outside of our control, outside our agency. We often cannot do much about them, and emphasizing their importance seems to increase or at least make us complicit in the unfairness that often characterizes the human condition. But, the fact that the contributions we make outside our control are of comparatively little importance and there is not much we can do about them anyway should not be confused with the very different claim that such contributions do not matter or have implications for our lives at all. Some of the things that fall outside the scope of our control and agency are extremely important, including our friendships and intimate relationships. A valuable life is one that includes, to some extent, close friendships and intimate relationships. We can influence whether someone is a friend, but in the end it is up to them.

Too narrow a focus on agency and tracing all value to that which flows from it also leaves one without an account of how things should go for those who are not autonomous. This implication is classically illustrated by the Kantian dilemma of explaining why it is wrong to torture (nonautonomous) animals. Yes, agency is important, but too great an emphasis on it raises ethical concerns of its own. Importantly, an account of how things should go for nonautonomous beings may have implications for how autonomous individuals ought to treat them. This is even more salient when we come to the question of the proper treatment of children. When we consider questions such as whether it is appropriate to enroll children in nonbeneficial pediatric research, we must extend our philosophical analysis beyond autonomous moral agents to determine what is important for other individuals, as well as for how we ought to treat them. And, to the extent that all of our lives include a phase of childhood, and many of our lives will include a phase of noncompetent dotage, an understanding of value at times when we lack agency necessarily is part of a complete account of the value of our lives.

Giving Comfort to Scoundrels?

The history of clinical research is littered with far too many examples of abusive studies, both with adults and with children. In these cases, the individuals' own interests were ignored in the pursuit of what were, or were perceived or claimed to be, societal benefits. In this regard, the claim that contributing to nonbeneficial research can be in children's interests, even when they do not decide for themselves to make that contribution, might seem to prove too much. Studies widely regarded as abusive may be seen as helping the children that we thought investigators were abusing, working for their interests rather than against them (assuming the abusive studies at least had social value).

The argument that contributing to nonbeneficial pediatric research is in children's interests may provide comfort to the perpetrators of previous abuses and increase the potential for future abuses: Those who object to being enrolled in a nonbeneficial research study simply misunderstand their own interests and should be enrolled, forcefully if necessary, over those objections. And investigators need have no scruples when enrolling individuals in research for the benefit of others, since doing so provides "participants" (here the term becomes ironic and especially inapt) the opportunity to contribute to a valuable project and, thereby, promote their overall interests.

This concern raises the possibility that, even if one is willing to grant that contributing to valuable projects can be in the interests of pediatric research participants, it does not necessarily follow that we should, as a matter of public policy, allow such research. We need first to evaluate the potential for abuse of such a policy. This task requires clarity on what constitutes a tragedy, and how we should understand abuses. Even many very low risk studies pose some chance of serious harm. Probabilities being what they are if investigators perform a sufficient number of research interventions that pose even a one in several hundred-thousand risk of death, a child sooner or later will die as a result. Such deaths will, without question, be tragedies and their foreseeability, even inevitability, does not make them less so.

Recognizing this, one might be tempted to retreat to the previously assayed position of simply prohibiting all nonbeneficial pediatric research, at least all research beyond simple interventions that seem truly to pose negligible risks, such as surveys that ask fairly innocuous questions and measurements of height and weight. Although this response is understandable, it is important to recognize that it is not one that will reduce, and likely would increase, the number of children who experience serious harm. A prohibition on nonbeneficial pediatric research would reduce our ability to improve medical treatments for children. As a result, a greater number of children would receive less effective and more toxic treatment. The effect of a prohibition, then, would be to shift the context in which these harms occur. Fewer children will suffer harm in the research context, but more will suffer harm in the context of clinical medicine.

The development of the rotavirus vaccines depended on the allowance of some purely research interventions, including interventions that posed a very low chance of serious harm. It is well and good to say that progress is optional, but one who takes that view must be clear about the kind of progress being optioned. It is the kind that may save the lives of hundreds of thousands of children who would otherwise have died before age 5, tragic deaths every one. Such examples highlight the fact that prohibiting nonbeneficial pediatric research would not reduce and most likely would increase the number of tragedies, understood as children experiencing serious harms.

Although the potential to help many children provides an important reason to allow nonbeneficial pediatric research, this consideration alone does not provide a definitive argument. To take an analogous case, a policy that allows organs to be harvested from some healthy children when doing so benefits a greater number of children would decrease the total number of children who suffer and die. Yet, no one takes this fact as sufficient reason to allow such a policy. As always, one needs to consider not just the outcomes, but the means by which the outcomes are realized. In the medical context, it is obviously tragic if children suffer and die as the result of receiving ineffective or even toxic medications. However, in these cases, the physicians who provide the medications are not responsible for the suffering and deaths of these children (assuming the harms are not the result of malpractice). In contrast, in the case of nonbeneficial pediatric research, the investigators *are* responsible for the risks the children face and any resulting harms they incur. It follows, one might argue, that these harms are not morally equivalent to the harms resulting in the context of clinical care. These harms are more problematic and should be avoided first.

This account of the moral difference between the harms that result in clinical research and clinical care recognizes that, in purely causal terms, the physicians and investigators who provide the interventions are equally responsible in both contexts. However, the physicians are acting in the clinical interests of the children. They are not morally responsible for the harms children experience due to toxic treatments. The fact of acting in the clinical interests of the children in effect clears the physicians of moral culpability. The point to notice, then, is that this argument assumes that investigators are morally culpable because they are acting contrary to the interests of the children who participate in nonbeneficial pediatric research. They cannot point to the medical interests of the children as justifying their interventions, and those interests are not present to clear them of moral responsibility in the event of harms.

By now we have a very different way of understanding the role of clinical investigators. Although enrolling children in nonbeneficial pediatric research is not in their clinical interests, it can be in their broader overall interests. This fact, of course, does not reduce the tragedy of a child who suffers harm in the context of nonbeneficial pediatric research. It does, however, change the analysis of the extent to which the investigators are responsible for those harms. Assuming the study is valuable, enrollment of children offered the opportunity for them to contribute to a valuable project. In addition, assuming the relevant safeguards are implemented, risks are minimized and compelling reason exists to enroll children who cannot consent, enrollment can be in the children's interests. Hence, the investigators are not acting wrongly and are not morally responsible for the harms which result (again assuming that the study was conducted properly).[12]

To put the point in a somewhat different way, children have a claim against others taking their organs, even when doing so leads to better consequences overall. One might argue that children have a claim, albeit a weaker one perhaps, against being enrolled in nonbeneficial pediatric research for the benefit of others. While many have taken that view, contributing to such research can be in the children's interests. Thus, the possibility of defeating the forced organ donation case is in terms of the claim that children have only a weak interest in contributing to important projects, one that can justify nonbeneficial pediatric research when the risks are sufficiently low, but not forced organ donation that will necessarily lead to serious harm or death. One might grant that this argument addresses the concern of drawing a distinction between nonbeneficial pediatric research and clear abuses, yet worry that, in practice, this distinction will be too thin to support adequate protections, since it depends on careful judgments, very difficult to make in practice, on how much an individual's interests are furthered by contributing to a research project designed to help others. This is the topic of the next section.

The Potential for Abuse

Any argument in support of and any policy to allow nonbeneficial pediatric research is subject to the potential for abuse. Prohibiting such research may not eliminate it, but seems likely to dramatically decrease the frequency with which it is conducted. Alternatively, a prohibition on nonbeneficial pediatric research may simply result in more research being packaged and approved as offering a prospect of clinical benefit. This, in the end, may have the deleterious effect of decreasing awareness of nonbeneficial pediatric research without significantly decreasing its occurrence.

As we have seen, prohibiting nonbeneficial pediatric research has serious drawbacks and could lead to worse outcomes for children in the medical setting.

Thus, unless one is willing to accept these costs, the best approach seems to be one of allowing such research, when it is ethical, and mandating safeguards to protect participants from abuse. Although the perpetrators of abuses may not be sensitive to the details of theoretical argumentation, it is worth remembering that contributing to even a very valuable project in a purely passive way has only minimal implications for one's interests. Thus, this consideration provides little added justification for abuses. At the same time, the importance of pediatric research and improving pediatric medical care can be seen as social incentives to enroll children in research and may increase the chances for abuse. The question, then, is whether justifying the research on some grounds rather than others may serve to increase or decrease the potential for abuse.

The extent to which a given contribution says something about an individual's life depends on the extent to which it is active rather than passive. This factor provides good reason to increase awareness of research participation on the part of the children and to engage them actively in the research, to the extent possible. In addition, the fact that passive contributions say very little about individuals' overall lives, and the inherent uncertainty over whether they will embrace the contribution, places a strict, if not fully specified limit on the risks to which children may be exposed. The downside one could argue is that determining whether a given study is ethical requires a precise evaluation of the extent to which contributing to that project says something valuable about the children's lives compared to the risks that the research poses to them. This evaluation is very difficult and there are no clear standards to apply, implying that final decisions in practice are subject to the vagaries of personal judgment. As a result, the social incentive to conduct such research may consciously or otherwise inflate in reviewers' minds the extent to which contributing to a given project is in the children's interests.

One alternative would be to argue that exposing children to research risks for the benefit of others is unethical, but to allow it in some cases, to "err bravely" as Ramsey puts it. Here the argument might be that regarding the research as unethical will place a strong brake on the liability of abuse. This approach in effect tries to make a protection out of cognitive dissonance, putting investigators, funders, and review committees in the position of regarding what they are doing as unethical to some extent. This approach could result in those who conduct the research continuing on, but in a cautious way that may mimic the safeguards one wants. Yet, there is an almost inevitable response to overt cognitive dissonance of taking steps to eliminate it. Hence, regarding such research as unethical but allowable may lead to the prohibition of all nonbeneficial pediatric research, with those serious consequences attendant to that approach that we have considered.

Alternatively, the practice of nonbeneficial pediatric research may continue and the practitioners may simply ignore the ethical concerns it raises. This result could be disastrous if it leads to the assumption that no risk limits need be placed on acceptable nonbeneficial pediatric research. Although these options do not seem better than the potential consequences of the present account, much of the debate here involves the psychological and social consequences of adopting one policy and justification for it rather than another. In this regard, theoretical analysis can take us only so far. Any final determination will require in-depth empirical analysis.

Worries about Distribution

The claim that contributing to a nonbeneficial pediatric research study can promote a child's interests seems to imply that contributing to many nonbeneficial pediatric research studies would promote the child's interests to even a greater extent. Even if one is willing to grant the present argument that enrolling a child in one or two studies for the benefit of others is not abusive, it seems clear that enrolling a particular child in an endless series of studies for the benefit of others would be abusive. This conclusion raises concern that the present analysis may be mistaken. How could more of what promotes children's interests be worse for them?

Enrolling a child in a nonbeneficial research study typically entails that many other activities are precluded during that time. Being in the study may prevent the child from playing with her friends, going to school, or taking music lessons. Such opportunity costs provide one reason why participation in many nonbeneficial pediatric research studies is not in a child's interests, even though participation in some nonbeneficial pediatric research studies may be in her interests. A flourishing human life involves many different pursuits, activities, and abilities, requiring parents and society in general to find an appropriate balance between all the things that contribute to children's present and long-term interests. We saw this previously with respect to altruistic acts by autonomous adults. Helping others to a certain extent is in the interests of competent adults, partly because it leads to a better life for them overall. Yet, a better life includes a balance of many ingredients, to the extent that too much of one, including helping others too often, may detract from the individual's life overall.

The importance of a fair distribution of the benefits and burdens of clinical research also places some limits on the extent to which participating in nonbeneficial pediatric research is in a given child's interests. Some contributions can be a benefit, but more contributions, at some point, constitute a harm. Consider the fact that it is a good thing for a life to have deep and committed, authentic personal relationships, and it can be a good thing for an individual to contribute to his friends and the maintaining of his relationships. One might conclude that making greater and more contributions to one's friends and one's friendships is always better; some is good, more must be better, without limit.

This conclusion does not follow because the distribution of the burdens that goes into helping each other and maintaining our relationships matter. One can do too much, especially when others are not doing enough or not doing anything at all. If my friend buys me dinner, she has done a good thing for me, and by contributing to our relationship there is a sense in which she has done a good thing for herself. Helping close friends is one of the most important contributions that one can make, and doing so deepens and gives value to one's life. But too much of a good thing, relative to the contributions made by the other friend, can become a bad thing. If my friend is always the one making the contributions, always the one helping me, and always the one maintaining and strengthening the relationship, there comes a point at which I start to take advantage of her, and she starts to be taken advantage of.

Determining precisely where to draw this line is difficult, and depends on many factors in addition to the number of people in the relationship.[13] Contributions to a relationship need not be exactly equal, but doing significantly more can be worrisome in many cases.[14] Parents should be willing on the present grounds to enroll their child in more trials, but not so many that their children are contributing far beyond their fair share. We need not come up with a precise figure; it will depend on too many incidental features of the case in question, but it is important to recognize that such considerations place another limit on the extent to which making a contribution to a project to help others can promote a given individual's interests.

TEN | Conclusion

Pediatric clinical research is critical to improving medical care for children, to ensuring current medications are safe and effective, and to finding new medications that are less toxic and more effective. Yet, the process of evaluating pediatric medical interventions inevitably requires interventions and studies that pose risks to the children who undergo them without a compensating potential for clinical benefit. This exposure to risks for the benefit of others seems a classic instance of exploitation, one that is especially worrisome with respect to children who cannot consent and to whom we have a special obligation of protection.

These very serious ethical concerns have led a number of commentators and courts to provide powerful and compelling arguments that nonbeneficial pediatric research interventions and studies are unethical. It is unethical, they claim, to expose those who cannot consent to research risks for the benefit of others. To date, commentators have developed at best partial responses to these arguments. This absence of a complete response places pediatric research in jeopardy and with it society's ability to improve medical care for children.

It is true that, under current regulations, nonbeneficial pediatric research may be approved only when it poses low risks and typically requires the permission of the child's parents or legal guardian. It is also true, in a liberal society, that we allow parents to expose their children to some risks for the benefit of others, free from state intervention. Although these points reduce the ethical concerns posed by nonbeneficial pediatric research, they do not fully address them. The limitation to low risks does not eliminate the chance of serious harms, even death. And obtaining parental permission does not necessarily imply that the activity in question is ethically acceptable, hence, does not support the involvement of clinicians and the support of society.

We considered attempts to justify nonbeneficial pediatric research that go through autonomous decision-making in some sense—the fact that children would consent to it if they could, or will accept what we have done to them once they are old enough to understand. We have seen that these attempts fail to provide an adequate justification, in large part because they fail to take seriously the fact that children are not autonomous. The potential for an alternative justification was suggested by the possibility that children may derive educational benefit from their participation in nonbeneficial pediatric research, in particular, it may teach children to be moral.

Although some children likely do derive educational benefit from some studies, the limited scope of this possibility points to the need for a more complete justification or to the unacceptability of much nonbeneficial pediatric research, including all nonbeneficial research with infants and young children. Despite these limitations, work on the potential for educational benefit underscores the crucial insight that children might benefit from participation in clinical research in nonclinical ways. This insight offers the possibility of meeting Ramsey's challenge that pediatric research can be justified only when it is in the interests of the participating children. To extend this work, we have considered the possibility of connecting children's interests more closely to the value of the study in question. This approach suggested that making contributions to valuable projects, including valuable nonbeneficial pediatric research studies, can be in children's interests by leading to a preferable or better life for them overall.

We began this investigation with three plausible conditions on any successful analysis of the acceptability of nonbeneficial pediatric research. First, the *risk allowance* condition holds that it can be acceptable to expose children to some research risks for the benefit of others. Thus, any analysis should explain why this can be acceptable despite the fact that children are not able to give their own informed consent and parents in particular and society more generally have a responsibility to protect and nurture children and help them to become mature adults. Second, the *risk threshold* condition states that there is a limit on the risks to which children may be exposed in research for the benefit of others. Put very generally, children may be exposed to only low risks, even when the study in question has great potential social value. Third, the *compelling justification* condition holds that children should be enrolled rather than competent adults only when a compelling reason exists to do so. This condition limits acceptable analyses to those that, in effect, do not prove too much. It excludes analyses that imply that there is no ethical concern at all with enrolling children to the point that no reason exists to prefer the enrollment of adults to the enrollment of children.

The present argument that participation in nonbeneficial pediatric research can be in children's interests to the extent that it involves their contributing to a valuable project or end and they later may come to embrace these contributions seems to capture all three conditions. First, the fact that making passive contributions can be in an individual's interests implies that parents can decide to enroll their child in a valuable nonbeneficial research study that poses some risks. The justification for exposing children to some risks for the benefit of others is that it can be in children's broader interests to contribute to valuable projects. This is the risk allowance condition. The claim here is not simply that enrolling children in such research is within the scope of parental authority. That claim might explain why parents can make this decision, but it would not account for why such decisions are consistent with parental responsibility to nurture their children. It also would not provide a justification for the involvement of third parties or for the support and endorsement of society in general. In contrast, the claim that such contributions can be in the children's overall interests implies that making these decisions can be consistent with parents' goal of helping their children to have a good and a valuable life.

Second, purely passive contributions say little about one's overall life and the possibility that young children eventually will embrace these contributions as adults is inherently uncertain. It follows that these contributions alone can justify only very low risks, thus satisfying the risk threshold condition. In this regard, we saw that the possibility of older children making more active contributions implies that it may be acceptable to expose them to greater net risks than younger children. Third, a contribution that goes through an individual's agency says a great deal more about that individual's life compared to a contribution made by a young child. Thus, while it can be acceptable to enroll a younger child in nonbeneficial research, it is better, when possible, to enroll individuals who can consent instead. This is consistent with the compelling justification condition that, when possible, nonbeneficial research should enroll those who can consent.

Finally, we are now in a position to explain the apparent ethical dilemma posed by nonbeneficial pediatric research. It seems that contributing to the rotavirus study necessarily involved taking advantage of some children because the participants were exposed to risks without their consent for the benefit of others. At the same time, there seems to be some sense in which the study was appropriate and it was acceptable to enroll children in it given that the study was important and the risks were very low. The present analysis suggests that this (apparent) dilemma traces to two different perspectives from which we evaluate the importance for an individual of making a contribution.

First, as in most standard philosophical analyses, one can evaluate the importance of the contribution for the individuals as persons or as moral agents. This perspective implies that what is of most importance for individuals is autonomously and actively pursuing their personal goals. It is from this perspective that the rotavirus studies appear necessarily unethical. The children did not make the decision to enroll in the trials and, furthermore, the ends or goals of the study were not ones that the subjects themselves shared. One can also evaluate these studies from the perspective of what is of value for an individual's life as a whole. This includes, but is not exhausted by, what is of value for the individual as an autonomous agent. From this perspective, contributing even passively to a valuable project can promote the interests of individuals. And it is from this perspective that contributing to the rotavirus studies can be understood as being acceptable on the grounds that contributing to valuable projects can promote the participants' interests, even when they make these contributions as infants, the decision to make them was their parents', and the contribution on the part of the infants was purely passive. Nonetheless, they did make a contribution to the study and doing so makes for a better overall life compared to the same life absent that contribution. The conclusion that these studies were acceptable is further supported by the possibility that these individuals might embrace the contributions when they become adults. The contributions may thus become personal attainments, in addition to being valuable human achievements.

It follows that participation in nonbeneficial pediatric research can promote children's interests, even the interests of infants and toddlers who contribute to the research without knowing what they are doing or choosing to do so. The possibility of even very young children contributing to clinical research studies provides the basis for my decision, described at the outset, to regard children in research as "participants" rather than "subjects." The view that nonbeneficial pediatric research involves taking advantage of children for the benefit of others implies that these children are subjects in the sense of being subjected to risks and burdens for the benefit of others. The present analysis does not change the fact that pediatric research involves exposing children who cannot consent to risks for the benefit of others. They are still subjects in this sense. The choice of the term "participant" is intended to highlight the central claim considered here that children who are involved in clinical research also are important contributors whose participation is vital to achieving the goals of the study.

How much a given contribution to a valuable project says about an individual's overall life, and the extent to which it promotes her interests, depends on at least 5 factors: the magnitude of her contribution, the extent to which it goes through her agency, the uniqueness of her contribution, the effort required, and the skill involved. These considerations point to the possibility of conducting nonbeneficial pediatric research that promotes the interests of the participating children, even when it poses burdens and some risks to them, and does not offer a compensating potential for clinical benefit. To realize this goal, it will be important for all those involved in pediatric research to recognize the extent to which children are exposed to risks for the benefit of others. It is not uncommon to downplay this aspect of pediatric research. The present analysis argues that we should instead work to increase children's and parents' awareness of the extent to which the children are helping others. This approach increases the extent to which the children's contribution is an active one, thus promoting the children's own interests in the process of improving health care for all children.

NOTES

Chapter 1

1. Although rotavirus also affects adults, it tends to be mild for them.
2. According to the website of a vaccine sponsor, rotavirus is responsible for approximately 250,000 emergency room visits among children younger than 5 years of age every year in the United States. See: http://www.rotateq.com/what-is-rotavirus.html.
3. This estimate comes from the Centers for Disease Control (CDC). See http://www.cdc.gov/ncidod/dvrd/revb/gastro/rotavirus.htm. Not surprisingly, estimates vary, from as low as 500,000 children a year to as high as 1 million children a year. See also Parashar UD, et al. Global illness and deaths caused by rotavirus disease in children. *Emerg Infect Dis* 2003; 9:565–572.
4. See: http://www.rotateq.com/what-is-rotavirus.html.
5. The earlier development of a rotavirus vaccine ended in an ethical dilemma. In 1999, it looked as though a successful vaccine had been identified until several infants developed a serious complication involving folding of the intestines (i.e., intussusception). It was estimated that the risk of intussusception from the vaccine was at most 1 in 2,500, and may have been significantly lower. Since rotavirus kills 1 in 200 children in the developing world, this seems an acceptable risk and one might assume that the vaccine deserved approval. However, this same risk of intussusception was considered unacceptable in the United States, where rotavirus kills very few children. Worries that it was unethical—employing a kind of double standard—to market a drug in the developing world that was too risky to be approved in the United States led to the vaccine being rejected, despite the fact that the background risks from rotavirus are dramatically different in the two places. For some of the story,

see Glass RI. New hope for defeating rotavirus. *Sci Amer* April 2006. Available at: http://www.cdc.gov/ncidod/dvrd/revb/gastro/sad0406Glas7p.pdf

6. Salinas B, Schael IP, Linhares AC, et al. Evaluation of safety, immunogenicity and efficacy of an attenuated rotavirus vaccine, RIX4414: A randomized, placebo-controlled trial in Latin American infants. *Ped Infect Disease J* 2005; 24:807–816; Vesikari T, Karvonen A, Korhonen T, et al. Safety and immunogenicity of RIX4414 live attenuated human rotavirus vaccine in adults, toddlers and previously uninfected infants. *Vaccine* 2004; 22:2836–2842; Ruiz Palacios GM, Perez-Schael I, Velazquez FR, et al. Safety and efficacy of an attenuated vaccine against severe rotavirus gastroenteritis. *N Engl J Med* 2006; 354:11–22. Recent data suggest that the vaccines' efficacy may be somewhat lower in at least some developing countries compared to what was seen in the clinical trials.
7. Glass RI, Parashar UD. The promise of new rotavirus vaccines. *N Engl J Med* 2006; 354:75–77. See also rotavirus vaccine program: http://rotavirusvaccine.org/index.htm.
8. The phrase used in much of the literature is research that does not offer a "prospect of direct benefit" to subjects. I avoid this phrase because the term "direct" benefit does not have an agreed-upon meaning and has been used in a number of different ways to address different concerns. Consistent with the literature, I assume that pediatric research needs special justification when it does not offer a compensating potential for *clinical* benefit. One might object that this account is too narrow, since children may benefit in other ways from their enrollment in research. They may, for example, be paid.
9. Katzman GL, Dagher AP, Patronas NJ. Incidental findings on brain magnetic resonance imaging from 1000 asymptomatic volunteers. *JAMA* 1999; 282:36–39.
10. Kim BS, Illes J, Kaplan RT, et al. Incidental findings on pediatric MR images of the brain. *Am J Neuroradiol* 2002; 23:1674–1677. For more on this topic see: Check E. Brain-scan ethics come under the spotlight. *Nature* 2005; 433:185; Illes J, Kirschen MP, Karetsky K, et al. Discovery and disclosure of incidental findings in neuroimaging research. *J Magn Reson Imaging* 2004; 20:743–747.
11. This topic was the focus of the summer 2008 issue of *The Journal of Law, Medicine and Ethics,* as well as a National Institutes of Health (NIH) workshop. On the latter see: Illes J, Kirschen MP, Edwards E, et al. Incidental findings in brain imaging research. *Science* 2006; 311:783–784.
12. Institute of Medicine. *Ethical Conduct of Clinical Research Involving Children.* Washington DC: National Academies Press, 2004, Chapter 2. Available at: www.nap.edu.
13. Nicholson RH. *Medical Research with Children: Ethics, Law, and Practice.* Oxford: Oxford University Press, 1986:40–60.
14. Roberts R, Rodriquez W, Murphy D, Crescenzi T. Pediatric drug labeling: Improving the safety and efficacy of pediatric therapies. *JAMA* 2003; 290: 905–911.

15. Caldwell PHY, Murphy SB, Butow PH, Craig JC. Clinical trials in children. *Lancet* 2004; 364:803–811.
16. Institute of Medicine. *Ethical Conduct of Clinical Research Involving Children*, pp. 25–26.
17. One example of a study of normal controls—and the review it received—as told from the investigator's perspective can be found at: Rosenfield RL. Improving balance in regulatory oversight of research in children and adolescents: A clinical investigator's perspective. *Ann N Y Acad Sci* 2008;1135:287–295.
18. See U.S. Food and Drug Administration. The pediatric exclusivity provision. Status report to Congress. January 2001. Available at: http://www.fda.gov/cder/pediatric.
19. Institute of Medicine. *Ethical Conduct of Clinical Research Involving Children*, pp. 66–72.
20. Ibid., pp. 68–70.
21. Institute of Medicine. *Ethical Conduct of Clinical Research Involving Children*, p. 71; Salvatoni A, Piantanida E, Nosetti L, et. al. Inhaled corticosteroids in childhood asthma: Long-term effects on growth and adrenocortical function. *Pediat Drugs* 2003;5:351.
22. Council for International Organizations of Medical Sciences (CIOMS). International Ethical Guidelines for Biomedical Research. Geneva: CIOMS; 2002, principle 14.
23. Berger WE. Reflections on law and experimental medicine. *UCLA Law Review* 1968;15(2): 438.
24. Edwards SD, McNamee MJ. Ethical concerns regarding guidelines for the conduct of clinical research on children. *Med Ethics* 2005; 31:351–354.
25. Kass L. Comments to The President's Council on Bioethics, April 2006. Available at: http://www.bioethics.gov/transcripts/apri106/session4.html
26. See May W. Experimenting on human subjects. *Linacre Quarterly* 1976; 43:73–84; Bartholome W. The ethics of non-therapeutic clinical research on children. In: Appendix to Report and recommendations: Research involving children. The National Commission for the Protection of Human Subjects of Biomedical and Behavioral Research. Washington DC: U.S. Government Printing Office, 1977:3.1–3.22; Ackerman TF. Moral duties of parents and nontherapeutic clinical research procedures involving children. *Bioethics Quarterly* 1980; 2:94–111; Kopelman L. In: Kopelman LM, Moskop JC, eds. *Children and Health Care: Moral and Social Issues*. Boston: Kluwer, 1989:89–99; Brock DW. Ethical issues in exposing children to risks in research. In: Grodin MA, Glantz LH, eds. *Children as Research Subjects: Science, Ethics and Law*. New York: Oxford University Press 1994:81–101; Ackerman TF. Nontherapeutic research procedures involving children with cancer. *J Ped Oncology* 1994; 11:134–136; McCormick RA. Experimentation in children: Sharing in sociality. *Hastings Center Report* 1976; 6:41–46; Ramsey P. The enforcement of morals: Nontherapeutic research on children. A reply to Richard McCormick. *Hastings Center Report* 1976; 6:21–30;

Fried C. Children as subjects for medical experimentation. In: Van Eys, J, ed. *Research on Children*. Baltimore: University Park Press, 1978:107–114.

27. This is not to say that all authors see the situation as presenting a dilemma. Some authors regard nonbeneficial research as clearly acceptable or unacceptable. Paul Ramsey, at least in most of his writings, falls in the latter group.
28. Murray TH. *The Worth of a Child*. Berkeley: University of California Press, 1996:74.
29. Fost N (professor of pediatrics and director of the Program in Medical Ethics, University of Wisconsin Hospital). Report to the President's Council on Bioethics, Thursday, December 8, 2005, Session 1: Bioethics and American Children. Available at: http://www.bioethics.gov/transcripts/dec05/session1.html
30. Sammons HM, Malhotra J, Choonara I, et al. Survey of pediatricians in Canada and Europe. *Eur J Clin Pharmacol* 2007; 63:431–436. A survey of the chairpersons of German research ethics committees also found a good deal of unease and discomfort regarding nonbeneficial pediatric research. Lenk C, Radenbach K, Dahl M, Wiesemann C. Non-therapeutic research with minors: How do chairpersons of German research ethics committees decide? *J Med Ethics*. 2004;30:85–87.
31. Bartholome W. Ethics of non-therapeutic clinical research in children. Appendix of the National Commission report on research with children, pages 3–17.
32. See Ackerman TF. Moral duties of parents and nontherapeutic clinical research procedures involving children. *J Med Human* 1980; 2:94–111.
33. See, for example, Nelson RM, Ross LF. In defense of a single risk standard. *J Pediat* 2005;147:565–566.
34. This approach is illustrated in a paper by Susan Wolf on happiness and meaning. She argues that a life has meaning to the extent that one is actively engaged with things of value: "A person who is bored or alienated from most of what she spends her life doing is one whose life can be said to lack meaning. Note that she may in fact be performing functions of worth." (In: Wolf S. Happiness and meaning: Two aspects of the good life. *Soc Philosophy Policy* 1997;14:211.) The requirement that the engagement be active seems to imply that the kinds of passive contributions we shall consider have no implications for how well an individual's life goes. However, the account Wolf is after seems clearly to be one of what qualifies as a meaningful life for us, that is, for autonomous adults.
35. A good deal of this critique has been developed by feminist philosophers. See, among many others, Noddings N. *Caring: A Feminine Approach to Ethics and Moral Education*. Berkeley: University of California Press, 1984; Noddings N. *Starting at Home: Caring and Social Policy*. Berkeley: University of California Press, 2002; Robinson F. *Globalizing Care: Ethics, Feminist Theory, and International Relations*. Boulder, CO: Westview, 1999; Tong R, Williams N. *Feminist Ethics, Stanford Encyclopedia of Philosophy,* 2006. Available at: http://plato.stanford.edu/entries/feminism-ethics/

36. The story is recounted at http://www.chicagotribune.com/sports/cs-13-cubs-bits-chicagoju113,0,6480204.story and also at http://chicago.cubs.mlb.com/news/gameday_recap.jsp?ymd=20080710&content_id=3105914&vkey=recap&fext=.jsp&c_id=chc.
37. Later we will consider in some depth what is required for a contribution to become part of one's life narrative in the relevant way. Here, one could press this point by asking whether the pitcher also contributed to the boy's injury. After all, it was his pitch that Lilly hit that injured the boy. To answer this question, we will need to consider when the causal interventions of others effectively "screen off" upstream contributors from making what we would regard as a personal contribution to the outcome in question.
38. Moral luck theorists argue that one way to establish the moral nature of one's action is to ask who should be held responsible for any costs associated with the resulting injury. When the resulting harms trace to a prior mistake—say, running over a child who darts into the street while knowingly driving with faulty brakes—one arguably should pay for the injuries that one causes. This does not seem to be the case here. Lilly should not be expected to pay the boy's medical costs.
39. Herman B. *Proceedings and Addresses of the APA* 2000. Volume 74:29–45:35.
40. Imagine, for example, that the world in which we do not contribute to the Nazi cause includes a (nonhuman) contribution that exactly replaces the loss of our contribution.
41. Darwall S. *Welfare and Rational Care.* Princeton NJ: Princeton University Press, 2002.
42. Griffin J. *Well-being*. Oxford: Oxford University Press, 1986:29.
43. Williams B. *Moral Luck*. Cambridge: Cambridge University Press, 1981.
44. Ibid., p. 23.
45. Ibid.
46. Williams calls this "constitutive" luck. *Moral Luck*, p. 20.
47. The reference is to Judith Thomson's essay on abortion (Thomson, JJ. A defense of abortion. *Philosophy Public Affairs* Autumn 1971; 1(1):47–66).
48. Williams B. *Moral Luck*, p. 23.

Chapter 2

1. Elliott C. Guinea-pigging: Healthy human subjects for drug-safety trials are in demand. But is it a living? *New Yorker*, Dept. of Medical Ethics, January 7, 2008.
2. For a nice overview of the history and ethics of pediatric research see: Diekema DS. Conducting ethical research in pediatrics: A brief historical overview and review of pediatric regulations. *J Pediat* 2006:149:S3–S11.
3. Levine RJ. Talk to the President's Council on Bioethics, April 20, 2006: http://www.bioethics.gov/transcripts/apri106/session3.html
4. This approach should be distinguished from one that insists research is acceptable only when it offers children a more favorable risk–benefit ratio than the available

alternatives. On that view, the question is not whether a clinician would be willing to have the child enroll on the grounds that the research does not conflict with the child's interests, but whether the clinician would positively recommend enrollment on the grounds that it would promote the child's medical interests (more than the available alternatives). The question of whether a single metric exists involves the question roughly of how expert clinicians make these judgments in individual cases. Do they reduce the various risks to some single metric and make the comparison on those grounds? Or do they (somehow) compare values of different types?

5. Phase 1 studies may pose this dilemma. They investigate medications that have undergone very little, if any, previous testing in humans. Typically, an experimental drug is introduced into Phase 1 studies on the basis of evidence in the laboratory and in animals that it may be useful in humans. At this point, the evidence may be insufficient to make a clear judgment regarding the potential that the new medication will benefit or harm humans, in which case individuals who have access to alternative treatments likely would be better off pursuing them. But what of an individual who has exhausted all standard treatment options? Is it in that individual's medical interests to enroll in the Phase 1 study of a new medication?
6. A complete analysis here would need to distinguish two different sources of uncertainty, one in which all the experts are unsure because the risks and benefits are very similar, versus one in which some are convinced that the risks are clearly unacceptable, but others disagree.
7. Lederer SE, Grodin MA. Historical overview: Pediatric experimentation. In: Grodin MA, Glantz LH, eds. *Children as Research Subjects: Science, Ethics and Law*. New York: Oxford University Press, 1994:19; also see Lederer SE. Children as guinea pigs: Historical perspective. *Account Res* 2003; 10:1–16.
8. Pappworth MH. *Human Guinea Pigs: Experimentation on Man*. London: Routledge & Kegan Paul, 1967.
9. Vollmann J, Winau R. Informed consent in human experimentation before the Nuremberg code. *BMJ* 1996; 313:1445–1449.
10. 1931 German Guidelines on human experimentation. Reprinted in: *International Digest of Health Legislation* 1980; 31:408–411.
11. Trials of war criminals before the Nuremberg military tribunals under Control Council law 10, v. 2 Washington, DC: U.S. Government Printing Office, 1949:181–182.
12. Indian Council of Medical Research. Ethical Guidelines for Biomedical Research on Human Participants, 2006. Available at: http://icmr.nic.in/ethical_guidelines.pdf.
13. SA Halpern. *Lesser Harms: The Morality of Risk in Medical Research*. Chicago: University of Chicago Press, 2004.
14. Ibid., p. 7.
15. U.S. Department of Health and Human Services. Code of Federal Regulations. 45 CFR 46.116.

16. U.S. Food and Drug Administration. Code of Federal Regulations. Title 21, 50.25. Volume 1, Revised April 1, 2005.
17. Nepal Health Research Council, Guidelines for Institutional Review Committees for health research in Nepal. Kathmandu, 2005.
18. Australian National Health and Medical Research Council, National Statement on ethical conduct in research involving humans. Available at http://www.hhs.gov/ohrp/international/HSPCompilation.pdf.
19. Guidelines for the Conduct of Health Research Involving Human Subjects in Uganda (1997), available at http://www.hhs.gov/ohrp/international/HSPCompilation.pdf; Tri-Council Working Group, Final Report of the Tri-Council Working Group on the Ethical Conduct for Research Involving Humans (1997). Available at: http://www.ethics.ubc.ca/code.html.
20. Available at: http://www.mrc.ac.za/ethics/values.htm.
21. National Council for Science and Technology. Guidelines for the Ethical Conduct of Biomedical Research Involving Human Subjects in Kenya. Nairobi, 2004.
22. Indian Council of Medical Research, Ethical Guidelines for Biomedical Research on Human Subjects.
23. See Kopelman LM. When is the risk minimal enough for children to be research subjects? *J Med Philosophy 1989;37:89–99; Fisher CB, Kornetsky SZ, Prentice ED. Determining risks in pediatric research. Am J Bioethics* 2007;7:5–10; Kopelman LM. Children as research subjects: A dilemma. J Med Philosophy 2000;25:745–764; Barnbaum D. Making more sense of minimal risk. *IRB: Ethics & Human Research* 2002;24(3):10–13.
24. This category is based on a recommendation by the U.S. National Commission. As discussed later, the recommendation did not gain unanimous support and led to the writing of an explicit dissent by two of the commissioners. This category continues to be controversial, in particular because it can be approved only when the research is likely to yield generalizable knowledge regarding the subjects' condition. There has been debate regarding what constitutes a "condition" for these purposes, but most agree that this requirement allows sick children to be exposed to greater risks than healthy children, thus the controversy.
25. Child health and the scope of research. Chapter 3 in Nicholson RH. *Medical Research with Children,* pp. 40–44.
26. Roberts R, Rodriquez W, Murphy D, Crescenzi T. Pediatric drug labeling: Improving the safety and efficacy of pediatric therapies. *JAMA* 2003;290: 905–911; Caldwell PHY, Murphy SB, Butow PH, Craig JC. Clinical trials in children. *Lancet* 2004;364:803–811.
27. See Ross LF. Children in medical research: Access versus protection. Oxford: Clarendon Press, 2006.
28. ICH, Guidance for Industry, E11, Clinical Investigation of Medicinal Products in the Pediatric Population. Available at: http://www.fda.gov/cder/guidance/4099fnl.pdf

29. NIH Policy and Guidelines on the Inclusion of Children as Participants in Research Involving Human Subjects, 6 March 1998. Available at: http://grants.hih.gov/grants/guide/notice-files/not98–024.Html.
30. FDAMA of 1997, Public Law 105–15, 111 Stat. 2296 (1997).
31. Children's Health Act of 2000, Public Law 106–310 (OCT. 17, 2000). Available at: http://frwebgate.access.gpo.gov/cgi-bin/getdoc.cgi?dbname=106_cong_public_laws&docid=f:pub1310.106.
32. Best Pharmaceuticals for Children Act, public law 107–109, 115 Stat. 1408 (January 4, 2002). Available at: http://www.fda.gov/opacom/laws/pharmkids/contents.html.
33. Goldkind S (bioethicist, Office of Pediatric Therapeutics, Office of the Commissioner, Food and Drug Administration). Presentation to the President's Council on Bioethics, Thursday, December 8, 2005, Session 4: Ethical Issues in Pediatric Research. Available at: http://www.bioethics.gov/transcripts/dec05/session4.html
34. See http://www.fda.gov/oc/initiatives/advance/fdaaa.html), and http://frwebgate.access.gpo.gov/cgi-bin/getdoc.cgi?dbname=110_cong_public_laws&docid=f:pub1085.110
35. See Murphy D (director, Office of Pediatric Therapeutics). Presentation, March 2007, Available at: http://www.fda.gov/oc/opt/presentations/LastVienna.ppt
36. Stephenson T. "Bonne Année," "Gutes Neues Jahr"? Will 2007 be a "Happy New Year" in Europe for children's medicines? *Arch Dis Child* 2007;92;661–663.
37. See http://www.emea.europa.eu/htms/general/contacts/PDCO/PDCO.html.
38. Permanand G, Mossialos E, McKee M. The EU's new paediatric medicines legislation: Serving children's needs? *Arch Dis Child* 2007;92;808–811.
39. Glantz LH. The law on human experimentation with children. In: Grodin MA, Glantz LH, eds. *Children as Research Subjects*, p. 127.
40. *Nielson v. Regents of the University of California et al.* No. 665–049 Civ. 8–9 (Super Ct. San Francisco, Cal. 23 Aug 1973).
41. TD Case. *T.D., et al. v. The New York State Office of Mental Health, et al.* 91 N.Y.2d 860, 690 N.E.2d 1259, 668 N.Y.S.2d 153 (1997). December 22, 1997.
42. The case is named for Erika Grimes, one of the children involved in the case.
43. Glantz L. Nontherapeutic research with children: *Grimes v. Kennedy Krieger Institute. Am J Public Health* 2002; 92:1070–1073; Mastroianni AC, Kahn JP. Risk and responsibility, *Grimes* v. *Kennedy Krieger*, and public health research involving children. *Am J Public Health* 2002;92;1073–1076; Lantos J. Pediatric research: What is broken and what needs to be fixed? *J Pediatrics* 2004; 144 (2):147–149.
44. Two very different explanations are consistent with this result: The court may have judged the case to be without merit, or the parties may have agreed to a settlement.
45. Maryland House Bill No. 917, 416th session, 2002 MD H.B. 917 (SN), enacted May 2002, effective October 2002; MD Health Gen. § 13–2001–2004.

46. See Va. Code Ann. § 32.1–162.20.
47. Doraine Lambelet Coleman J. The legal ethics of pediatric research. *Duke Law J* 2007;Vol. 57, No. 3.

Chapter 3

1. Note that the title is *The Patient as Person* (Ramsey P., New Haven: Yale University Press, 1970). Chapter 1 is titled "Consent as a canon of loyalty with special reference to children in medical investigations," pp. 1–58.
2. Ramsey P. The enforcement of morals: Nontherapeutic research on children: A reply to Richard McCormick. *Hastings Center Report* 1976;6:21–30.
3. Ramsey P. Children as research subjects: A reply. *Hastings Center Report* 1977;7:40–42.
4. Ramsey P. *The Patient as Person*, pp. 11–12.
5. Ibid., p. 14.
6. Ibid., p. 37.
7. Ibid., p. 37.
8. Hurd HM. The moral magic of consent. *Legal Theory* 1996;2:121–146; Alexander L. The moral magic of consent (II). *Legal Theory* 1996;2:165–174.
9. Some might object that whereas informed consent is vital to clinical research, consent to playing sports (and perhaps many other activities in daily life) need not be informed, or not so informed. The activity and one's participation in it is considered acceptable provided one is a competent adult who agrees to participate. One need not be informed, unless one insists on being informed. My own view is that some level of information is assumed in essentially all cases of consent. This need not require a formal consent process, with explanation and written forms, as occurs in the context of clinical research. Yet, one has to understand some things in order to give consent even to playing sports. Often the information that one needs to understand is minimal and may be assumed when the individual in question is a competent adult and the activity is a familiar one.
10. *Prince v. Commonwealth of Massachusetts.*, 321 U.S. 158 (1944). 321 U.S. 158. *Prince v. Commonwealth of Massachusetts*. no. 98.
11. It is common, but a mistake nonetheless, to think that an individual's full consent can render any treatment of him acceptable. This is a mistake because there are at least two additional conditions on our ethical treatment of others. First, to some extent, we have an obligation to protect the interests of others. Thus, if an individual provides full consent to something that is dramatically contrary to his interests, that fact itself provides good reason for us not to perform the action. Second, as mentioned previously, there are ethical constraints on the actions of actors that do not depend on the interests of the recipients.
12. For present purposes, we need not consider the case in which the individual refuses to consent.

13. This case differs from nonbeneficial pediatric research in an important way. The present case involves the potential for immediate benefit in the face of clear and imminent danger to a present and identified individual. Nonbeneficial pediatric research, in contrast, typically involves the potential for benefit in the future to presently unidentified, and possibly not-yet-existing individuals. Although I will not consider the point here, this difference may influence the extent to which it can be acceptable to expose nonconsenting individuals to risks for the benefit of others. It may be acceptable to expose individuals to greater risks when the benefits are immediate, essentially certain, and for an identified individual. However, the satisfaction of these conditions does not seem necessary for exposing nonconsenting individuals to some risk. Imagine while on vacation you hear what you think is a young child falling into water and calling for help. Due to an injury you are unable to get up. The only other means of assistance is your 12 year old daughter. In at least some cases, especially when the risks to your daughter are low, it seems perfectly acceptable to send her to check on the situation. Here you are exposing her to some risks for the chance of helping some as yet unidentified and possibly not even existing individual. Those factors may influence the level of risks to which you can expose your daughter compared to the risks to which you can expose the thin man. But it does not imply that exposing your daughter to some risks for the benefit of some possible other is unethical. I also will not consider here the possibility that the potential to immediately help an identified individual may allow Utilitarian tradeoffs of interests of the kind we do not accept in the context of nonbeneficial pediatric research.
14. Charles Fried points out that Ramsey argues from the prohibition on unconsented touching of competent adults to the general principle: "do not intentionally impose upon another without that person's consent." (Fried C. Children as Subjects for Medical Experimentation. In: Van Eys J, ed. *Research on Children: Medical Imperatives, Ethical Quandaries, and Legal Constraints*. Baltimore, University Park Press, 1978:107–114.)
15. Millions of children participate in charitable activities each year that involve their being exposed to risks for the benefit of unidentified others: collecting money, digging wells, planting crops. For the relevance of these practices to clinical research, see Wendler D. Protecting subjects who cannot give consent: Toward a better standard for "minimal" risks. *Hastings Center Report* 2005;35:37–43.
16. Transplant cases involve physicians directly exposing one child to risks for the benefit of another child. However, as we have seen, most courts argue that transplantation involving children as donors is acceptable only to the extent that it can be shown that it is in the interests of the donor, either because of the good being done or because of the possibility of allowing the donor to avoid some harm (e.g., the loss of a sibling). The case of the German measles (Rubella) vaccine provides an example closer to nonbeneficial pediatric research. German measles poses very high risks to fetuses, including risks of profound cognitive deficits, malformations of the heart and eyes, and possibly deafness. The primary reason to

vaccinate young children against German measles is to protect the fetuses of pregnant women with whom the children may come into contact. To this extent, vaccination of children against German measles looks a good deal like nonbeneficial pediatric research. This example is complicated by the fact that children do get German measles and, although it is not devastating for them, it does produce symptoms in some individuals, including possible fever, swollen and tender lymph nodes, rash, and sometimes headache, loss of appetite, and pain and swelling in the joints. Avoidance of these rare symptoms by receipt of the vaccine offers some clinical benefit to vaccinated children.

17. Charitable activities represent a kind of middle case. The responsible individuals are not directly exposing individuals to risks in the way of much clinical research. Yet, responsible adults establish the activities and invite children to participate. Compare this to cases in which adults allow children on the other side of the world to experience harm by simply going on with their daily lives. Charitable activities thus suggest that the examples typically cited in discussion of the active/passive distinction may represent ends of a continuum of responsibility.

18. I note that given present concerns about the ethical appropriateness of nonbeneficial pediatric research developing a justification for it has the prudential virtue of providing a response to its present critics. The present analysis of the ethical concern posed by nonbeneficial pediatric research is consistent with the fact that most regulations allow research without consent in a number of other cases. Research with cognitively impaired adults also involves exposing some to risks without consent for the benefit of others. In addition, most regulations allow some, typically minimal risk, research to be conducted without the consent of competent adults. Briefly, nonbeneficial research with incapacitated adults (for instance, adults with severe Alzheimer disease) can be justified by the fact that it is consistent with the participants' competent preferences and values. Consent for research with competent adults can be waived when the risks are minimal and obtaining consent is, in the words of the U.S. regulations, 'impracticable'. One might object that the fact children cannot consent implies that obtaining their consent is impracticable as well. Although this is true, the impracticability in the case of research with competent adults typically traces to the fact that the investigators are not interacting with these individuals. For example, consent may be waived for research on individuals' medical records, in which the investigators never interact with them. The claim is that the need for consent is greater when one is the proximate cause of the risks. Thus, it is important to obtain consent when one inserts a needle in a child's arm, but not when one conducts research on the medical records of competent adults. It is also more plausible, as considered below, to argue that adults have an obligation to contribute to medical research from which they have agreed to benefit.

19. For a summary of how the debate between Ramsey and McCormick influenced the thinking of the National Commission, and its recommendations, from one who was there, see Jonsen AR. Nontherapeutic research with children: The Ramsey versus McCormick debate. *J Pediatr* 2006;149(1 Suppl):S12–14.

20. A number of authors have made similar arguments, essentially justifying the parents' decision to enroll children on substituted judgment grounds. Worsfold argues that children should be permitted to participate in research to which the reasonable child would approve in retrospect. When the child develops "rational powers, he will accept our decision on his behalf and agree with us that we did the best thing for him" (Worsfold V. A philosophical justification of children's rights. *Harvard Edu Rev* 1974;44:142–157, 154–155). Stephen Toulmin similarly argues that children could not reasonably object to being enrolled in important research when the risks are low (Toulmin S. *Fetal experimentation: Moral issues and Institutional Controls*. National commission for the protection of human subjects of biomedical and behavioral research, research on the fetus, appendix. Washington DC: U.S. Government Printing Office, 1976, DHEW Publication No. (OS) 76–128, section 10, 10–7, 10–8).
21. Although we might assume that this is the justification for resuscitating unconscious adults, there is a slightly different argument, one that we will consider below. It is not that we assume that the patients would consent to the efforts. Rather, we assume that the efforts promote their medical interests and, thus, barring any reason to think that either this judgment is mistaken or reason to believe that the individual does not want us to further his medical interests, in this way in this case, we resuscitate him. One might respond that we proceed in this case because we assume that individuals will choose what is in their interests. But that ignores the plausible possibility that promoting the individual's medical interests is an independent and valid goal that does not require consent. Of course, when the person can consent, that ability introduces an independent consideration that must be balanced against his best interests.
22. This argument was suggested to me by Paul Litton.
23. Ramsey P. *The Patient as Person*, p. 14.
24. McCormick RA. Proxy consent in the experimental situation. *Perspect Biol Med* 1974;18:2–20.
25. McCormick RA. Experimentation in children: Sharing in sociality. *Hastings Center Report* 1976;6:41–46.
26. Murray T. *The Moral Worth of a Child*. Berkeley: University of California Press, 1996:94.
27. Council of Europe. Additional Protocol to the Convention on Human Rights and Biomedicine, concerning Biomedical Research, 2005. Available at: http://conventions.coe.int/treaty/en/Treaties/Html/195.htm.
28. Medical Research Council of the U.K. Available at: http://www.mrc.ac.uk/pdf-ethics_guide_children.pdf#xml=http://www.mrc.ac.uk/scripts/texis.exe/webinator/search/xml.txt?query=risks+in+children&pr=mrcall&order=r&cq=&id=44b886ec2.
29. Curran WJ, Beecher HK. Experimentation in children. A reexamination of legal ethical principles. *JAMA* 1969;210:77–83.

30. Fried C. Children as subjects for medical experimentation. In: Van Eys J, ed. *Research on Children: Medical Imperatives, Ethical Quandaries, and Legal Constraints*. Baltimore, University Park Press, 1978:75.
31. Fried C. Children as subjects for medical experimentation. In: Van Eys J, ed. Thomas Murray in *The Moral Worth of a Child* suggests a similar view. He claims that nonbeneficial pediatric research is acceptable when the risks are minimal or not undue. The kinds of risks he considers, a "small bump on the head" (page 84), the possibility of a sleepy infant getting a little less sleep (page 85), seem to assume that minimal risk research does not pose any risk of serious harm.
32. At one time, the British Paediatric Association used the concept of "negligible" risk to children (British Paediatric Association. Guidelines to aid ethical committees considering research involving children. *Arch Dis Child* 1980;55:75–77). Nicholson estimated that this category of risk is roughly equivalent to the U.S. standard of minimal risk and that both allow research procedures that pose a risk of death, provided that risk is less than 1 in 1 million (Nicholson RH. *Medical Research with Children: Ethics, Law, and Practice*. Oxford: Oxford University Press, 1986:119).
33. See, for example Freedman B, Glass KC. *Weiss v. Solomon*: A case study in institutional responsibility for clinical research. *Law Med Health Care* 1990;18:395–403.
34. Ethical dimensions of experimental research on children. In: Van Eys J, ed. *Research on Children,* p. 61.
35. In this sense, psychologically healthy individuals are not Bayesians with respect to the risks they face in daily life.
36. Tversky A, Kahneman D. The framing of decisions and the rationality of choice. *Science* 1981;211:453–458; Slovic P. Perception of risk. *Science* 1987;236:280–285; Weinstein N. Optimistic biases about personal risks. *Science* 1989;246:1232–1233.
37. Freedman B, Fuks A, Weijer C. In loco parentis: Minimal risk as an ethical threshold for research upon children. *Hasting Center Report* 1993;23:13–19.
38. Also see Fisher CB, Kornetsky SZ, Prentice ED. Determining risk in pediatric research with no prospect of direct benefit: Time for a national consensus on the interpretation of federal regulations. *Am J Bioethics* 2007;7:5–10, 7.
39. Available at http://brightfutures.aap.org/web/healthCareProfessionalstoolsAndResources.asp.
40. For an estimate from industry, see http://us.gsk.com/health/faqs.htm#5.
41. See Levine RJ. Children as research subjects. In: Kopelman LM, Moskop JC, eds. *Children and Health Care*. Dordrecht: Kluwer, 1989:73–87.
42. Fried C. In: Van Eys J, ed., p. 113.
43. *Protecting Human Research Subjects: IRB Guidebook*. Washington DC: Government Printing Office, 1993.
44. The National Commission for the Protection of Human Subjects of Biomedical and Behavioral Research. *The Belmont Report*. Washington DC: Department of Health, Education and Welfare, 1979.

45. Wendler D, Martinez R, Fairclough D, et al. Proposed regulations for clinical research with adults unable to consent: What are the views of those most likely affected? *Am J Psychiatry* 2002;159:585–591.
46. Council of Europe. Convention for the protection of human rights and dignity of the human being with regard to the application of biology and medicine: Convention on human rights and biomedicine. Article 17. Available at: http://conventions.coe.int/Treaty/EN/cadreprincipal.htm.
47. Ramsey responded to the present argument as follows: "For if a child loves his or her grandmother at least as much as his or her peers, I see no reason why that child may not be entered as a partner in geriatric research" (In: Van Eys J, ed., p. 65).

Chapter 4

1. Critics of the U.S. regulations might point out that the 407 category does not have a strict limit on risk level, but requires only that the "research will be conducted in accordance with sound ethical principles." Although I will not argue it here, this requirement does not seem a Utilitarian one but includes an implicit risk limit. Even if one does not accept this argument, the fact remains that the other categories are not strictly Utilitarian, nor are the many non-U.S. regulations that do not include an analogous category.
2. This account may have difficulty explaining why it can be acceptable for individuals other than parents to enroll children in research.
3. Ross LF. *Children, Families and Health Care Decision Making*. Oxford: Clarendon Press, 1998.
4. Ibid., pp. 39–44.
5. Ibid., p. 10.
6. Ibid., p. 47.
7. Raz J. *The Morality of Freedom*. Oxford: Clarendon Press, 1986:425.
8. See, for instance, Feinberg J. The child's right to an open future. In: Aiken W, LaFollette H, eds. *Whose Child? Children's Rights, Parental Authority, and State Power*. Totowa, NH: Littlefield, Adams, 1980:124–153.
9. Ross LF. *Children, Families and Health Care Decision Making*, p. 49.
10. Ibid., p. 23. It is worth noting that the disagreement may not be as stark as all this. Commentators often focus on what parents should do, how ideally they should raise their children. Ross may have no objection to the claim that parents should raise their children to have a wide range of life plans. Her focus instead is on the limits of state intervention in the family context. What obligations do parents have to their children such that failure justifies state intervention?
11. Ibid., pp. 92–93. One noteworthy implication of Ross's view is that she would not require, contrary to the view of many regulations and commentators, pediatric *assent* for nonbeneficial pediatric research that poses minimal risk. In her view, the independent determination of the extent to which the child has a say in whether

he participates in minimal risk research represents an improper infringement on parental decision making for their children.

12. Ibid., p. 97.
13. Ibid., p. 95.
14. Ibid., p. 93.
15. Ross LF. *Children in Medical Research: Access Versus Protection*. Oxford: Clarendon Press, 2006:22.
16. This discussion recalls the distinction between what Buchanan and Brock call guidance principles and intervention principles. See Buchanan AE, Brock DW. *Deciding for Others: The Ethics of Surrogate Decisionmaking*. New York: Cambridge University Press, 1989:10–11. The thought that best interests is the correct guidance principle does not imply that any deviation from this principle justifies intrusion by the state or others to block parental authority. Several reasons for this exist, most notably, the fact that state intrusion poses many costs.
17. For discussion of this point, see Ackerman, TF. Fooling ourselves with child autonomy and assent in nontherapeutic clinical research. Clin Res, 27 (5), 345-8, 1979.
18. See Curran WJ, Beecher HK. Experimentation in children a reexamination of legal ethical principles. *JAMA* 1969;210:77–83.
19. Bartholome WG. Central themes in the debate over involvement of infants and children in Biomedical Research: A critical examination. In: Van Eys J, ed. *Research on Children: Medical Imperatives, Ethical Quandaries, and Legal Constraints*. Baltimore: University Park Press, 1978:73–74.
20. Ibid., p. 74.
21. Grodin MA, Glantz LH, eds. *Children as Research Subjects: Science, Ethics and Law*. New York: Oxford University Press, 1994, p. 89.
22. Alternatively, one might argue that parental obligations go beyond the child's own best interests to include raising the child to be a better person. Here one would need to explain the basis for this obligation. If the obligation is a social one, one wonders whether the same account might imply that children have an obligation to participate in some research, thus obviating the need for the intermediate step of the child's learning to be moral.
23. Cumbo KB, Vadeboncoeur JA. What are students learning?: Assessing cognitive outcomes in K-12 Service-Learning. *Michigan Journal of Community Service Learning* 1999 Fall:84–96.
24. McPherson K. Service learning: Making a difference in the community. *Schools in the Middle* 1997 Jan/Feb: 9–15.
25. Fertman CI. Linking learning and service: Lessons from service learning programs in Pennsylvania. *ERS Spectrum* 1996 Spring:9–15.
26. Carter KG, Winecoff HL. Across the country: Community schools' involvement in service learning. *Community Education J* 1998 Fall/Winter:5–9.
27. For argument and citations, see Wendler D, Shah S. Should children decide whether they are enrolled in non-beneficial research. *Am J Bioethics* 2003;3:1–7.

28. Gaylin W. Competence: No longer all or none. In: Gaylin W, Macklin R, eds. *Who Speaks for the Child: The Problems of Proxy Consent*. New York: Plenum Press:27–54.
29. Bartholome WG. Ethical issues in pediatric research. In: Vanderpool HY, ed. *The Ethics of Research Involving Human Subjects: Facing the 21st Century*. Frederick MD: University Publishing Group, 1996:356–361.
30. See Diekema DS. Conducting ethical research in pediatrics: A brief historical overview and review of pediatric regulations. *J Pediatr* 2006:149:S3–S11.
31. Ross LF. *Children in Medical Research: Access Versus Protection*, p. 97.
32. Veatch RM. *The Patient As Partner: A Theory of Human-Experimentation Ethics*. Bloomington: Indiana University Press, 1987:57.
33. Caplan AL. Is there a duty to serve as a subject in biomedical research? *IRB: Ethics and Human Research* 1984 Sep–Oct;6:1–5.
34. Ibid., p. 4.
35. Harris J. Scientific research is a moral duty. *J Med Ethics* 2005;31:242–248.
36. Ibid., p. 246.
37. Ibid., p. 7.
38. For a discussion of the application of contract theory to participation in clinical research and the resulting generational problem, see Heyd D. Experimentation on trial: Why should one take part in medical research? *Jarhrbuch for Recht und Ethik (Annual Review of Law and Ethics)* 1996;4:189–204.
39. Brock DW. Ethical issues in exposing children to risks in research. In: Grodin MA, Glantz LH, eds. *Children as Research Subjects*, p. 95.
40. This argument, as Brock acknowledges, implies not simply that clinical research is acceptable, but that individuals have an obligation to participate in it. That is, it implies that adults are obligated to participate in clinical research, although for practical reasons we might refrain from forcing them to do so.
41. The classic formulation of this concern was voiced by Ronald Dworkin (Dworkin R. The original position. In: Daniels N, ed. *Reading Rawls*. Stanford, CA: Stanford University Press, 1989:16–53, especially pages 17–21). Cynthia Stark tries to fend off this "standard indictment" of hypothetical consent by arguing that hypothetical consent does not yield obligations but rather provides one with a moral reason for acting in accord with the decision that one would have made in the hypothetical context (Stark C. Hypothetical consent and justification. *J Philosophy* June 2000;97(6):313–334).
42. One could, if one is uncomfortable with the implicit assumption of 100% efficacy, adjust this figure. The conclusion here would be unaffected as long as the vaccine is at least somewhat effective and would be widely available. Rawls claims that individuals in the original position do not have access to probabilities: "the veil of ignorance excludes all knowledge of likelihoods. The parties have no basis for determining the probable nature of their society, or their place in it. They have no basis for probability calculations" (Rawls J. *A Theory of Justice*, revised edition. Cambridge, MA: Belknap Press, 1999:134). Leaving aside the question of whether individuals in the original

position have any basis for determining probabilities, it is unclear how one could insist on this limitation in the present case and yet still use the original position to determine the appropriate policy with respect to nonbeneficial pediatric research. It seems unclear, for example, how one would go about deciding whether to allow nonbeneficial pediatric research without knowing anything about the probabilities of its leading to harm and benefit, for example.

43. A similar problem faces a recent attempt to justify nonbeneficial research with adults who are not able to provide informed consent (e.g., adults with severe Alzheimer disease). The argument is that nonbeneficial research using incompetent adults is ethical because such individuals are better off in a world that allows such research to proceed. The overall benefits to individuals of allowing such research justify the risks they face of being enrolled in specific nonbeneficial studies. The author responds to the present concern by arguing that high-risk research would subject individuals to significant burdens that could well outweigh the benefits from research conducted with those who cannot consent. The HIV challenge studies illustrate the problem with this response: it depends on the details of the case and the specific number of individuals who will benefit. Yet, the intuition that the challenge studies are unethical is not a function of the number of people who will benefit. See Coleman CH. Research with decisionally incapacitated human subjects" an argument for a systematic approach to risk-benefit assessment. *Indiana Law Journal* Summer 2008; 83:743.
44. Rawls J. *A Theory of Justice*, p. 133.
45. The three special features are that a) the veil of ignorance excludes all knowledge of likelihoods (see footnote 41); b) the choosers have a conception of the good, leading to their caring "very little, if anything, for what he might gain above the minimum stipend" (p. 134); and c) the alternatives have outcomes that "one can hardly accept" (Rawls J. *A Theory of Justice*, pp. 133–135).

Chapter 5

1. Note that I focus here only on the conditions specific to nonbeneficial pediatric research. Failure to mention other conditions, such as independent review and the value of the research are not intended to imply that they are inapplicable, but that they are applicable to clinical research generally.
2. The phrase "reflective equilibrium" to describe this process comes from Rawls. See Rawls J. *A Theory of Justice*, revised edition. Cambridge, MA: Belknap Press, 1999:18.
3. Scanlon TM. *What We Owe to Each Other*. Cambridge: Belknap Press, 2000:125.
4. Harman G. *Explaining Value and Other Essays in Moral Philosophy*. Oxford: Oxford University Press, 2000:154, especially Chapter 9, Human Flourishing, Ethics, and Liberty.
5. Scanlon TM. *What We Owe to Each Other,* p. 131.
6. Rawls J. *A Theory of Justice*, p. 54.

7. Ibid, p. 348.
8. See, for example Huber J, Payne JW, Puto C. Adding asymmetrically dominated alternatives: violations of regularity and the similarity hypothesis. *J Consumer Res* 1982; 9:90–98; Simonson I, Tversky A. Choice in context: Tradeoff contrast and extremeness aversion. *Marketing Res* 1992; 29:281–295.
9. Redelmeier DA, Shafir E. Medical decision making in situations that offer multiple alternatives. *JAMA* 1995;273(4):302–305.
10. Scanlon TM. *What We Owe to Each Other*, p. 109.
11. Raz J. The role of well-being. *Philosophical Perspectives* 2004;18:269.
12. Scanlon TM. *What We Owe to Each Other*, p. 112.
13. Shelly Kagan provides a distinct argument from that presented here on how doing the morally right thing, "living in pursuit of the good," can be in an individual's interests. In considering the tension between promoting one's own interests and promoting the good, Kagan points out that most philosophers, in effect, take the agent's own interests as fixed and then insist that the demands of morality can have pull on the individual only to the extent that they are seen to be consistent with those interests. Kagan argues that a kind of integrity comes with eliminating the tension between self-interests and the claims of morality. And this, Kagan points out, can be realized by adapting one's aims and goals to the demands of morality, adopting as one's own goals what morality demands, rather than holding one's own interests and goals constant and insisting that morality be molded to them. See Chapter 10 in Kagan S. *The Limits of Morality*. Oxford: Oxford University Press, 1989:386–393.
14. Parfit D. *Reasons and Persons*. Oxford: Oxford University Press, 1984:4. See also Hurka T. *Perfectionism*. Oxford: Oxford University Press, 1993.
15. See, for example Overvold M. Self-interest and getting what you want. In: Miller HB, Williams WH, eds. *The Limits of Utilitarianism*. Minneapolis: University of Minnesota, 1982; Overvold M. Self-interest and the concept of self-sacrifice. *Can J Philosophy* 1980;10:105–118; Sumner LW. The subjectivity of welfare. *Ethics*, July 1995;105(4):764–790; Sobel D. On the subjectivity of welfare. *Ethics* Apr 1997;107(3):501–508; Rosati CS. Internalism and the good for a person. *Ethics* 1996;106:297–326.
16. Hare RM. *Moral Thinking*. Oxford: Clarendon Press, 1981:Chapter 12.
17. Griffin J. *Well-being*. Oxford: Oxford University Press, 1986:33.
18. This articulation recalls, but does not depend on, Stephen Darwall's account of interests and welfare.
19. Plato (4th century BCE). Protagoras: 351 c, page 343 of *Plato, Collected Dialogues*, edited by Hamilton E, Cairns H. Princeton: Princeton University Press, 1980. Also available online in English, from The Perseus Digital Library, Gregory Crane, ed.
20. Bentham J. *An Introduction to the Principles of Morals and Legislation,* 1789.
21. For a classic account of evolutionary fitness, see Sober E. *The Nature of Selection: Evolutionary Theory in Philosophical Focus*. Cambridge, MA: MIT Press, 1985.

22. One might think that the kinds of beings we are for the purposes of determining our interests is fully exhausted by the nature of our minds. However, our interests likely are determined by additional considerations, including our history.
23. For an interesting debate on one aspect of the question of who we are and who is us, see: Kumar R. Permissible killing and the irrelevance of being human. J of Ethics 2008; 12:57-80, and McMahon J. Challenges to human equality. J of Ethics. 2008; 12:81-104.
24. Raz J. The role of well-being. *Philosophical Perspectives Ethics* 2004;18:269.
25. Griffin J. *Well-being*, p. 67.
26. Nozick R. *Anarchy, State, and Utopia*. Oxford: Basil Blackwell, 1974:43.
27. Depression is a good example here. The diagnosis of clinical depression involves a finding that an individual does not care about the things he should care about.
28. Perhaps the most famous and literal use of this perspective occurs in Leo Tolstoy's novella *The Death of Ivan Ilyich,* written in 1886. The technique is also used, although not quite so literally, in Thornton Wilder's play *Our Town.*
29. Sumner LW. *Welfare, Happiness and Ethics*. Oxford: Clarendon Press, 1996.
30. Ibid., p. 35.
31. David Sobel points out that Sumner provides two different accounts of subjective theories of welfare. A "necessary condition" account holds that having a pro attitude toward an option or state of affairs is a necessary, although not a sufficient condition on its being beneficial for one or promoting of one's welfare. Mind-dependent accounts of subjectivity hold that the goodness of an option for an agent, at least sometimes, depends on the agent having a pro attitude toward the option, and that this is something objective accounts deny (Sobel D. On the subjectivity of welfare. *Ethics* Apr 1997;107(3): 501–508). The present account is subjective on the mind-dependent definition since the agent's attitudes are relevant in some cases, but not on the necessary condition view of subjective accounts. In some instances, what is in an agent's interests does not depend on her having a pro attitude toward it.
32. Sumner LW. *Welfare, Happiness and Ethics*, p. 1.
33. Ibid., p. 20.
34. Ibid., p. 172.
35. Ibid., p. 171.
36. I have been assuming that something is in an individual's interests when it is the case that, holding all else constant, providing that thing improves the life of the individual in question. In some cases, however, it seems that satisfying one of an individual's biological needs will not improve his overall life. Imagine that we satisfy a biological need of an individual who is in a permanent coma: perhaps we increase his body temperature to normal or feed him. If the individual remains in the coma, it is not clear that satisfying this need has improved his life at all. If this is right, it follows that satisfying a given biological need is not always in an individual's interests in the sense of improving his overall life. Joseph Raz concludes, in contrast, that simply satisfying one's biological needs does not

contribute to one's well-being, but rather only provides necessary conditions for one to pursue one's well-being (see Raz J. *Ethics in the Public Domain*. Oxford: Clarendon Press, 1994:7–8).

37. Skevington SM. Investigating the relationship between pain and discomfort and quality of life, using the WHOQOL. *Pain* 1998;76:395–406; Atkinson JH, Slater MA, Patterson TL, et al. Prevalence, onset and risk of psychiatric disorders in men with chronic low back pain: A controlled study. *Pain* 1991;45:111–121.
38. Sumner LW. *Welfare, Happiness and Ethics,* p. 112.
39. The long-term consequences of a given contribution may intrude here and require a more complicated account. What if I make a contribution that saves the life of an infant? This appears on the face of it to be a valuable contribution. But, to take the most science-fiction version of the example, what if the infant grows up to be Hitler and the rest is history as we know it? One option would be to retreat to different ways of describing the contribution. Described as an act of saving the life of an infant it has value, but described as an act of saving Hitler perhaps not, although one might want to dig in even here and say that saving the life of an infant is always a valuable act and does not depend on the way in which that individual goes on to live his life.
40. Darwall S. *Welfare and Rational Care*, p. 97.
41. It may be that what we might think of as superhuman health and well-being are not in individuals' interests, or at least not nearly to the same extent as the curing of cancer say. Thus, it may be that contributing to clinical studies that aim to improve health and well-being beyond some human or normal range, ones that would allow everyone to run faster and jump higher than current world-class athletes, would not involve valuable achievements, or at least not to the same extent. For the present purposes, we need not resolve this issue, taking as our paradigm trials that are designed to avoid, ameliorate, or eliminate disease. One area of current study for which this issue may be relevant is studies into senescence and increasing the human life span. One can think about this in terms of the treatment/enhancement distinction, if one prefers. But those skeptical of the possibility of making a clear distinction on those grounds can simply think of the difference between improvements in health and well-being that clearly promote individuals' interests versus those that may not promote their interests.
42. Griffin J. *Well-being*, p. 23.
43. Sumner LW. *Welfare, Happiness and Ethics,* p. 127.
44. Ibid., p. 175.
45. Parfit D. *Reasons and Persons*, p. 494.
46. Griffin J. *Well-being,* p. 22.
47. The skeptical view traces largely to Hume's famous challenge to identify anything in the causal relationship beyond temporal priority of the cause, spatiotemporal contiguity of the cause and effect, and constant conjunction over time of the cause followed by the effect (Hume D. *1739–1740, A Treatise of Human Nature*, edited by Selby-Bigge LA. Oxford: Clarendon Press, 1888). Counterfactual accounts

attempt to provide an analysis of causality consistent with Hume's claim that nothing exists beyond the temporal and logical relationships between cause and effect. Roughly, these accounts determine whether X is a cause of Y by asking whether Y would have occurred if X had not occurred. If X's occurrence is a necessary condition for the occurrence of Y, then X is a cause of Y. Counterfactual accounts of causality have the virtue of doing without any additional connection or relationship between cause and effect. They have difficulty, however, with a number of cases, including overdetermination, in which two inputs are sufficient to cause Y. Both inputs seem to be causes despite the fact that Y would still have occurred even if one of them did not occur. These accounts also seem to imply that shields, which allow causal interactions to occur, themselves count as causes—the absence of the shield would have allowed for an interfering input, which would have kept Y from occurring. Classic accounts of the counterfactual approach include Aronson J. On the grammar of cause. *Synthese* 1971;22; and Mackie J. *Cement of the Universe*. Oxford: Oxford University Press, 1974.

48. Salmon WC. A new look at causality. In: Salmon WC, ed. *Causality and Explanation*. New York: Oxford University Press, 1998:17. This work is a follow-up to Salmon's *Scientific Explanation and the Causal Structure of the World*, Princeton: Princeton University Press, 1984.
49. Fisher and Ravizza make the same point using cats and vases; see Fischer JM, Ravizza M. *Responsibility and Control*. Cambridge: Cambridge University Press, 1998.
50. For a summary of the relationship between causal responsibility and moral responsibility, see Sartorio C. Causation and responsibility. *Philosophy Compass* 2007;2:749–765.
51. This example is taken from Beebee H. Causing and nothingness. In: Collins J, Hall N, Paul LA, eds. *Causation and Counterfactual*. Cambridge MA: MIT Press, 2004:291–308. The proposed counterexample there involves the Queen of England.
52. Of course, if we take this route we are left with the puzzle of how to account for the fact that we describe people as causes of outcomes when they should have acted so as to prevent the outcome in question, but didn't. I think that the correct response to these cases is to recognize that we often use the word "cause" or apply the concept in different ways. In casual conversation we regard individuals as the cause of a given outcome when they are (partially) responsible for that outcome. And one can be responsible by being part of the causal process that led to the outcome. This is the sense of cause we are considering here. One also can be responsible for an outcome in the sense of being morally responsible for it. This can happen even when one is not causally responsible; most obviously, when one is morally responsible for not acting. Keeping distinct these two uses of the term "cause" obviates the need to develop an account of causality that captures the possibility that we can be causal agents through our failures to act. Schaffer points out that such an account, one in which omissions cannot be causes, implies that a great deal

of what we describe as causes are not causes in the final analysis. He points out that many apparent causes operate through intervening absences. The paradigm case here is of killing: I shoot you, the bullet hits your heart, your blood supply is depleted, and your brain ceases to function in the absence of a sufficient supply of blood. (See Schaffer J. Causation by disconnection. *Philosophy of Science* 2000;67:285–300.) Sartorio suggests, on the basis of this argument, that we should allow that omissions can be causes (Sartorio C. Causation and responsibility. *Philosophy Compass* 2007;2:749–765). I suggest instead that we need to know more about the causal facts, and it may turn out that many causes are causes in the "responsible for" sense without being part of the causal process. At least some states in the United States define death in terms of the permanent cessation of cardiopulmonary function. In these states, the bullet destroying the heart, assuming the destruction is permanent in the relevant sense, would imply that the bullet caused the person's death. In a jurisdiction where death is defined by the permanent cessation of brain function, the bullet would be an agent of the person's death only as a result of the intervening absence of blood to the brain. The distinction between one's being morally responsible and one's being causally responsible blurs when we consider acts that are causally responsible for states of affairs that inevitably lead to a further state of affairs. Imagine that by touching you with my magic wand I remove all the blood from your body, but otherwise leave you untouched. My action does not directly influence your brain, but it does eliminate the supply of oxygen that keeps your brain alive. Here the moral and causal responsibility for the death of your brain (and you) are very close.

53. Griffin J. *Well-being*, p. 64–68.
54. See Portmore DW. Welfare, achievement and self-sacrifice. *J Ethics Social Philosophy* 2007;2(2).
55. See Scanlon TM. *What We Owe to Each Other*, p. 120; Portmore DW. Welfare, achievement and self-sacrifice, p. 3.
56. Portmore labels the related achievementist views "hard core" achievmentists (Welfare, achievement and self-sacrifice, p. 3).
57. A great deal more could be said about the differences here, and many different distinctions would need to be made. One example is the distinction between acts and activities. Acts are single contributions at one time, activities are contributions that extend over time. See Raz J, Morality and self-interest, Raz J. *Engaging Reason: On the Theory of Value and Action.* Oxford: Oxford University Press, 1999.
58. Portmore accepts the investment principle, which holds that the significance of our achievements depends on the amount we invest in them (see Welfare, achievement and self-sacrifice). He argues that we should understand the level of investment in terms of how much the individual sacrifices, not in terms of how much effort he expends. However, the fact that the level of effort expended influences the significance of the contribution, even when one enjoys the effort—enjoys the painting or the running—implies that the level of effort is an

independent consideration. Part of the significance of running a marathon is determined by how much effort it requires. Expending that level of effort is significant, independently of how much a sacrifice it is for the individual (e.g., how much he enjoys it, what implications it has for what he has to forego for lack of energy).

Chapter 6

1. Slote M. *Goods and Virtues*. Oxford: Clarendon Press, 1983.
2. Joseph Raz uses this kind of dependence to argue for what he calls a "variable pattern" view of well-being. See Raz J. The role of well-being. *Philosophical Perspectives Ethics* 2004;18, especially pages 276–281.
3. Slote M. *Goods and Virtues,* p. 17.
4. Ibid., p. 14.
5. Ibid., p. 15.
6. For this reason, Slote argues that even though it might be the case that, once I am older and retired, it would be good for me to achieve success as a champion shuffleboard player (page 19 of *Goods and Virtues*), the value of that accomplishment for me then does not provide a transtemporal reason for action. It does not provide me now with a reason to practice my shuffleboard skills, even if it is true that practice now would increase the chances of my becoming a shuffleboard champion then.
7. This might not be true for individuals who end up pursuing a life of monastic self-reflection and come to regard all aesthetic pursuits and accomplishments as anathema. The possibility of such exceptions serves as a reminder that judgments of the value of a given accomplishment for one's life must take into account that life as a whole.
8. For differences in pediatric and adult evaluations of risks see, for example, McCarthy AM, Richman LC, Hoffman RP, Rubenstein L. Psychological screening of children for participation in nontherapeutic invasive research. *Arch Pediatr Adolesc Med* 2001;155:1197–1203; and Lantos J, Mukherjee D. Witches, pubertal development, and "minimal risk." *Arch Pediatr Adolesc Med* 2001;155:1195–1196.
9. Parfit D. *Reasons and Persons*. Oxford: Oxford University Press, 1984; especially pages 298–302.
10. Parfit D. *Reasons and Persons,* p. 301.
11. Parfit argues for this conclusion by pointing out that we regret not having memories of our youth, and we would regret ceasing to love those we now love, or ceasing to care about the things for which we now care. He regards this regret as implying that we have less reason to prudentially care about the person who has those memories, loves, and goals. That person is, in a fundamental sense, a different person. Although we care about some degree of unity in this regard, it

is not clear that this value implies something about the boundaries of our (now) lives as opposed to something about what we value within our lives.

12. Susan Wolf points out that even if one accepts Parfit's reductionism with respect to personal identity, the question remains what implications that acceptance has for how we should conduct our lives, for how we should treat ourselves, and others. See Wolf S. Self-interest and interest in selves. *Ethics* 1986;96:704–720.
13. In the United States, an IRB could approve the participation of healthy children (those without a condition) in such a study only if the risks were no more than minimal. An IRB could approve the enrollment of children with a condition provided the risks do not exceed a minor increase over minimal. Nonbeneficial studies that pose higher levels of risk may be conducted only following review and approval by the Departmental Secretary using the process described in section 407 of the regulations.
14. See, for example, Ondrusek N, Abramovitch R, Pencharz P, Koren G. Empirical examination of the ability of children to consent to clinical research. *J Med Ethics* 1998;24:158–165; Chou KL. Effects of age, gender and participation in volunteer activities on the altruistic behavior of Chinese adolescents. *J Genetic Psychol* 1998;159:195–201; Eisenberg N, Miller PA, Shell R, et al. Prosocial development in adolescence: A longitudinal study. *Dev Psychol* 1991;27:849–857; Harbaugh WT, Krause K. Children's contribution in public good experiments: The development of altruistic and free-riding behavior. *Economic Inquiry* 2000;38:95–109; Lew C, Lewis M, Ifekwunique M. Informed consent by children and participation in an influenza vaccine trial. *Am J Public Health* 1978;68:1079–1082; Leikin S. Minors' assent, consent, or dissent to medical research. *IRB* 1993;15:5; Susman EJ, Dorn LD, Fletcher JC. Participation in biomedical research: The consent process as viewed by children, adolescents, young adults, and physicians. *J Pediatr* 1992;121:547–552; Weithorn L, Campbell S. The competency of children and adolescents to make informed decisions. *Child Dev* 1982;53:1589–1598.
15. For a similar view, see Darwall (Darwall S. *Welfare and Rational Care*. Princeton NJ: Princeton University Press, 2002:97), where he focuses on what he calls virtuous activity, using the example of a concert pianist. Darwall focuses on virtues and considers examples of individuals engaging in value through their great skills. Although these contributions seem especially important, the connection to value does not require them.
16. Consideration of other examples reveals that things here can get more complex. What if a person adopts different goals at different periods of her life? How do we decide overall how her life went? Achieving goals at the time one has them seems to count for something in itself, but what of overall considerations in general? Also, what of an individual who has the wrong goals, but successfully achieves them, perhaps setting out to do wrong under the mistaken view that she is doing right. The actual wrongs that the person commits under this mistaken impression certainly do not count in favor of her overall life, but what of the fact that at this

point in her life she set goals, faithfully pursued, and successfully achieved them? Does that fact have any positive implications for an overall assessment of her overall life? Is steadfast pursuit of a goal which lacks value valuable at all, ever?

17. UNESCO. Report of the International Bioethics Committee of UNESCO, 2008. See the case of John on page 30. Of note, the report uses this possibility to argue not that participation in the study benefits the child, but for a kind of presumed consent justification for his participation. Available at: http://unesdoc.unesco.org/images/0017/001781/178124e.pdf.
18. Redmon RB. How children can be respected as "ends" yet still be used as subjects in non-therapeutic research. *J Medical Ethics* 1986;12:77–82.

Chapter 7

1. Bracketing this issue has the implication that the present analysis is silent on research using such infants. This approach has practical importance when we consider the question of nonbeneficial research with nonviable infants. Interestingly, the U.S. federal regulations do not allow nonbeneficial research with nonviable infants that poses any net risks to them ("there will be no added risk to the [nonviable] neonate resulting from the research"; 45 CFR 46.205 c3), a stricter standard than that applied to viable infants. Although a good deal of analysis would be required to consider whether this approach makes sense, one might regard it as following from a substantive answer to the present issue. That is, one could argue that viable infants have interests in contributing to valuable projects whereas infants that will not make it to adulthood do not have such interests, hence, less justification exists for enrolling them in nonbeneficial research.
2. One way to understand this conclusion would be in terms of the claim that the fact of making a contribution has value independent of the individual's agency. It is a good thing to make even passive contributions to valuable projects, and increasing the extent to which the contributions go through the individual's agency increases the extent to which they are relevant to an overall assessment of the individual's life. Although the present example supports the conceptual independence of the value of making a contribution and the extent to which it goes through the contributor's agency, other examples undermine this independence when it comes to competent contributors. Imagine that a competent individual is forced to contribute to a good cause. Forcing the individual clearly wrongs and possibly harms them in virtue of failing to respect them as autonomous beings. What, then, should we conclude about the positive contribution itself? Do we say that the forcing was wrong, but the contributing is a good thing for the individual's life, and then defend the claim that we ought not to force competent individuals to do good things for their own good on the grounds that the wrong of forcing them outweighs the positive implications that come from their having made a valuable contribution? That is one possibility. However, it also seems plausible that the

fact of forcing the individual may eliminate the extent to which his making the contribution says something valuable about his life. To take a related possibility, pitched at a slightly different level of analysis, it may be that we do not want *to say* that making the contribution itself promotes the individual's interests since espousing that view provides comfort to scoundrels. To avoid that possibility, we say that the contribution does not have positive implications for his life overall (but does saying this imply that the contribution does not say something valuable about his life, or only that we do not want to admit that it says something valuable; in effect, what hold do our preferences and views have on the facts of the matter?). Consider a case in which an art collector is forced to allow public access to his collection. Assuming that this contribution to the public weal is a good thing, it seems to say something valuable about the collector's life, even though the collector was forced to make the collection public. Here it might be that we are willing to say the contribution, though forced, says something valuable about the contributor's life because we have the prior active and voluntary act on his part of having assembled a valuable art collection in the first place. An actual example to consider in this regard is the life of Albert Barnes, a Philadelphia physician who amassed during his lifetime one of the great private collections of paintings in the world. Barnes also had a very particular view of art education and how his paintings should be arranged and viewed. Barnes' stipulations on the treatment of his collection following his death have been progressively modified to allow money to be raised to protect the collection and to allow greater public access to it. For details on Barnes life, see http://www.barnesfoundation.org/h_bio.html.

3. Empirical research finds that we tend to underestimate our ability to adapt to disease and disability, hence, overestimate the magnitude of harm associated with disease and disability. See, for example, Ubel PA, Loewenstein G, Jepson C. Whose quality of life? A commentary exploring discrepancies between health state evaluations of patients and the general public. *Qual Life Res* 2003;12:599–607.
4. Bernard Williams considers the view that what counts are only those actions and their consequences that go through my agency, and these count only to the extent that I could do something about the actions or their consequences. I do my best, and that's all that counts from my point of view; the rest is luck. He notes: "my involvement in my action and its results goes beyond the relation I have to it as an ex ante rational deliberator." I want to say that he's right, but that he takes this only to cover the results of my intentional acts that go beyond what I intended and what was in my control. I want to go further and say that this line of reasoning takes us beyond rational agency to the possibility that the mere fact that I physically make a contribution to a cause or outcome can have implications for my overall life, independent of the extent to which it went through my agency.
5. Knopp G (translated by Angus McGeoch). *Hitler's Children*. Phoenix Mill: Sutton Publishing, English translation 2002, originally published in German in 2000; 180.

6. Ibid., p. 229.
7. Ibid., p. 183.
8. Kater MH. *Hitler Youth*. Cambridge MA: Harvard University Press, 2004:265.
9. Kurzem M. *The Mascot: Unraveling the Mystery of My Jewish Father's Nazi Boyhood.* New York: Viking Books, 2007.
10. Hunt IA. *On Hitler's Mountain.* New York: Harper Collins, 2005; pages 5 and 74.
11. A recent antismoking advertisement provides a positive example of a reluctant propagandist and a different (nonresearch) context for the possibility of exposing children to some risks for the benefit others. In the commercial, a 3-year-old boy is upset by his mother's brief disappearance. As the camera zooms in on the boy, he begins to cry. The point of the commercial is to graphically highlight the impact on children of their parents smoking and dying prematurely. If the commercial is successful, the child will have been an important, albeit unwitting, and somewhat distressed, contributor to reducing the number of smokers and, presumably, the number of children who lose a parent prematurely. See: http://www.msnbc.msn.com/id/30027473/
12. Raz J. *The Role of Well-being,* p. 274.
13. The fact that we regard negative contributions as more significant for our evaluation and treatment of actors may trace to the fact, if it is a fact, that, in some sense, it is worse to experience negative events than it is beneficial to experience positive events. Susan Wolf considers a related asymmetry concerning the fact that discussions of morality and free will tend to focus on cases in which individuals are influenced by external forces to do something wrong (thereby calling into question whether the person acted freely and is to blame) and comparatively little attention on cases in which individuals are influenced by external forces to do the right thing. Wolf suggests that this difference may trace to the fact that cases of blame are of greater social importance because they raise the possibility of punishment. Although that seems right, it raises the question of why the mechanisms in place to punish are more developed than those to praise. Treating people negatively in response to wrong actions (e.g., putting them in jail for killing) presumably deters them from acting wrongly. Although that seems plausible, it also seems plausible that treating people positively for behaving well (e.g., giving people a vacation for saving a life) would encourage them to act charitably. See Wolf S. Asymmetrical freedom. *J Philosophy* March 1980;77(3):151–166.
14. Thomas Murray considers a related example: parents who have been asked to bring their (now) sleeping baby to a church they had visited only once to fill in as baby Jesus for a child who is sick. He concludes that doing so "falls within the compass of permissible moral discretion" (Murray TH. *The Worth of a Child.* Berkeley: University of California Press, 1996: 85). He bases this conclusion in part on the claim that the child faces only minimal risk. It is not clear from the example whether this includes any chance of serious harm. See consideration of his view earlier in the text.
15. Thanks to Dennis Thompson for emphasizing this point.

16. Bartholome W. Ethical dimensions of experimental research on children (In: Van Eys J, ed. *Research on Children: Medical Imperatives, Ethical Quandaries, and Legal Constraints*. Baltimore: University Park Press, 1978: 57–68; page 67).
17. Ramsey P. *The Patient as Person*. New Haven: Yale University Press, 1970:14.
18. Wendler D, Glantz L. A new standard for assessing the risks of pediatric research: Pro and con. *J Pediatr* 2007;150:579–582. The legal reference is to *In re Richardson*, 284 So. 2d 185 (La. App. 1973).
19. Although not widely noted, these two standards can come apart in actual cases, for example, when an individual has a phobia that prevents him from deciding consistent with his own preferences and values.
20. See, among others, Matsui K, Kita Y, Ueshima H. Informed consent, participation in, and withdrawal from a population-based cohort study involving genetic analysis. *J Med Ethics* 2005;31:385–392; Hoeyer K, Olofsson B, Mjorndal T, Lynoe N. The ethics of research using biobanks: Reason to question the importance attributed to informed consent. *Arch Int Med* 2005;165:97–100;165:652–655; McQuillan GM, Porter KS, Agelli M, Kington R. Consent for genetic research in a general population: The NHANES experience. *Genet Med* 2003;5:35–42; Stegmayr B, Asplund K. Informed consent for genetic research on blood stored for more than a decade: A population based study. *BMJ* 2002;325:634–635; Malone T, Catalano PJ, O'Dwyer PJ, Giantonio B. High rate of consent to bank biologic samples for future research: the eastern cooperative oncology group experience. *J Natl Cancer Inst* 2002;94:769–771.
21. Wendler D, Glantz L. A new standard for assessing the risks of pediatric research.

Chapter 8

1. Again, this is not to imply that all passive contributions have implications for one's life, nor that all scenarios in which one plays a causal role involve one's making a contribution. In particular, the involvement of others sometimes screens off my causal input (i.e. renders it a noncontribution as far as my life is concerned) to the end in question. Imagine that an individual is reared his entire life to react in a violent way to a particular and particularly ordinary brand of shoes. Further imagine that the first such shoes he encounters following this (successful) training happen to be on my feet, leading the individual to rage and the subsequent harming of others. While I have a (passive) causal role in the resulting harm, it seems that the outcome may not become part of the narrative of my life. It may instead be entirely about the individual in question and especially about those who so trained him.
2. For more on the importance of obtaining assent in pediatric research, see Joffe S, Fernandez CV, Pentz RD, et al. Involving children with cancer in decision-making about research participation. *J Pediatr* 2006; 149:862–868; Kon AA. Assent in pediatric research. *Pediatrics* 2006;117:1806–1810; Rossi WC,

Reynolds W, Nelson RM. Child assent and parental permission in pediatric research. *Theor Med Bioeth* 2003;24:131–148.

3. The National Commission for the Protection of Human Subjects of Biomedical and Behavioral Research. *The Belmont Report: Ethical Principles and Guidelines for the Protection of Human Subjects of Research*. April 18, 1979. Available at: http://ohsr.od.nih.gov/guidelines/belmont.html.
4. See also Gidding SS, Camp D, Flanagan MH, et al. A policy regarding research in healthy children. *J Pediatr* 1993;123:852–855.
5. Bartholome W. Ethical dimensions of experimental research on children. In: Van Eys J, ed. *Research on Children: Medical Imperatives, Ethical Quandaries, and Legal Constraints*. Baltimore: University Park Press, 1978: 57–68.
6. The National Commission for the Protection of Human Subjects of Biomedical and Behavioral Research. *The Belmont Report*, p. 137.
7. Ramsey P. *The Patient as Person*. New Haven: Yale University Press, 1970:25.
8. Some critics of clinical research assume that all participation is, in some sense, degrading to the extent that one is a passive subject being exposed to risks by others for the benefit of third parties. The point of the present analysis is that this is only one way to characterize research participation. And, as a general characterization, I think it is largely false. This, of course, does not preclude the possibility that one could imagine studies for which this would be the case. To consider one possibility briefly, imagine that investigators designed a study to evaluate the effects of schoolyard bullying by bringing children into the hospital and subjecting them to bullying by research staff. Such a study could, in principle, gather socially valuable information about bullying and methods for blunting its effects. Despite this value, participation in such a study might not be in the overall interests of the participating children (even bracketing the obviously harmful psychological impact). It might be that this type of contribution is not one that is valuable for individuals to make, despite the social value of the information to be gained.
9. It is tempting to embrace the irony here and argue that participation in these studies is in children's overall interests precisely because it is not in their interests. This does seem possible in certain cases. For some individuals, the value of doing something very stressful, like running a marathon, may be precisely the fact that doing so is (otherwise) contrary to the individual's interests. Similar are cases in which one learns a valuable lesson as the result of going through a harmful experience. The harm is a necessary condition for the benefit. In these cases, the benefit, at the second level as it were, depends on the fact that the activity is not beneficial at the first level. That is a necessary condition for one learning the valuable lesson. Here, the benefit typically requires that the individual realizes the reasons against the activity and then decides to participate in the face of that knowledge. In the case of pediatric research, in contrast, the valence need not be contradictory at the two levels of analysis. It is the fact that children are contributing to helping others that involves them making an important contribution,

and this possibility exists even in the context of studies that offer a compensating potential for clinical benefit.

10. One may regard the moral obligations on clinicians to be even stronger than I am representing them. One might argue that clinicians in particular have a strong obligation to act in the best interests of the patient in front of them. Some take this to imply that it is wrong for clinicians to conduct nonbeneficial research, especially with those who are unable to consent. This common approach rests on two assumptions, both implausible. The first is that in the context of research clinicians are subject to the obligations that bear on them in the standard clinical setting; that the research context, the fact that it is research, does not make a substantive difference to their moral obligations. The second assumption is that in the standard clinical setting clinicians are obliged always to act in the best interests of the patient in front of them. There are numerous counterexamples to this common view.
11. The use of EMLA cream may increase the overall distress of needles for some children by alerting them to the impending injection.
12. McCarthy AM, Richman LC, Hoffman RP, Rubenstein L. Psychological screening of children for participation in nontherapeutic invasive research. *Arch Pediatr Adolesc Med* 2001;155:1197–1203.
13. For an analysis of this tension from a philosophical point of view see Merritt M. Moral conflict in clinical trials. *Ethics* 2005;115:306–330.
14. Miller M. Phase 1 cancer trials: A collusion of misunderstanding. *Hastings Center Report* 2000;30:34–43.
15. The apparently common failure to distinguish the methods and goals of clinical research from those of clinical care has been coined the "therapeutic misconception." A voluminous literature exists on this phenomenon. For the pioneering work, see Appelbaum PS, Roth LH, Lidz C. The therapeutic misconception: Informed consent in psychiatric research. *Int J Law Psychiatry* 1982; 5: 319–329; Appelbaum PS, Roth LH, Lidz CW, et al. False hopes and best data: Consent to research and the therapeutic misconception. *Hastings Cent Rep* 1987;17:20–24. For more recent work on the topic, see Appelbaum PS, Lidz CW, Grisso T. Therapeutic misconception in clinical research: Frequency and risk factors. *IRB* 2004;26:1–8; Horng S, Grady C. Misunderstanding in clinical research: Distinguishing therapeutic misconception, therapeutic misestimation, and therapeutic optimism. *IRB* 2003;25:11–16; Henderson GE, Churchill LR, Davis AM, et al. Clinical trials and medical care: Defining the therapeutic misconception. *PLoS Med* 2007;4:e324.
16. National Health and Medical Research Council, National statement on ethical conduct in research involving humans. Available at http://www.hhs.gov/ohrp/international/HSPCompilation.pdf.
17. Nepal Health Research Council. Guidelines for Institutional Review Committees for health research in Nepal. Kathmandu, 2005.

18. Department of Health and Human Services. Code of Federal Regulations. 45 CFR 46.116.
19. Food And Drug Administration. Code of Federal Regulations. Title 21, 50.25. Volume 1 Revised April 1, 2005.
20. See Kopelman LM, Murphy TF. Ethical concerns about federal approval of risky pediatric studies. *Pediatrics* 2004;113:1783–1789; Nelson RM, Ross LF. In defense of a single standard of research risk for all children. *J Pediatr* 2005;147:565–566. Whether these shortcomings lead to children being exposed to excessive risks *in practice* is unknown.
21. Kopelman LM. Minimal risk as an international ethical standard in research. *J Med Philosophy* 2004; 29:351–378. Nelson RM. Minimal risk, yet again. *J Pediatr* 2007;150:570–572.
22. Ross LF, Nelson RM. Pediatric research and the federal minimal risk standard. *JAMA* 2006;295:759.
23. Thompson K. Kids Risk Project. Harvard University. Unpublished data available at: http://www.kidsrisk.harvard.edu.
24. Tauer C. The NIH trials of growth hormone for short stature. *IRB* 1999;16:1–9; Gidding SS, Camp D, Flanagan MH, et al. A policy regarding research in healthy children. *J Pediatrics* 1993;123:852–855.
25. Ackerman TF. The ethics of drug research in children. *Paediatr Drugs* 2001; 3:29–41.
26. For more on this approach, see Wendler D. Minimal risk in pediatric research as a function of age. *Arch Pediatr Adolesc Med* 2009;163:115–118. One might take the argument even further: The fact that older children can provide competent consent implies that investigators ethically may expose them to whatever level of risks they agree to take on. Although I will not argue the point here, I do not think that this view applies even to research with competent adults. The fact that a competent adult provides informed consent does not imply that investigators may expose him to any level of risks, for any reason. By exposing the participants to risks, the investigators gain an independent obligation to make sure that the decision on the part of the competent adult makes sense, or at least is not wildly contrary to his overall interests. The fact that a competent adult asks me to kill him does not imply that it necessarily is ethical for me to do so. This point has even more resonance when we consider research with children. Because children are inexperienced and part of a family, with parents, we typically are even less willing to take their consent, even when competent, as sufficient reason to treat them in a particular manner.
27. For additional details on the 407 review process, see Office for Human Research Protections (OHRP). Special Protections for Children as Research Subjects: Guidance on the HHS 45 CFR 46.407 ("407") Review Process, May 26, 2005, Available at: http://www.hhs.gov/ohrp/children/guidance_407process.html

28. Ross LF. Convening a 407 panel for research not otherwise approvable: "Precursors to diabetes in Japanese American youth" as a case study. *Kennedy Institute of Ethics* 2004;14:165–186.
29. Wendler D, Varma S. Minimal risk in pediatric research. *J Pediatr* 2006; 149:855–861.
30. Kopelman LM, Murphy TF. Ethical concerns about federal approval of risky pediatric studies. *Pediatrics* 2004;113:1783–1789.
31. McWilliams R, Hoover-Fong J, Hamosh A, et al. Problematic variation in local institutional review of a multicenter genetic epidemiology study. *JAMA* 2003; 290:360–366; Shah S, Whittle A, Wilfond B, et al. How do IRBs apply the federal risk and benefit standards for pediatric research? *JAMA* 2004;291:476–482.
32. The National Commission for the Protection of Human Subjects of Biomedical and Behavioral Research. *The Belmont Report*. Available at: http://ohsr.od.nih.gov/guidelines/belmont.html.
33. Canadian Tri-Council Policy Statement: Ethical Conduct for Research Involving Humans, Article 2.5. Available at: http://www.pre.ethics.gc.ca/english/policy-statement/policystatement.cfm.
34. CIOMS, Guideline 14. Available at: http://www.cioms.ch/frame_guidelines_nov_2002.htm. The Indian Council of Medical Research (ICMR) guidelines include the same statement on research with children, Ethical Guidelines for Biomedical Research on Human Participants, 2006, section IV, ii. Available at: http://www.icmr.nic.in/ethical_guidelines.pdf.
35. Sauer PJ. A report of the Ethics Working Group of the Confederation of European Specialists in Paediatrics (CESP). Research in children. *Eur J Pediatr* 2002;161:1–5.
36. Indian Council of Medical Research. Guidelines, section IV, ii.
37. The National Commission. Recommendations for research with children. Also see: Jonsen AR. Research involving children: Recommendations of the National Commission for the Protection of Human Subjects of Biomedical and Behavioral Research. *Pediatrics* 1978;62:131–136.
38. Iltis A. Pediatric research posing a minor increase over minimal risk and no prospect of direct benefit: challenging 45CFR46.406. *Accountability Res* 2007;14:19–34. Also see Nelson RM, Ross LF. In defense of a single standard of research risk for all children. *J Pediatr* 2005;147:565–566.
39. A number of studies have found differences early on in the brains of those who later develop Alzheimer disease, as well as those who have a gene that increases the risk of Alzheimer disease. One fascinating project follows a group of nuns who religiously record their daily activities. The early writings of those who went on to develop Alzheimer disease were found to have significant differences, suggesting that the brains of those who develop the disease are different at a relatively early age from those who do not. These differences might indicate independent brain changes that put these individuals at risk for the disease. Or, the changes might be

very early symptoms of the disease process itself. To exclude this possibility, investigators might be interested in studying the brains of individuals before they develop any of these changes, which, depending on how early in life these changes are manifest, might require enrollment of children. See Snowdon DA, Greiner LH, Mortimer JA, et al. Brain infarction and the clinical expression of Alzheimer disease: The Nun Study. *JAMA* 1997;277:813–817.

40. Jonas H. Philosophical reflections on experimenting with human subjects. *Daedalus,* Spring, 1969.
41. I am bracketing the debate over whether investigators should prefer to enroll those who can consent in research that offers the potential for medical benefit. Is it better to enroll competent adults rather than adults with dementia in a trial that offers the same potential for medical benefit to both groups? I have argued that even in this case there are important reasons to prefer enrolling competent adults. My colleagues routinely inform me that they find my arguments for this position unconvincing. See Wendler D. When should "riskier" subjects be excluded from research? *Kennedy Institute of Ethics Journal* 1998; 8:307–327.

Chapter 9

1. One might imagine the case of an individual who is not himself concerned with his own autonomy. Perhaps he adopts a lifestyle that downplays or ignores the importance of making his own decisions. Would it be acceptable to force this individual? It depends. As always we first would need to make a determination of whether ignoring his own interests in this way is a mistake for him. If it is, we should not act in accord with his wishes in this regard, even though he considers it to be for the best (this case takes on aspects of the paradigmatic case of whether an individual should be allowed to use his autonomy to place himself in slavery).
2. Compare campaigns regarding cigarettes and trans fats. One lesson here is that there are different ways to try to get competent adults to do certain things and avoid others. Although both practices involve attempts to influence behavior, there is a great deal of practical difference between denying competent adults access to something we perceive as bad for them versus forcing them to ingest something we consider good for them. But here too the details make a difference. Compare, for example, force feeding some competent adults spinach versus fluoridating their water by fluoridating everyone's water.
3. One of the primary dilemmas one must address in developing an analysis of this topic is how individuals should be treated when their current preferences and values conflict with the preferences and values they expressed while competent. See, for example, Dworkin R. *Life's Dominion: An Argument About Abortion, Euthanasia, and Individual Freedom*, 1st ed. New York: Knopf, 1993; Jaworska A. Respecting the margins of agency: Alzheimer's patients and the capacity to value. *Philos Public Aff* 1999;28:105–138; Dresser R. Life, death, and

incompetent patients: Conceptual infirmities and hidden values in the law. *Ariz Law Rev* 1986;28:373–405.

4. See, for example, Shiffrin S. Autonomy, beneficence, and the permanently demented. In: Burley J, ed. *Dworkin and His Critics: With Replies by Dworkin*. Malden, MA: Blackwell Publishing, 2004:195–217.
5. For simplicity I will focus on reasons that pertain to the child alone. Although this is the common approach to assent and dissent, the claims of others also are relevant. For example, independent of the distress on the child, forcing an objecting child to undergo a research procedure can be problematic for the research staff.
6. While analytic philosophers often seem to ignore this point, it has a very long history in Western philosophy. See *Nicomachean Ethics*, Book 1, lines 1099a30–1099b10.
7. The problem of moral luck, related to the present concerns, presses whether this is an adequate response or whether similar concerns arise even within the scope of moral agency. For the classic accounts, see Nagel T. Moral Luck, in his collection *Mortal Questions*. Cambridge, UK: Cambridge University Press, 1979; Williams B. Moral Luck, reprinted in his collection *Moral Luck*. Cambridge, UK: Cambridge University Press, 1981. Barbara Herman offers a response along similar lines to that offered here, focusing on the claim that morality can be unfair, blaming us for things beyond our agency. Or, perhaps, blaming us for things that our agency reaches which are beyond our control. She focuses on the importance of building just and proper social and political institutions: "And in more modern work, Rousseau clearly, but also Kant, and then Hegel and Marx, insist on this same co-development of state and soul. Their collective message might be put this way: without a politics of the right sort, we lack normative space sufficient for confident and correct moral action" (Herman B. Morality and everyday life. *Proceedings and Addresses of the American Philosophical Association* Nov 2000;74(2):29–45, on page 36).
8. Nussbaum MC. *The Fragility of Goodness: Luck and Ethics in Greek Tragedy and Philosophy*. Cambridge NJ: Cambridge University Press, 1985.
9. Ibid., p. 19.
10. Raz J. *Ethics in the Public Domain*. Oxford: Clarendon Press, 1994:3.
11. Ibid., p. 4.
12. This fact does not preclude the possibility that they may feel more responsible. Presumably, there is a greater opportunity to feel responsible when one is directly or proximately the cause of a harm than if one is not. This emotional response, although important, does not imply moral culpability, assuming the relevant safeguards were in place and accepted practices were followed. Similarly, surgeons likely feel more responsible for bad outcomes when they directly cut the wrong artery, say, than do physicians who prescribe the wrong medication, even when the resulting harms are identical.
13. It is an interesting fact, if it is one, that certain close personal relationships have independent conditions on what counts as an acceptable level of contribution to

the relationship. In particular, it seems, at least in some cases, that each party must make some minimum level of contribution to the relationship, but not make too great a contribution, independent of the respective party's ability to do so. Consider a friendship between the billionaire and the pauper. Relative to their saving and ability to contribute, and the cost to each of them of contributing, the billionaire it seems could and perhaps should make all the monetary contributions to the relationship, buying all the dinners and even a house for the pauper friend. At some point, such relationships become untenable, suggesting that there are more objective thresholds and limits on the respective contributions that each party should make to a given relationship.

14. Here too the facts matter, and they can vary across cases, as illustrated by the example mentioned previously of so-called "long-term nonprogressors," individuals who have had HIV disease for years without suffering any of the ill effects typically associated with the disease, despite receiving no treatment. The members of one important group all contracted HIV as the result of receiving blood from the same donor who was HIV+. For a decade at least, none of these individuals developed symptoms of the disease. Such a cohort is of immense scientific importance, potentially holding the key to how the immune system can fend off the ravages of the disease. These individuals were asked to contribute to many studies assessing ways in which they might be winning the battle against the disease. Their unique situation makes it the case that they can contribute to a significantly greater number of studies than average before we want to start saying that they are contributing too much relative to others and are being taken advantage of.

INDEX